Constructing Musical Healing

of related interest

Music Therapy
Intimate Notes
Mercedes Pavlicevic
ISBN 1 85302 692 1

Music Therapy in Context
Music, Meaning and Relationship
Mercedes Pavlicevic
Preface by Colwyn Trevarthen
ISBN 1 85302 434 1

Music Therapy in Palliative Care
New Voices
Edited by David Aldridge
ISBN 1 85302 739 1

Music Therapy Research and Practice in Medicine
From Out of the Silence
David Aldridge
ISBN 1 85302 296 9

Music Therapy with Children – CD Rom
David Aldridge
ISBN 1 85302 757 X

Music for Life
Aspects of Creative Music Therapy with Adult Clients
Gary Ansdell
ISBN 1 85302 299 3 pb ·
ISBN 1 85302 300 0 CD

Music and People with Developmental Disabilities
Music Therapy, Remedial Music Making and Musical Activities
F.W. Schalkwijk
ISBN 1 85302 226 8

Music Therapy in Health and Education
Edited by Margaret Heal and Tony Wigram
Foreword by Anthony Storr
ISBN 1 85302 175 X

Clinical Applications of Music Therapy in Psychiatry
Edited by Tony Wigram and Jos De Backer
ISBN 1 85302 733 2

Clinical Applications of Music Therapy in Developmental Disability, Paediatrics and Neurology
Edited by Tony Wigram and Jos De Backer
ISBN 1 85302 734 0

Making Music with the Young Child with Special Needs
A Guide for Parents
Elaine Streeter
ISBN 1 85302 187 3

Constructing Musical Healing
The Wounds that Heal

June Boyce-Tillman

Foreword by Paul Robertson

Jessica Kingsley Publishers
London and Philadelphia

Figures 2.2 and 5.4 are reproduced by kind permission of Arts Access Aoteroa, a New Zealand arts organisation providing access to the arts for people who currently have limited access.

Figure 3.1 is reproduced courtesy of the Ralph Rinzler Folklife Archives and Collections, Centre for Folklife and Cultural Heritage, Smithsonian Institute.

Frontispiece, figures 4.1, 4.2, 4.3, 4.4 and 4.6 are reproduced by kind permission of the Tonalis Centre for the Study and Development of Music.

Figure 5.3 is reproduced courtesy of the Gurukul Institute of Indian Classical Music.

Figure 6.3 is reproduced courtesy of the Council for Music in Hospitals.

First published in the United Kingdom in 2000 by
Jessica Kingsley Publishers Ltd,
116 Pentonville Road,
London N1 9JB, England
and
325 Chestnut Street,
Philadelphia, PA 19106, USA.

www.jkp.com

© Copyright 2000 June Boyce-Tillman

Library of Congress Cataloging in Publication Data
A CIP catalog record of this book is available from the Library of Congress

British Library Cataloguing in Publication Data
A CIP catalogue record of this book is available from the British Library

ISBN 1 85302 483 X

Printed and Bound in Great Britain by
Athenaeum Press, Gateshead, Tyne and Wear

Contents

Acknowledgements

This book represents the interaction of a circle of people with an interest in this area, drawn from a variety of different disciplines. I am particularly grateful to the following.

The people with whom I conducted formal interviews: Dr Akin Euba, Dr Elaine Barkin, Richard Bolton, Michael Deason Barrow, Jennifer Fowler, Jan Hughes-Madden, Carole Killick, Lorin Panny, Chris Southall, Olu Taiwo, Saulius Trepekunas, Roger Watson, Liz Wilcock.

King Alfred's, Winchester, which gave me a sabbatical semester to write it, and the Research Centre for Community and Performing Arts who have supported me, especially the director, Dr Stevie Simkin.

Janet Topp-Fargion at the National Sound Archive for the material on shamanic and spirit possession cults.

Groups who have given me a chance to test my ideas, especially Holyrood House and Elizabeth and Stanley Baxter, Chris Dodd and the Sophia Centre for Health Promotion, St Michael's Convent, Ham, Dr Antoniou of the Royal Hampshire Hospital, the Psychology Research Centre at King Alfred's and Dr Helen Ford, a holistic practitioner.

Elaine Wisdom, Tonalis and Arts Aoteroa who provided me with photographs.

People who helped in the formulation of the ideas and the revision of the writing: The Rev Canon Ian Ainsworth-Smith, Frankie Armstrong, Dr Carol Boulter, Professor Chris Clarke, Malcolm Floyd, Professor Mary Grey, Marian Liebmann, Myra Poole, Professor Paul Robertson, Dr Frances Silkstone and Dr Jan Walker.

People who gave me advice and encouragement during the process: Peri Aston, Penelope Eckersley, Professor Mike Hart, Ianthe Pratt, Stefan Narkiewicz, Jean Powell CGA, Professor Elizabeth Stuart and the Rev Andrew Todd.

All the people who returned questionnaires after my performances.

Alma Smith and Andrew Parker who transcribed the tapes.

Jessica Kingsley for inviting me to write the book.

Helen Parry and Emma Woolf for their patience and forbearance in editing the book.

My sons, Matthew and Richard, for believing in me. My daughter-in-law Andrea for her support.

The book is dedicated to Professor Michael Finnissy and the late Professor Mike Llewellyn, who always had faith in the ideas and enabled me to keep faith in them too.

June Boyce-Tillman
London, January 2000

Foreword

This lovely and engrossing book makes a very significant contribution towards establishing an important new musical paradigm. Drawing on an immense and impressively diverse musical knowledge, June Boyce-Tillman beautifully integrates a vast gamut of different musical cultures into an entirely relevant contemporary context.

By skilfully orchestrating ancient myth and traditional story-telling with personal experience and scholarship, she has created a compelling work as engrossing to the general reader as it is significant to the professional music-maker.

For anyone for whom music has given a glimpse of the transcendent, this book offers special insights and rewards. I anticipate returning to it with continuing pleasure for many years to come.

Professor Paul Robertson
Sussex, March 2000

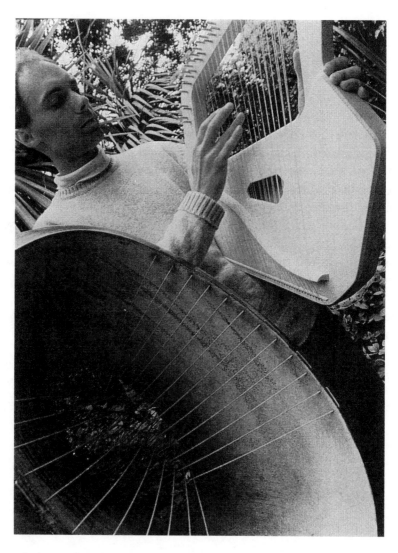

Lyre (maker: Hofstetter) interacting with Barbara Hepworth stringed sculpture
Reproduced courtesy of the Tonalis Centre for the Study and Development of Music

CHAPTER ONE

Setting the Scene

La Trapera

Deep in the desert there lives an old woman. She is secret and private. She is a crower and a cackler; she is fat. She lives in a dark, hidden cave. And her task is the gathering of bones, which is why they sometimes call her 'La Trapera' – the one who gathers. She creeps around the desert collecting whatever bones she can find – deer, birds and snakes and other animals that are likely to die out; but she specialises in the bones of wolves, which is why sometimes she is called 'La Loba' – the wolf woman. And she brings the bones back to her deep, dark cave and lays them out on the rocky floor. And when she has a complete beautiful skeleton she starts to find the right sound for the bones. And she sits by the fire exploring all the lost sounds of the world. And when she has found it, she starts to sing. And gradually the bones come together. And she sings and she breathes. And gradually the bones grow flesh. And she sings and she breathes. And gradually the flesh grows fur. And she sings and she breathes, breathes life into the creature. And the creature opens its eyes and stands and starts to walk. It prances right out of the darkness of the cave. And whether by leaping and prancing or whether by a flash of sunlight or a splash of water, that creature becomes a laughing, dancing human being.

So if you are lost and wandering in the desert, maybe La Trapera will find you and will sing you one of her songs. (The main source is Pinkola Estes 1992, pp.27–28)

This myth from South America illustrates not only the ancient connection between music and healing but also the philosophical framework that underpinned it. This was bound up with the central power of music to make connections – within the body, human being to human being, humans to the natural world, human beings and the natural world to God or the spiritual. The ethics of most world religions show a love of peaceful connectedness.[1] This is the reason for the centrality of music in religious ritual, whether it is the pagan rites celebrating the turning of the seasons or the seven offices of the monastic day.

Ways of knowing

In an increasing movement in the late twentieth century the West has been endeavouring to restore a rift that has developed in its intensely rationalistic culture. In some societies the relationship between music and healing would be self-evident. But it is not by accident that the story of La Trapera attributes to the musical healer (who was almost certainly a shaman) a number of qualities that Western culture has marginalised – fatness, the older woman, crowing, cackling and intuition. Western post-Enlightenment culture, still the dominant culture, sees reason as paramount and this has coloured the way in which music is regarded. Order and clarity and a desire to see the world as defined by scientific reality – 'as it really is' – have been the ultimate goals. The chaotic, the imaginary and the obscure have been seen as enemies – indeed, requiring of a cure that can be achieved largely by reason. In line with this, musicians have been marginalised by the community in which they once played a central role. Their art has been seen as an escape from the real world. It is interesting to reflect that a dichotomy between two worlds exists in shamanic thought, but here it is less clear which is the 'real' world – that of the every day reality or that of the altered state of consciousness (see Chapter Three).

Stan Gooch (1972) in his book *Total Man: Towards an Evolutionary Theory of Personality* defines two systems of thought, which co-exist in the human personality and have the potential for development. The favoured characteristics of one system (System A) are activity leading to products, objectivity, impersonal logic, thinking and thought, detachment and discrete categories of knowledge which is based on proof and scientific evidence. The other system (System B) favours being, subjectivity, personal feeling, emotion, magic, involvement, associative ways of knowing, belief and non-causal knowledge (Gooch 1972, p.522). He suggests that the Western world has chosen to value the first of these value systems. The second has therefore

---

1   Hildegard of Bingen (1098–1179) called this connection justice. 'God,' she said, 'has arranged all things in consideration of everything else.'

become devalued. I have called the ways of knowing that characterise System B subjugated ways of knowing.

One of the characteristics of postmodernity is an increasing acknowledgement that these subjugated ways of knowing are important. This view has been seen in such diverse fields as quantum physics or cybernetics (Van Nieuwenhuijze 1998), feminist theory (Belenky et al. 1986; Braidotti 1994), and certain branches of psychology (Csikszentmihalyi 1993; Redfearn 1992). Music, clearly, will have a greater value within a System B society. The distrust of rationalism, awareness of the feminine and ecological, quest for a post-materialist quality of life, return to spirituality, sense of dispersal and disillusionment with Utopia that characterises post-modern sensibility are strands leading to a re-evaluation of the role of music.

This is linked with a greater valuing of intuition. Intuition is important not only in music but also in ordinary discourse. Work in communication studies shows how important the non-verbal is. Our sensitivity to other people is carried by a multitude of non-verbal links; these embrace music in its widest sense, including such areas as the pitching and tone colour of the voice and the rhythm and pace of the words. At both an individual level and a cultural level we need to recognise our own rhythms and melodies and those of other people and races so that we can relate our patterns to theirs.

Western society has tended to deny the notion of otherness, the spiritual, the transcendent. The result is the reduction of artistic products to the level of status symbols and marketable commodities. But there are hopeful signs. Once science, spirituality and music would have been inextricably entwined (James 1993, pp.3–19) and there are signs of reconnecting them. Also, as psychiatry is honestly addressing its own limitations, doctors and psychotherapists are turning to musicians for any remedies they might offer for the sicknesses of contemporary society. Community musicians are being welcomed in health-care establishments. There is an acknowledgement of an an-aesthetic quality in current medical practice, a rediscovery of the deep human need for the aesthetic and a rebirth of interest in many different areas (including among professional musicians, medical practitioners, psychotherapists, New Age practitioners) of music's potential to heal. All of these are indicators of a desire to explore other ways of knowing.

There is an inextricable relationship between the individual and the society in which he or she lives. Theories of personality like the inventory of the Myers–Briggs Type Indicator (Myers 1993; Myers and McCaulley 1985), based on the work of Jung, classifies personalities in terms of types. It is a system that is based on four polarities within the personality. Where a person falls on these scales is rated by questionnaire, indicating whether he or she is introverted or extroverted, favours thinking or feeling, sensation or intuition, and finally whether he or she prefers a degree of organisation or 'going with the flow'. Two of these are clearly rated to Gooch's systems described above. One is 'thinking–feeling' and people are rated as to whether they tend to make decisions on the basis of feeling or thinking. It is clear that 'thinking' types are likely to be more in tune with prevailing Western values. Another scale is 'sensation–intuition', which distinguishes those who rely on the material, practical world from those who trust the intuitive flash of insight.

Although the two systems – the cultural analysis of Gooch and the personality types of Myers–Briggs – do not completely marry, it is possible to see that we can identify certain individuals as Type A; that is, those who are happy acting on the logic and scientific reasoning which are part of System A. Others can be called Type B and will favour System B, acting intuitively and valuing belief and magic. It is clear that the Type A people will feel more at ease than Type B in Western society. Type B people are more likely to exhibit signs of dis-ease, and, indeed, to be classified as 'abnormal' by the surrounding society, than Type A. However, Type A people will also have the Type B characteristics within themselves and these will require exploration to achieve a fully rounded humanity. Similarly, Type B people can use the prevailing values in the culture to develop the less-favoured aspects of their personality. This analysis may appear simplistic and does not do justice to the complexity of the Myers–Briggs Indicator. The notion of culture is not so simple in contemporary society. All of us are now in a globalised world in which we are required to operate within a number of different cultures, each with their own version of these value systems. However, the analysis does serve to highlight the relationship between the individual personality and society and the roots of some human dis-eases.

So Western society has embraced one set of values. Other value systems exist which are reflected in other cultures. These are subjugated within Western culture. Individual people have a preference for a particular way of knowing, although all the ways of knowing exist within the human psyche. In a society where the individual's way of knowing is in tune with that of the society, the person is more likely to be seen as well-adjusted and will suffer less stress and dis-ease. He or she is more likely to see the surrounding culture as a safe, womb-like structure. Those who don't have a good 'fit' are more likely to see culture as a cage, limiting their choices and their potential. These people are more likely to become sick simply from this mismatch between themselves and their surroundings. This is dis-ease, certainly in a psychological sense. What underpins this book is that all the ways of knowing lie within each individual, and that they can be validated through music-making. Music-making potentially becomes a way of challenging the dominant value system, as well also of supporting it.

Notions of well-being

Work within a culture will tend to encapsulate the dominant values of the society. Studies of leisure in Western society do indicate that people use leisure time to create some sort of balance within themselves. In leisure people 'compensate' for their work practices (Wilensky 1960, pp.32–56). Studies of leisure like Stebbins (1992) (summarised in Haworth 1997, p.12) identify distinctive features like perseverance, the development of knowledge, training and skill, personal enrichment including a sense of identity, improved self-image and identification with a group.

Studies of conditions at work conducive to well-being indicate that collective effort and a sense of identity are significant (Jahoda 1982, summarised in Haworth 1997, p.16). Some of these are clearly attempts to provide a balance to the dominant value system. Warr (1987) (summarised in Haworth 1997, pp.17–18) draws on similar categories in defining

'principal environmental influences' which interact with different 'enduring' characteristics of individuals to influence well-being…

These principal environmental influences include a sense of being in control, a chance to use skills and the opportunity for interpersonal contact.

The notion of well-being has been systematically explored by Mihalyi Csikszentmihalyi who sees enjoyment as central. In defining his notion of 'enjoyable flow' which is at the heart of his theory, he identifies the following characteristics:

- intense involvement
- clarity of goals and feedback
- deep concentration
- transcendence of self
- lack of self-consciousness
- loss of a sense of time
- intrinsically rewarding experience

- a balance between skill and challenge. (Csikszentmihalyi and
  Csikszentmihalyi 1988, as summarised in Haworth 1997,
  pp.84–85)

So there is within these theories evidence of theorists attempting to balance
the prevailing value systems of the West. These are often connected with
leisure activities which can become a place where people explore other
aspects of their personality. Certain qualities are identified as characterising
well-being. Many of these involve interpersonal contact in some way – a
sense of community (often as a counterbalance to a predominantly individualistic work culture). There is also a fostering of a sense of self, often through
a balance of using and affirming existing skills with acquiring new skills. The
notion of transcendence or the loss of a sense of time is identified as
important, sometimes attained by activities that are physical in character.
Variety – a balance of activity and relaxation – also features.

Healing as process

So, on the one hand 'health' might be perceived as being in an environment
that suits you; on the other hand, in the dynamic process of living, a dis-ease
may be seen as a call to explore other parts of one's own psyche.

How are the words 'healing', 'health' and 'therapy' related? The words
have become polarised, annexed by particular groups, each with its own
particular emphasis. Two of them are nouns, and one is much more closely
related to a verb.

The nouns 'health' and 'therapy' have acquired much more clearly
defined meanings in the late twentieth century. Health in the UK has become
associated with 'the Health Service', which in general has concentrated on
the physical, and in the area of psychology has concentrated on medication-based solutions. There are now real attempts to broaden this notion,
whether in the attempts by GPs to explore arts activities at their surgeries or
in imaginative schemes for health promotion.

Health and therapy can be seen as enabling people to become 'normal'.
This resonates with the ideas already discussed on the relationship of the
individual to the surrounding society. The concept of therapy as power sets
out a model for therapy as an instrument for changing people so that they
adopt the values of the dominant discourse. A norm for health will be established by the dominant discourse and people will be edged towards it by a
variety of techniques:

For the ancient wisdom of oriental medicine, religion and science are integrated; there is no antithesis, therefore no synthesis is necessary. For the Western doctor, oriental medicine is pre-Hippocratic; it is full of superstition, formalism and magical thinking… [S/He] traces his professional ancestry, as he traces back many of the noble and rational liberating attitudes of our civilisation, to the ancient Greeks. (Redfearn 1992, p.191)

Therapy in Western society's discipline of psychology has become linked into a methodology based on psychoanalytic or behavioural techniques. At the end of it the patient will be better 'adjusted' to life in the surrounding society. In a physical sense, therapy has been associated with acute conditions like the malfunction of a limb, as in the case of physiotherapy. When the limb can perform its 'normal' functions the therapy ceases. In both of these examples 'wellness' is defined at the point where the person can function according to what is defined as 'normal'. But to define a moment of health in our lives is difficult. The model associated with the word 'health' seems to have lurking in it somewhere the notion that we are working towards a point when we shall be healthy; then the task will be to maintain ourselves in that state. The implication in this notion is that then we should live the rest of our life in some sort of sterile bubble, free from influences that make us ill.

Anthony Giddens in his 1999 Reith lecture, 'Tradition', suggested that the growth in the therapy and counselling industry in the contemporary West is part of a search of personal identity in a society that no longer provides that identity within its own structures. Here people find their identity by story-telling. He suggests that it is part of the process of globalisation in which we all have a greater range of choice than before. He sees psychotherapy as a method for the renewal of self-identity, in the early stages of a detraditionalising culture (Giddens 1999). This is a process model of the construction of self-identity, which is much wider and more dynamic than the more product-based model described earlier.

'Healing', a term derived from a verb, is more closely associated with the *process* of living. The transpersonal psychologist Jean Achterberg (1985) defines eight concepts of healing, all of which are more process than product based:

- A journey to wholeness which may take a lifetime

- A remembering of one's connection with God/the Cosmos

- An accepting of what is feared

- The opening of blockages in the self
- The experiencing of the transcendent
- A feeling of creativity, passion and love
- The expressing of the self fully and authentically
- Learning to trust the processes of living.

At a macro level, healing is the process of dealing with major traumas over a lifetime; at a micro level, it is the clearing the decks of 'rubbish' at the end of each day. It is more like the functioning of the immune system to which it is linked: the ongoing process of strengthening and sifting our experiences, selecting and rejecting in an ongoing process of balancing, which is the ongoing process of living. The process of living is a process of encounter with a variety of experiences, some of which appear more helpful than others. Events which at the time appear devastating can, if they are handled well, produce rich fruits; events that seemed wonderful at the time can lead up blind alleys. Apparently negative events can be turned around to positive ends; *but this is not always so.* The reasons why some suffering is apparently productive, redemptive and other suffering is not is perhaps the greatest mystery at the heart of life, and it is the starting point for the religious or spiritual quest. It is at the heart of the great world religions. The question 'Why do we suffer?' is one common to them all. The answers that each gives is different.

The process of living is that of being able to process experiences productively. Healing is associated with a dynamic model of wellness, which is wider than the curing of individual illnesses. It encompasses the realisation of the full potential of the self within the context of the prevailing value system. This may mean that some people will find it important to challenge these value systems.

We find here some themes that we have already encountered, such as notions of transcendence and the creation of an identity. This is extended here to include the notion of acceptance of other parts of the persona, so creating a sense of diversity within the self. There is a desire for freedom and expression which is linked with a sense of wholeness that includes widening the range of personal experience.

Models of health

Cecil Helman (1994), in his book *Culture, Health and Illness,* describes three models that underpin thinking about the health of the body. These are:

- The *balance/imbalance* model – 'the healthy working of the body is thought to depend on the harmonious balance between two or more elements of forces within the body'. (Helman 1994, p.21)

- The *plumbing* model – 'the body is conceived of as a series of hollow cavities or chambers, connected with one another, and with the body's orifices, by a series of "pipes" or "tubes"... Central to this model is the belief that health is maintained by the uninterrupted *flow* of various substances...between cavities, or between a cavity and the body's exterior via one of the orifices.' (Helman 1994, pp.24–25)

- The *machine* model – 'the conceptualization of the body as an internal combustion engine, or as a battery-driven machine, has become more common in Western society'. (Helman 1994, p.26)

John Foskett (1984), dealing with mental health, identifies five models:

- The *medical* model – which sees it as the result of a chemical deficiency.

- The *psychodynamic* model – based on the work of analysts like Freud.

- The *behavioural* model – which deals in cause and effect and is influenced by experimental psychology and learning theory.

- The *social* model – which emphasises the effect of social deprivation.

- The *medieval* model – which sees it as the work of the Devil or an evil spirit.

The present book is based on the model of healing – physically, psychologically and spiritually – as balancing. It draws on Helman's balance/imbalance model of bodily health and the psychodynamic model of mental illness (although the medieval model is encountered in Chapter Three in relation to traditional healers).

The music therapist David Aldridge illustrates the model of health as balance with musical improvisation. He sees the need for a balance between stability and change, conventional and unconventional. He concludes:

Creativity is a process which exists within a framework of the aesthetic. The status of health is the striving for creative realisation. Within the individual the ability for self-regulation is based upon a repertoire of improvisational possibilities. While it is essential to have a standard repertoire of responses for everyday life, it is also necessary to improvise solutions when necessary. This is true of the biological, as it is of the musical, as it is of the existential. There exists a balance between stability and change; both the conventional and the unconventional lie in a healthy tension. For example, the music therapist talks about the patient's ability to maintain the logic of a sustained melodic line alone. For the patient…this is her melody according to her inner logic. We can assume that this is part of therapeutic change in that the patient finds and expresses her own inner logic. Yet this individual expression is contained within the context of a relationship. The personal and the social are balanced. Health is a statement about an ecology. (Aldridge 1996, pp.16–17)

The notion of health or healing as balance removes it from being exclusively in the hands of health practitioners and restores it to a place in the web of society and culture. In contemporary society people are becoming dedicated to being healthy which is perceived as being much more than simply not being sick. The notion of being a healthy person is now an important part of identity, and publications promoting a healthy lifestyle proliferate. Health strategies include a range of practices including diet, exercise, aesthetic pursuits, psychological techniques and spiritual practices. These are bound up with the construction of a 'healthy' identity for oneself. It pursues more than emotional well-being and is a real embodiment of health.

So, the model of healing as balancing is linked with debates about work and leisure, which in turn are linked with relationship of the individual to the surrounding culture. Healing is a process of rebalancing the system and can be attained through creative activity. This is not necessarily achieved only through the operations of health practitioners but may also be reached by means of a pattern of activities chosen with a degree of self-awareness.

Creativity and well-being

In the middle of the twentieth century there was a great upsurge in writing on creativity, much of which linked it with personal development. The ancient concept of creativity, which saw it as originating in the Divine, was intertwined with the post-Enlightenment concept of human creativity, which posited an independent life linked with the *controlling* of nature. In the US in the 1930s came the Progressive Education Movement in which teachers and parents observed children's natural curiosity, experimenting and exploration. Such spokesmen as William James (1900), John Dewey (1910, 1934),

William Heard Kilpatrick (the leader of the movement), Francis Parker, Boyd Bode, George Counts and others challenged traditional educational methods in favour of methods allowing children to develop through the processes of discovery and self-motivated play (Lieberman 1967). This was extended to the wider population. Through being creative, people would realise their human potential. An area of psychology called the Human Potential Movement came to be developed, encouraging lateral thinking and right-brain activity, with exponents like Eric Fromm, Carl Rogers (1970, 1976), Abraham Maslow (1958, 1962a, 1962b, 1967, 1987) and Rollo May. These concepts also came to be linked with industrial and military progress, especially in the Cold War between the US and the USSR. Techniques for producing 'original' solutions to problems were developed by writers like Brian Ghiselin (1952, 1956), Paul Torrance (1970) and J. P. Guilford (1962). With the advent of New Age philosophies the notion of an element of the Divine or spiritual came to be reintroduced into the notion.

In this literature the notion of the creative individual as a 'self-actualising' person is very strong. There is great stress on freedom as a necessary part of the creative process. This is often linked with a return to the processes of childhood, especially play. The arts are seen as a place where adults can play, where they are free to explore their own subconscious and also to make mistakes. They are, therefore, important arenas of self-development. There is a notion of rebellion, a challenging of the conventions of society in the exploration of the new ideas implicit in the free play of the creative process.

This process is seen (Sparshott 1981; Stein 1967; Wallas 1926) as including various phases (which are adjusted, fine-tuned and restructured by various writers). These include preparation (the exploration of possibilities and generating of ideas), incubation (which involves less conscious activity), illumination (the 'eureka' experience) and elaboration (the working out of the project in a tangible form). Importantly, a descent into the personal unconscious or subconscious with its somewhat chaotic nature is seen as an important component of the incubation phase. Particularly creative people have strategies for handling this phase and where it is possible for all to enter into the process (particularly the idea-generating first phase), how far they proceed is often limited by their level of skill (Hindemith 1952). Arthur Koestler (1964, 1981) developed a theory of bisociation as central to this process in which two previously unconnected domains of the mind come together to produce the new outcome. The process is seen as part of the flow of living and important for growth and change. It involves a degree of courage on the part of the person, who needs to be free to enter playful processes in order to achieve what is seen as a re-ordering of personality. The result is a sense of empowerment, which can be nurtured by encouragement and an environment that encourages acceptance and spontaneity. Philosophers and psychologists have linked creativity to states of ecstasy and transcendence although creativity always involves some bodily action.

The main themes which emerge from this literature are those of freedom, often involving playfulness, the need for acceptance, creativity as a universal human trait leading to growth and change, the necessity for a measure of chaos in the process and a notion of transcendence as part of a 'peak experience' in the creative process.

Musical development

The educational implications of this thinking were worked out in the UK in particular in the 1960s and 1970s by the development of composition/improvisatory activities in the classroom. Aspects like freedom, playing, the production of new ideas, often from the association of previously unconnected ideas (Loane 1984), the importance of an accepting environment and the notion of music as self-expression were found in the writings of the time (Paynter 1977; Tillman 1976). Children exploring sounds freely in groups characterised what came to be known as creative music-making. My own work (Swanwick and Tillman 1986; Tillman 1987) charted how pupils developed musically in this environment. It shows how the youngest children explore sound freely as part of wider sensory exploration of the world and how the development of the ability to control bodily movements is linked with the ability to control sound. The developing capacity for self-expression through music is clearly seen and needs supporting by a sensitive and authoritative teacher. It shows how children need at certain times to experiment freely and at other times to be part of traditions. It shows that a time of embracing a tradition may well be followed by one of breaking the boundaries that were once freely accepted. In this need for both tradition and experimentation a balance is maintained between freedom and containment. Children become increasingly able to handle musical ideas and motifs (musical gestures) in the construction of musical form. Developing self-awareness can lead to the use of music as a form of self-development and self-regulation. Musical ability nurtured represents not only musical empowerment but also a personal empowerment in other areas. In a project in which children with chronic anxiety were given 'creative' music lessons (Boyce-Tillman 1998d), their symptoms decreased. At some time pupils want to experiment on their own and at other times they want to be part of shared music-making activities. These often helped to create communities within which diversity is valued (Boyce-Tillman 1996a). Involvement in a deep way with the interlocking areas of materials, expressive character, construction (form) and valuing by the process of improvising/composing can lead to a measure of transcendence, called 'spirituality' in this figure:

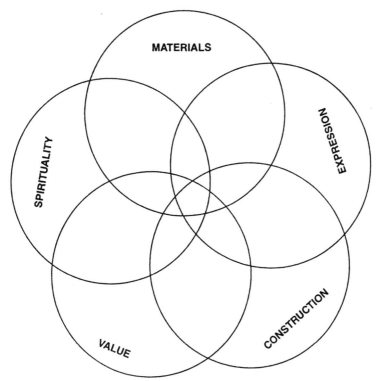

Figure 1.1 The interlocking areas of musical experience

This research maps the balance implicit in musical development. It includes such elements as freedom and containment, the importance of bodily gesture in the creation of sound and the possibility of transcendence, the desire for self-expression and the need for nurture as well as challenge in development.

My own experience

My own exploration into this world represented an embracing of a musical freedom that I could not find in classical training that ended in a music degree at Oxford University. This degree study consisted of history and analysis and written composition in the style of composers from 1550–1900. My grandfather had been the village dance band pianist in a New Forest village and played by ear; but he wanted his granddaughter to enter the world of classical music (epitomised by his 78rpm recording of Jose Iturbi paying Chopin's *Fantaisie Impromptu*). I was too young when he died to realise what I had lost by not learning his skills. In fact, as a child, I was glad of the containment of the classical tradition. I knew where I was by learning how to read the notes and enjoying the poise and elegance of Mozart and Haydn, who were my favourites at that time. I was terrified of improvisation in any form. The printed notes offered a security that I needed. It was through exploring sound with children in school that I found that freedom and this was followed by playing folk guitar and (much later) buying a djembe (a drum found in some African traditions). Twenty-five years after leaving Oxford I dared to improvise in public and felt that I could claim that musical freedom.

Although I composed a few original pieces at Oxford (not as part of the academic course) I wrote few classical pieces for the next 20 years. Oxford had taught me that composers were usually male, German and dead. It was during a prolonged illness that I started to compose again and became aware that this process was actually part of my own healing process, that in combining and recombining the ideas musically I was actually changing parts of myself.

At this point composing was essentially an individual activity done at the piano or on paper, as I had been taught. I was a pianist, and a piano is an essentially individual instrument. I enjoyed accompanying but the examination system dictated that I was always examined as an individual. My parents could only afford for me to learn the cello in a class so advanced orchestral playing was not available. Choral singing was the only communal music-making experience open to me. Playing folk guitar for large gatherings in the 1960s offered me an experience of communal music-making that had largely been denied.

My route into the musical profession consisted largely of a set of challenges called examinations and as a child I remember my musical life as a series of hurdles. No sooner was one surmounted than the next one loomed on the horizon. The notion of using music for relaxation was not a possibility and indeed was discouraged by teachers of musical analysis who despised what they called 'wallpaper' music and set listening up as something to engage the whole mind, and certainly never to be indulged in while doing something else. It took the discovery of therapeutic massage to introduce me to the use of music to nurture and heal, as an accompaniment to other activities.

My discovery of other approaches to music was achieved by means of moving from the classical tradition into other musical traditions. At first this was the protest song movement and I can remember the sense of rebellion in going back to Oxford to sing at my college and using a song entitled O that Greedy Landlord which I accompanied myself on the guitar in my essentially classical programme. The scene was set for the embracing of musical diversity as a way of exploring different parts of my own psyche. It has led me through various New Age groups, into ethnic traditions and an exploration of the tenets of music therapy. At first I was concerned about the diversity and discrepancies between what was the dominant tradition for me – classical music – and the other ones. Now I rejoice in the diversity and realise that each represents a different aspect of my persona and can be respected in the same way as I teach respect for difference in the course in world musics. This is as true internally as it is externally in terms of society.

Through these other traditions – especially the drumming – I discovered a much greater awareness of the role of my body in music-making. Although I necessarily spent much time on technical exercises in learning the piano and was aware of how the state of my physical health affected my singing, the tradition I was being initiated into did not show a great concern for the role of the body in the tradition and concentrated largely on the role of the mind which was seen to be the ruler of the body. I sang in church for as long as I can remember, and was a deeply religious child. Up to the age of 12 I could not sing in the choir, which was all male, and when I did sing in a choir that included girls, I found that most of the church choir had little sense of the religious meaning of music (less so often than the congregation). It took explorations into Hinduism and New Age to discover a group of people who genuinely believed in the transcendent power of music and, indeed, sometimes linked this with the embodied art of dancing.

This is a brief summary of my entry into the experience of music, which was essentially a process of self-discovery, self-construction and reconstruction. Various themes run through it – such as containment and freedom, individualism and communal music-making, the challenging nature of the classical tradition, the embracing of diversity and the place of the body and transcendence in music-making.

Establishing the polarities

Certain themes emerge from these various fields. Themes like community, freedom, expression, empowerment, transcendence (not necessarily linked with a religious affiliation) and the presence of physical activity recur with different emphases. It is from these that I have drawn the list of 7 polarities that make up the dynamic model of the self on which the book is based. These are:

- community/individualism
- containment/freedom
- expression/confidentiality
- unity/diversity
- challenge/nurture
- excitement/relaxation
- embodiment/transcendence.

They are expressed as polarities which mirror the process of living and can be related to the nature of music. They represent continuums within the self. Philosophers have often dealt in related polarities. Aristotelian thought,[2] for example, identified a number of dualities which included:

- limited/unlimited
- male/female
- rest/motion.

He regarded the first as most important: 'To establish a rational and consistent relationship between the limited (man [sic], finite time and so forth) and the unlimited (the cosmos, eternity, etc.) is not only the aim of Pythagoras's system but the central aim of all Western philosophy' (James 1993, p.28).

In Hegelian dialectic it is represented by the thesis, antithesis, synthesis model. The triangle was central to Pythagorean thought and in this model the apex of the triangle was perceived as the balancing point of the dualities. This gave a possibility of synthesis without denying the polarities but including them in different proportions. Women have had little input into philosophical and theological principles that have shaped Western culture and many feminist writers have opposed such dualistic thinking. Yet within

2   Aristotle, *Metaphysics.*

the model set out below the polarities are always in relationship. In this dynamic process of balancing process the self is exploring different patterns of being.

So the notion of polarities has been part of Western philosophy. In the Pythagorean thought model:

- they are in a dynamic relationship

- we need to explore both ends of the spectrum and this will be easier in some societies than others

- full personhood is to be realised by exploring a wide range of human experience.

A model of the self

First of all we must conceive of the interrelationship of these polarities. To do this I have shown these within a circle. The enclosure within the circle shows how these polarities are all interrelated within the person. They are shown in Figure 1.2 as linked together.

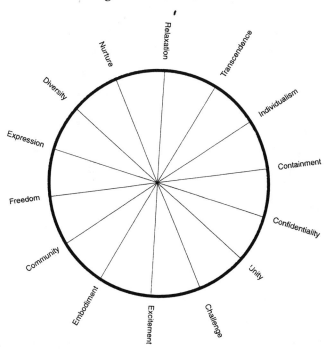

Figure 1.2 The polarities within the self

The polarities are also interlinked themselves. Notions of individualism, especially within Western culture, are linked with notions of self-expression and challenge (as we shall see in Chapter Two). Challenge and excitement are closely related. Relaxation and nurture are linked together in New Age thinking (as we shall see in Chapter Four) and are related to the body, especially in such complementary therapies as massage and aromatherapy. Notions of community and nurture are linked, particularly in cultures where shamanism and spirit possession are established forms of therapy and here they are linked with the body (as we shall see in Chapter Three). In Figure 1.3 the dotted lines show other potential links that may be made.

Each polarity has a point of synthesis:

- The balancing of community/individualism is individuation

- The balancing of containment/freedom is incarnation[3]

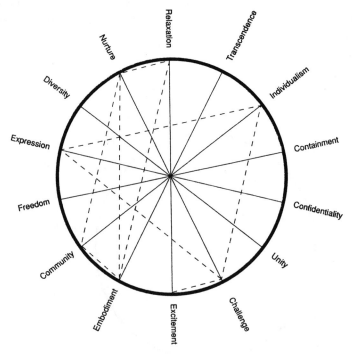

Figure 1.3 The interconnections between the polarities

3 The idea of incarnation – the process of encoding an idea in the form of sounds – is taken from Dorothy Sayers' ideas in *The Mind of the Maker* (London, Methuen, 9th edition 1947, first published 1941). She developed it in relation to her own writing, as she describes the way ideas take shape as a play or novel is written.

- The balancing of expression/confidentiality is maturity
- The balancing of unity/diversity is creativity
- The balance of challenge/nurture is growth
- The balance of excitement/relaxation is rhythm
- The balance of embodiment/transcendence is wisdom.

These points are similar to the points of synthesis in psychosynthesis. In Figure 1.4 I have used the triangle favoured by Robert Assagioli to illustrate this.

Assagioli (1994) uses the triangle shape to differentiate between compromise and synthesis: 'The two elements are absorbed into a higher unity endowed with the qualities which transcend those of either. The difference between such synthesis and a mere compromise is fundamental' (pp.101–103).

He illustrates this by distinguishing between calm and serenity. Calm is a compromise between excitement and depression, but the two are synthesised into the higher unity in serenity. When, for example, we are beginning to achieve individuation the pole of individualism becomes solitude and that of community becomes togetherness. We are equally happy with both. It is, however, difficult to represent such subtleties in a single model. Therefore, in the interests of clarity, I have plotted them as points along the lines (Figure 1.5).

From this it can be seen that the balance point is not necessarily the mid-point of the lines. It can be at any position on the line and will constantly be moving until we are content in any position. As we explore the various positions of balance we become more at ease with them and achieve a synthesis of the polarities.

Now they can be mapped onto the circular model to give different shapes for the self (Figure 1.6). Here is a shape that has a sense of transcendence and individuality, that is quite contained and likes confidentiality, that feels quite united, enjoys challenge and is a little excited. This shape is quite in tune with the values of Western society.

Another self-shape (Figure 1.7) shows a very different value system. Here the person is quite relaxed and enjoys nurture, has some sense of diversity within it, enjoys freedom and expression within a community and has a real sense of the body. This might be less at ease in Western society.

The model of the musical self is a dynamic and fluid model in which extremes can be explored freely. Personal wholeness in the model is the ability to undergo human experience in a way that is productive and fruitful. It is a process of continual balance, not avoiding the extremes but able to move to them aware of where you are. As Chopra (1991) points out, 'The play of opposites... cannot be abolished. But opposites can co-exist without challenging each other – and that is the secret. For wholeness to be a living reality one must learn to expand beyond the field of duality encompassing the most diametrically opposed qualities of life' (pp.253–254).

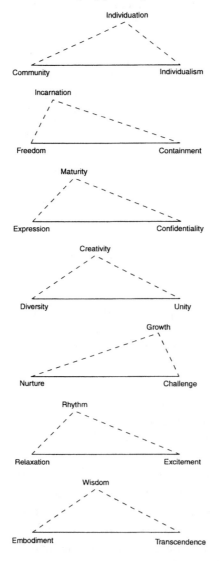

Figure 1.4 Balancing the polarities in triangular form

Balance is not a premature calm but a search for a whole humanity that we can compose for ourselves, making living more like a symphony and less like a machine (Aldridge 1996).

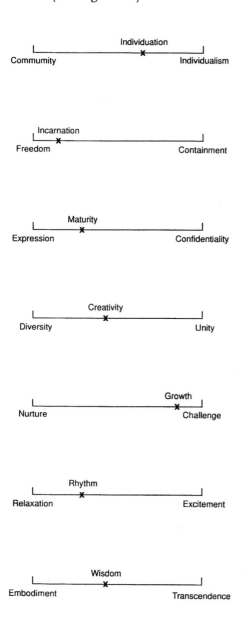

Figure 1.5 Balancing the polarities in linear form

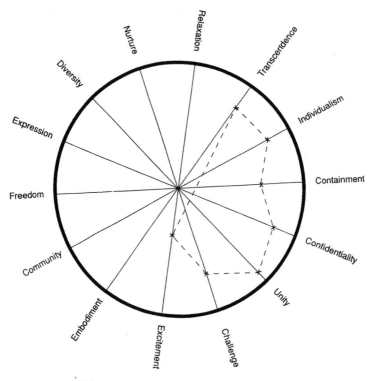

Figure 1.6 A self-shape

The self-shapes using the model are drawn using a process not unlike the process of category generalisation that characterises grounded theory methodology. It also has some similarities with George Kelly's (1955) personal construct theory, using a spatial conceptual structure for the data.[4] Certainly the way the polarities were constructed and their positioning on the circle is similar to the cluster analysis within Kelly's approach. The model, like Kelly's original theory, may prove useful in helping people to a greater degree of self-awareness in the way in which they use music in their lives.

Music and the model of the self

The present book examines how various musical traditions have synthesised the polarities. It necessarily takes an essentially functionalist approach to music, even within the Western classical tradition. My own background and

---

4   There are limitations in the process of model making, since no model can depict the
     totality of human knowing.

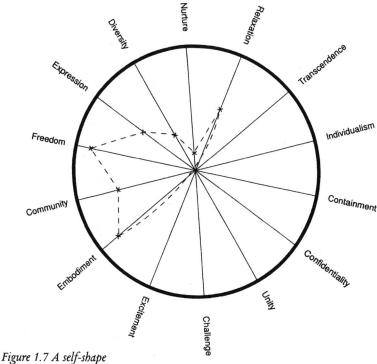

Figure 1.7 A self-shape

experience have dictated the areas examined, which are the Western classical tradition, the shaman and spirit possession cults, the New Age and music therapy. There is no systematic study of the area of Western popular music or jazz, except when New Age ideas have influenced it (as in some areas of trance and rave music).

Anthony Storr (1992) sees music as having a balancing function. He cites a close link between the functions in the ear of perceiving sound and the ability to balance physically. It is not by accident that the two distinct systems are located close together.

The model of the self relating to music is based on the notion that music is a complex art form. The elements of music are the fundamental elements of human communication. Music is therefore intimately involved in the general interactions of everyday living as well as with the aesthetic moment:

> Sequence, order, phrasing, the fundamentals of musical form are vital elements in maintaining coherence whether in physiological systems, personal development or interpersonal relationships ... The basis of... mutual knowledge is both physiological, in that we share common

physiologies, and cultural. The forces which bind us together, which are the essence of our mutuality, are musical ... If musical elements are essential to communication, then the improvised musical playing for people may make manifest both underlying pathology and possibilities of growth and change. (Aldridge 1996, pp.51–55)

The literature about music can almost be divided into that which deals with the nature of music as a freestanding art form and that which concentrates on the roles that music can play personally and culturally. Traditional musicology rooted as it is in Western Enlightenment philosophy has dealt largely with the 'objectivity' of music – the nature of the sounds, their patterns, and the way the individual sounds combine. Ethnomusicology and studies in popular music have dealt largely with the relationship of music to culture, while the 'therapeutic' literature has concentrated on the personal meanings of music (bearing in mind also that it is difficult to separate a person from their culture).

The scope of the book

My aim in this book is to examine how these polarities are associated with the healing/therapeutic properties of music and how they are reflected in different musical traditions. I will examine different emphases, different perspectives, different languages and conceptual frames. My intention is to see whether there are common elements or themes which may be disguised by the different technical languages. The book is structured in one dimension by the source of the material, as the chapter headings indicate; in the other dimension it is structured by tracing the themes of the polarities through the different traditions.

In general, it will concentrate on music intended for therapeutic purposes. The notion of music as therapy will also be explored particularly in relation to traditions where notions of healing are not explicit.

The notion of the musician is fluid too. The 'average' person in the West usually uses the word for others. They refer to the great performers (who are usually alive) and the great composers (who are usually male and dead). The West (and it is not alone in this trend) has developed a very elite notion of the musician – the one set apart, the master. The dilemma in any philosophy of the healing nature of music is that these people are often seen as the most suffering of all humanity. Theories about this will be developed. These will link with the construction of 'madness' in the West, the notion of the scapegoat and the notion of the shaman.

The construct of music in the West implies the public making of music. The increasing ranks of music therapists are often shy to call themselves musicians because their art is private and practised in the confidentiality of the client–patient relationship. This book includes music therapists alongside shamans, classical composers and New Age musical practitioners.

The book is also intended for the discriminating and understanding listener – the owners of personal stereos calming themselves on the commuter train coming home from work with a piece of Mozart or Pachelbel's *Canon*, accompanied by sounds of the sea. There will be reference too to community music-making activities – the local choral society singing *The Messiah* every Easter and *The Sound of Music* at Christmas. These can be likened to ancient musical rituals and may be the last remaining example of seasonal ritual in our society. The New Age has deliberately breached the elitism of the dominant culture. Now there are groups of overtone chanters with their singing bowls who meet in an open space to enjoy an hour of music-making each week. Their intention often includes healing.

My aim is not to define the notion of the musician but to explore the process of music-making as healing. As such, it is open to anyone, for it involves the private as well as the public, the amateur as well as the profes-sional, the listener, the performer and the composer/improviser. Indeed, the processes described in this book may be more accessible to the non-professional than the professional, for whom the act of music-making may be constrained by issues of economics, established reputation, precon-ceptions of an established public and notions of excellence as constructed by a particular tradition.

Leslie Bunt (1994) summarises the range of music-making included in this book when he writes:

> What are the connections between us and music? The answers include: the pleasure gained from listening; the warmth and friendship from being part of a group making music; the stimulus and satisfaction from regular practice and rehearsal; the intellectual delight from exploring the intricacies of musical forms and structures; the physical energy released within us by both playing and listening to music, inspiring us often to move and dance. (p.1)

So the book adopts a functionalist approach to music and concentrates on traditions that are designed to heal. However, reference will be made to ways in which other music operates as therapy. The rest of this chapter will consider the nature of the polarities that underpin the model of self used in this book and how they might relate to music. Each polarity will be illustrated by a case study.

Community/individualism

I have chosen to use the word 'community' rather than the term 'collectivism' more commonly used in sociological literature. This is because in certain traditions within this notion is included an element of belonging to the natural world and the wider cosmos, including a spiritual element.

The need of human beings for community is to be found in many sources today – political, psychological and religious, to name but a few. The legacy in the UK of the Thatcher years is one of fragmentation and an excessive emphasis on the individual. But it is a process that started with the Enlightenment and its rediscovery of the epic of the heroic journey. The male hero narrative (based on Homer's *Odyssey* and Virgil's *Aeneid*) is of one who asserts his individuality and 'finds himself' through the undertaking of a journey. This is usually without a permanent companion (although with many temporary travelling associates who are often either embraced or killed). After this, he returns home as a mature man, assured of his personhood. This particular myth is at the very heart of Western civilisation.

Kathleen Fisher (1996), drawing on the work of Jordan *et al.* (1991), designates it the 'Lone Ranger' model of meeting challenges:

According to this model, we evolve through a series of crises in which we achieve a sequence of separations from others. Autonomy and independence, rather then intimacy and closeness, become the touchstones of maturity … When personhood is founded on independence and autonomy, whole groups – older people, women, racial and ethnic minorities, the poor – can be seen as less than fully human. Life development becomes a process toward a peak with an upward and downward slope on either side. (Fisher 1996, p.14)

The heroic journey model is essentially a lonely journey and is characterised by a search for absolute independence, the ability 'to stand on one's own feet' as the saying goes. Its dangers lie in an abrogation of responsibility for anyone but oneself, a denial of any responsibility for the results of one's actions and a confusion between the private and the public. The results have been a fragmentation of communities as the pole of the individual is stressed and fostered. John Foskett (1984) sees a correlation between this and the incidence of mental illness.

The heroic journey was not open to large numbers of people in Western civilisation – the poor and women, to name but two groups. This has only in the last part of the twentieth century been questioned by such people as the theologian Mary Grey (1989) and the psychiatrist Jean Baker Miller and her colleagues (Jordan *et al.* 1991) at the Stone Centre for Developmental Research and Services at Wellesley College, US. Their work has shown women's patterns are moving from attachment to continued connection, so that the self emerges within a web of complex relationships. Many women in particular have sensed the need for this in the nurturing and rearing of children. For them the heroic quest was never a possibility and they felt torn apart by a double standard – a society that prized the individualism that characterised the heroic search and their own sense of a deep need for community and stability for the sake of their children or their family. As individualism progressed, families broke up, men pursued their heroic quest (less successfully in an era of high unemployment) and traditional communities were fragmented by various social trends.

The heroic journey myth underpins some psychotherapeutic models: 'The overly rationalistic model of modern psychiatry is itself an imaginal construction, a fantasy based on the image of a heroic ego whose task is to conquer a resistant reality' (Levine 1997, p.10). This construct of the individual self led to a greater stress being laid on the knowledge of the boundaries of the self than on the ability to let down the barriers to be at one with other people. This experience of deep unity not only with other humans but with the cosmos as a whole has been re-evaluated by the New Age. It forms an important part of the healing elements in the accounts of people who have been part of the audience in my presentations, in which they are asked to sing or dance as a group. Redfearn (1992) distinguishes between the world of action and the world of conscious awareness: 'I am contrasting (opposing) the world of action with the world of containment, reflection and conscious awareness… In the world of action, differences and boundaries usually must be clear-cut or even emphasised; in the world of holding, unity, joining, and intercourse prevail' (1992, p.174).

Jung's concept of individuation contained notions of connection at the most profound level. Whereas we all have our own personal histories we are united by a common store of archetypes that find expression in myth, folklore and the arts. As Csikszentmihalyi (1993) says, 'Personal identity is only achieved through the balancing of these polarities in the process of individuation' (p.252). And yet individuation and individualism have often been confused. The model of the impassive analyst who gives nothing of him or herself away is now balanced by a more connected model of a nurturing relationship and even friendship.

The unity of many communities has been maintained by music. Levi-Strauss (1970) classified societies into 'hot', who have a sense of historical time, and 'cold', who perceive the past and the present as in parallel and are more a-temporal. In the 'cold' society music and ritual are likely to be seen as having an important role in bringing the community together.

In the 'hot' Western traditions, the concept of individualism in music appeared most clearly in the growth of romanticism. The heroic journey and its associated isolation was an important notion in the construct of the genius or master composer: 'For the first time in cultural history the desiring imagination is given priority over forms of the community' (Gans 1994a, p.48). And yet Anthony Storr (1992, p.23) sees parallels between religious and warfare rituals and Western coronations and state funerals.

To understand how the collective unity develops we can draw on the notion of 'entrainment'. The observations of Huygens, a Dutch scientist, in 1665 showed that two pendulum clocks placed side by side would develop a synchronicity through means of a shared beat. In later scientific work it was called the 'mutual phase-locking of two oscillators' or 'entrainment'.

We are vibrating (oscillating) beings. Harmonious activity, having a shared pulse such as singing and marching, produces an experience of 'entrainment' (Leonard 1978). It actually makes those participating more like one another. The same can happen in a concert when a performer has such power that he or she can create a unity such that the audience members are breathing 'in sync' with one another (Ortiz 1997).

The process of entrainment starts with the music being roughly at the common pulse of the group (or the individual in a one-to-one situation). This process has been used practically to create a common pulse for a group of diverse individuals involved in synchronised action such as rowing or hauling ropes (as in sea shanties).

The process of entrainment is why regular rites, rituals and family gatherings included music prominently. John Blacking (1987) links music and dance together and gives them a central place in the inculcation of human values: 'Human attitudes and specifically human ways of thinking about the world are the results of dance and song' (p.60). So the relation of the composer/performer to the audience is potentially a close one. It is formalised in the Western classical tradition into clapping at the end of a piece. In the folk tradition there is a subtle relationship between performer and audience: 'The song, after all, is one expression of whatever is going on at that particular social gathering' (Carson 1986, p.50). The relationship between player/composer/improviser is much more overt and carried by a wide range of subtle signals incomprehensible to the listener outside of the tradition:

> The inexperienced punter [in an Irish pub] may be somewhat discon-certed by the custom whereby little whoops and screams are uttered while the music is in progress. These expressions of appreciation may not be as random as they seem. An attentive punter may, for example, make a little yelp at that point where the tune has been played once and is now to be played again (tunes are played at least twice round), indicating a) that he knows where a tune ends and b) that he would like to hear it again, which he will anyway. On the other hand, the yelp may come at a point in the tune which is determined by the punter's perception of a particularly fine melodic variation; to the musician who just played it, it may have been a mistake. Or it may not. (Carson 1986, p.56)

The preference of Western society for an individualised, discrete view of knowledge and its love of scientific knowing has also led to a stress on tools that will support these values and a marginalisation of areas of knowing that might support more communal ways. The pole of separation has been stressed by the emphasis on literacy and numeracy in UK schools. Lessons requiring corporate action have been downplayed in favour of the acquisi-tion of individual skills, often learned by exercises performed individually (such as silent reading). Children are tested individually.

Words divide but sounds unite. The task of words is to distinguish one group of objects or people from another, to further divide them into subsets and then into individual objects or persons by detailed descriptions of individual names. When a group of people makes music together their unity is restored. The chief loss resulting from the decline of Judaeo-Christian theology in our culture may not be the theology but the whole community coming together once a week to make music. No Sunday morning DIY activity done by a single person in an individualised dwelling can replace the community-building power of the hymn or worship song. This may be the attraction of the retention of the school assembly. It is a chance for the whole school to sing together once a day. In the last 50 years the nature of the song may have changed but deep in the psyche of educational planners (although often not acknowledged publicly) is the wisdom that retains this central act of music-making in the school curriculum.

There is an increasing interest in the function of musical elements in the first relationship a person makes as an infant. The discourse of mother and child has been carefully analysed, showing how the rhythm of the relation-ship is established by non-verbal vocalisations that show subtle interrelationships developing in the utterances of mother and child (Stern *et al.* 1975). The creation of relationship through music (Pavlicevic 1997) is central to music therapy.

At different times in our lives we may be closer to community and at others we may need more solitude. Gianluigi di Franco (1993) links the notions of fusion and individualisation with foetus in the womb and individualisation with the pursuit of identity: 'The relationship between the tendency towards fusion and the one towards individualisation will become a "playing", sometimes a "dramatic playing", which will determine the effort of balancing these two opposite variables' (p.84).

The re-establishment of communities based on kinship or geographical location may now no longer be a possibility. Ken Roberts (1997), writing on work and leisure in young people's lives in the UK, concludes that various trends in this area including unemployment, the growth in part-time employment and a variety of patterns of studying

> are leading to prolonged adolescence and an increase in individualisation – an increase in individual experience and more variety within all social categories, while not necessarily diminishing the differences associated with social backgrounds and gender. Each individual nowadays tends to have an individualised network of relationships, and the youth population is linked through interlocking webs rather then clearly divided into groups, all with distinctive subcultures, between which there is little contact. Individuals may feel strong attachments to groups, but often only fleetingly. They may feel that their opportunities, achievements and problems are personal; rather than shared by large numbers of peers. Individualisation is also seen as coupled with increasing uncertainty and risk, and that it is impossible for today's teenagers to know the types of adults they will become, and when transitions have ended… Prolonged transitions, uncertain prospects and individualised predicaments are normal facts of life for young people in the 1990's, and can be simultaneously liberating and threatening. (Roberts, summarised in Haworth 1997, p.9)

Music plays an important part in the establishment of these informal networks. One of the main agents of this is the personal stereo. This phenomenon allows people the possibility of an individualised musical experience (for the first time in music's history) which nonetheless makes them part of a community of people who are also listening to the same CD. The establishment of communities of musicians by means of radio stations and the Internet is a new and exciting late twentieth century phenomenon which enables people both to individualise and socialise in a single act.

The development of greater ecological concern has opened up the possibility of a wider view of community. The connection of the natural world and music was deep in pagan traditions. In these traditions people sang to apple trees so they would increase their yield and animals were encouraged to give up milk with songs. This was lost in Christianity with its concentration on domination over nature and on the humanity of God. In the classical tradition, romanticism in the nineteenth century often saw nature as God. But the flow was seen as one way – it was seen as an inspiration. There was no notion that the natural world was in turn affected by the music. Ideas that the material world could be influenced by sound disappeared post-Enlightenment as scientific realism gained sway.

It has resurfaced in the New Age. It has rediscovered ancient notions that music is vibration and that the whole of the natural world is in vibration. In this system it is not seen as surprising that music will affect the natural world. The walls of Jericho could have fallen if Joshua found the right note, and sound can shatter glass. In concentrating on the destructive potential of music, the possibility of using music to create and build in the natural world has deliberately been ignored or ridiculed. This is counter to the dominant culture. Music and healing in the New Age are now being related in a cosmic context. Humans are healed by being restored to a relationship not only with other humans but to relationship with the natural world.

Case study

Roger Watson runs a community music organisation entitled Traditional Arts Projects. He has a strong sense of the importance of rooting people in their own indigenous culture. His prevailing concerns are with the English folk tradition and how, from this base, he can enable people to become creative and reach out to other cultures. He runs a group called Millan in which he plays his accordion and joins with people from various Eastern traditions to see what they can share to create group pieces. Roger is interested in personal authenticity and integrity as the starting point for peace-making. His approach is essentially democratic and is concerned with allowing people freedom to make their own decisions in the improvisatory groups that he runs. He does have a wider view of community which includes the natural world, especially in the area of the materials from which the musical instruments are made. His work provides an interesting reconciliation of the polarity between personal authenticity and community-building through music.

Summary – community / individualism

Each person will at any time be closer to a community or closer to being alone. Sometimes this community is thought to include the whole of the cosmos. Jung called the balancing of these poles and the ability to move with ease between them individuation. This can be done through the medium of music. The classical tradition offers models of individual performance linked to the heroic journey, while religious rituals and community music-making (and now contemporary phenomena such as music radio stations and the Internet) offer exploring community through music. Such phenomena show music being used to balance the pole of separation that characterises the values of Western scientific rationalism.

Containment/freedom

The development of depth psychology in the twentieth century made accessible, indeed encouraged, access to the deepest recesses of the human personality. In it, at its crudest, were found to lurk some very powerful emotions often associated with trauma in the early years of life. Accessing this area was difficult; but the analytical methods developed by Freud and Jung opened up the dark abysses and Jung in particular used human imagination (the root of artistic activity) in this process. He is reported to have encountered a concert pianist called Margaret Tilly who in a single session convinced him of the potential power of music:

> This opens up whole new areas I'd never dream'd of. Because of what you have shown me this afternoon – not just what you have said but what I have actually felt and experienced. I feel that from now on music should be an essential part of every analysis. This reaches the deep archetypal material that we can only sometimes reach in our analytical work with patients. This is remarkable. (Jung, quoted in Jensen 1982, pp.125–128)

Controlling these emotions once accessed became a problem. It was like unblocking a dam and then not knowing where to channel the water: 'The coming-together of opposites generates subjectively intense psychic energy which is often difficult or impossible to contain or harness' (Redfearn 1992, p.171). The primacy of language is well established in the Western world and the analytical traditions embraced it as a valuable tool. There are many now who see the potential of music in this area as an essential adjunct to, or replacement for, verbal therapy.

Music has always been aware (at some times more than others) of its relationship with human feeling but has always had the other pole of musical form to manage the feelings in some way. Suzanne Langer (1953) entitled her significant book on the philosophy of music *Feeling and Form: A Theory of Art*. In it she examined this complex relationship. It is a mysterious process – that of the embodiment or containment of feeling in formal structures – and few have attempted to chart the process successfully. The process of encoding feeling in the materials of sound is one of containment.

This polarity of the free expression of emotion or feeling and its encoding in musical structures features highly in the literature on music. There is a freedom about music in every mode of encounter with it. The thoughts of the listener fly freely over a wide range of images, the performer enters a wide range of feeling states and the composer/improviser is able to explore the unspeakable. The development of particular musical traditions has often been the story of the development of methods containing these potentially destructive feelings within musical forms and structures. Some traditions permit more freedom than others.

This process of exploring the deepest emotions can in some psychological models be seen as a return to childhood. Yet the very process of music-making from these deep sources is also a containment of potentially overwhelming feelings and emotions. A local head teacher newly appointed to a difficult school introduced drumming lessons as a significant part of her strategy of turning the disrupted atmosphere around. It was a strategy that worked. The aggressive feelings of the disruptive elements were contained by the process of drumming.

An essential part of the shamanic training in traditional societies was a visit to the Underworld with the guiding of a more experienced traveller (see Chapter Three). The exploration of the Underworld could be equated with the exploration of the unconscious. In this tradition it is regarded as another world (the Other World).

Various musical traditions have included improvisatory practices within them to a greater or lesser degree, and these have been controlled to a greater or lesser extent. There has sometimes appeared to be a dichotomy between the freer traditions of improvisation and the more fixed and rigid high art traditions allowing improvisation within certain culturally and tradi-tion-governed boundaries. But even the more improvisatory traditions have constraints. Topi Jaërvinen (1997) describes these restraints well: 'Improvisa-tion is an interesting musical activity, because it imposes strict temporal con-straints on the creation of music. For while improvising one cannot go back and revise some past event that in retrospect appears unsuitable' (p.157). This constraint of time, however, means that there is a greater concentration within the tradition on the process which is synonymous with the product. Jaërvinen's (1997) paper also examines how tonality and metre are used as containing structures for the tradition. So within improvisatory traditions there are restraints on freedom operating culturally and personally.

Case study

Jan Hughes-Madden is a community musician who runs a community choir and works with people with special needs, mental health users, cancer patients, people in the spinal unit and Alzheimer sufferers in local hospitals. Her own story shows how she was freed by discovering her voice with practitioners such as Frankie Armstrong (see Chapter Four). In an interview in 1998 she talked about her own history and how important music was as means of expression, particularly at difficult times:

> I used to live on the road amongst the travellers ... I came very very close to death on many occasions and it was at that point in my life that I actually found music. I didn't know that I could sing till I was 23. I couldn't play an instrument. I had no musical history or background. I discovered that I was able to sing and therefore to join in and then started to play the ... [I went] on from that to working with the choir and forming it out of nothing. That is, for me, without a doubt, a spiritual experience. It's a better high than any drug I ever took ... It's real, uniting those people vocally like that ... I don't believe I do that ... I think it comes through me ... I think I am a channel and I think that's the most important for me – if I can keep expressing and keep the channel open then it can come through me.

She is motivated by her desire to pass this freedom that she has discovered onto others. Some of her work is for REACH, an organisation set up to promote and run projects involving people with disabilities and mental health problems. One of REACH's aims is to integrate these people with the wider community and release their potential through expression. Her work shows how the discovery of one's natural voice is a liberating phenomenon in personal development and how it can be used to contain very difficult feelings.

Summary – containment/freedom

The depth psychology of the early psychoanalysts opened up the deepest recesses of the human personality. Intense human emotions were scrutinised and released. Some of these are associated with childhood experiences, and they need some form of containment. Music has always been related to human feelings and emotions. Each piece of music-making manages to incarnate these – that is, to put them into audible form. Musical form behaves like a container. Music-making activities are places where adults can play safely and lose some of the restraint imposed by Western society – letting out some of the most unruly areas of the personality. (Sometimes these unruly areas are called the Underworld or the Other World). In some traditions the formal aspects of music-making has been more emphasised than others. Musical traditions have included a greater or lesser degree of improvisation and managed it in various ways. This has led to a greater stress on process rather than product, which necessarily challenges the values of a capitalist society where the notion of a product is central to the notion of the market-place.

Expression/confidentiality

This follows logically from the exploration of containment/freedom and relates to the public and the private. The fundamental basis of psychotherapy is to give a space for reflection on feelings, thoughts, dreams and emotions. 'Better out than in' is an old adage and the problems involved in 'bottling up' significant events and associated emotions are well documented. Western society, in its desire to control the material world, has devalued the imagination and dreaming and has had difficulty in accepting its existence. It is located in the private sphere although the popularity of the chat show is relocating it.

Healing the West is often a private affair. The model of treating illness in Western society is to remove the sick person from the surrounding society into hospitals or institutions where healing can take place away from the main society. Words are used as the main discourse for psychotherapeutic encounters. So the process of healing, whether psychological or physical, is one of confidentiality. This is particularly true of psychotherapy. This is necessary with the explicit medium of words. It may never be appropriate to express certain emotions publicly in words or it may take a great deal of therapeutic work. Other societies have less private models of healing, especially those that value the arts more highly in the healing process.

There is a profound difference between words and music as a means of expression: 'In verbal dialogue an issue is focused on a common meaning. In music the expression itself is meaningful' (Kortegaard 1993, p.61). Sadly, elitism disenfranchises people from their natural expression through the medium of music. But not all cultures are elitist. Messenger (1958) writes of the Anang Ibibo tribe in Nigeria where he searched in vain for the 'unmusical' person:

> We were constantly amazed at the musical abilities displayed by these people, especially by the children who, before the age of five, can sing hundreds of songs, both individually and in choral groups, and, in addition, are able to play several percussion instruments and have learned dozens of intricate dance movements calling for incredible muscular control. We searched in vain for the 'non-musical' person, finding it difficult to make enquiries because the anang language possesses no comparable concept. (p.20)

Western music therapy and the New Age has opened up the world of music-making to everyone. Its use in conjunction with conventional therapy has been to recall past events, contact 'lost' emotions and communicate these to others. Some regard music as one of the most direct routes to the unconscious (Erdonmez 1993). The strength of music is not only to recall the event but also the associated emotions. Because music validates the expression of negative emotions, it is therefore more able to access and express the previously inaccessible negative emotions associated with unpleasant events.

To make a musical sound is to externalise some aspect of the personality; it is an icon of the psyche. Therefore it is important that this is accepted by others. Music has this built into its structures with clapping (or sighing in Renaissance Europe) or whistling and calling and laughing in other contexts.

Music has certain qualities that make it useful as a public means of expression. It is a 'veiled' medium. Particularly in instrumental music the meaning is not specific, the original events or emotions are veiled with a diaphanous cloak of unclear meaning which both reveals and hides them simultaneously. As Levi-Strauss (1970) writes:

> Music is a language by whose means messages are elaborated ... Since music is the only language with the contradictory attributes of being at once intelligible and untranslatable, the musical creator is a being comparable to the gods, and music itself the supreme mystery of the science of man. All other branches of knowledge stumble into it, it holds the key to their progress. (p.18)

Music is both a public and private medium, where each listener decodes the meaning in his or her own way and is unlikely to come up with specific details of events and happenings. Indeed, structuralists have seen the main difference between musical and spoken language as who decides on the nature of the message. In spoken language it is the sender who decides; in music it is the listener (Leach 1996). It is well illustrated by the work of Benjamin Britten. Only when Britten's diaries were released after his death did the world know the extent of his suffering and yet it had been encoded in piece after piece which dealt with the loss of innocence (even including pieces with words) (Carpenter 1992).

Anthony Kemp (1996) in his book *The Musical Temperament* finds the quality of introversion prevalent in musicians, and suggests that this is an important aspect of communication for this personality type (one suited to the classical notion of the composer and performer in particular). Kemp also suggests that what is important is the element of control that makes the medium so attractive for this personality type, but I think it is because of the 'veiled, different to penetrate' quality of the medium of communication.

It is this quality that allowed the shaman in some societies to practise his or her art of therapy publicly. Much traditional healing with music was done in the context of communal gatherings. Using music, healing did not need to be a private act. The community could be involved, so there was then less problem in getting the community to accept the cured person back into the community. Where the process of healing has been private, the community has no proof that the person has been healed.

Also, particular pieces will have acquired particular meanings for particular people. Pachelbel's *Canon*, for example, is almost universally regarded as peaceful and uplifting. I visited a special school where it was used every morning to keep the school calm. But for one person it was associated with a particular personal tragedy, which interrupted its culturally determined mood. Cecil Sharp, the collector of English folksongs, tells the story of how he searched for a particular fiddle tune. After a difficult search, he came across a fiddler (the only one) who knew it; but the fiddler had last played it at the funeral of a close friend, and had vowed that he would never play it again. He refused Sharp's persuasion and the tune was lost forever because of its individual associations for that particular person.

Case study

Carole Killick is a therapist who uses the Bonny method of Guided Imagery and Music. This was a system developed by Helen Bonny who was a musician, psychotherapist and music therapist. It is a way of therapy that involves getting people to image while listening to music. She developed it originally in the 1960s as a way of treating drug addiction, when the sessions would sometimes be 16 hours long, replicating the drug 'trip'. It is described in Killick's publicity leaflet (see Appendix II) as: 'A humanistic and transpersonal psychotherapeutic approach involving listening to very carefully sequenced choices of classical music designed to be congruent with the subject's mood or state of mind and leading towards resolution on inner conflicts.'

In the Bonny method clients are asked to allow the images to form in their mind while the music is playing and tell them to the guided imagery therapist. It concentrates on the emotional component of music, although the pre-prepared tapes that are used show careful planning of both the expressive and the structural areas of music. Only classical music is used. The form and content of particular pieces are related to the needs of a client. Although the same tapes are used for many clients, each client will have a different set of images. The tapes are designed to start where the client is and take them gently to different places. The composer is regarded as a co-therapist (the process is rather like a shamanic journey) with the trained therapist whose role is to guide. The training involves an interrelated mixture of psychology and music. It is conducted, in general, in a one-to-one setting where expression is in the context of a sense of confidentiality. The method shows clearly how a single piece of music will produce different reactions in many people and also how this has been embedded in the confidential structures of Western psychotherapy.

Summary – expression / confidentiality

Western medicine has a confidential model of healing. Sick people are taken out of the wider society, treated and then returned. In psychotherapy where words are the main tool, confidentiality is regarded of supreme importance. Music has the capacity to express and awaken hidden aspects of the personality and has elements of both public and private because its meaning cannot easily be read. It is therefore a way of gaining a wider acceptance of painful private areas of human experience and aids the process of maturity: to know how to use music to express private events publicly can lead to maturity.

Unity/diversity

The Western Enlightenment model of the self stresses unity above diversity, often using words like integration and disintegration. These terms are tightly bound up with systems that value order above chaos, which they attempt to eliminate or suppress. The notion of therapy as integration is deep within the therapeutic literature, following Jung. The notion of the united or integrated self is deep in the Western psyche. People presenting themselves as 'ill' often present symptoms of disintegration. Yet there is a rhythm to the integration and de-integration. With its roots in Platonic philosophy, the desirability of unity has, in general, underpinned much of Western philosophy: 'Unity is the integration of a dis-integrated totality, the overcoming of alienation. In Kant and Hegel, in particular, we see this notion of unity as integrative overcoming of difference' (Levine 1997, p.18). However, the theologian Jurgen Moltmann (1967), also drawing on Hegel, stresses the need for contradictions as a necessary condition for living: 'A thing is alive only when it contains contradiction in itself and is indeed the power of holding contradiction within itself and enduring' (p.337).

The work of the philosopher Gillian Rose is similarly based on Hegel and her notion of working in what she calls 'the broken middle' has within it the necessity of living with the contradictions:

> Her work seeks to retrieve the experience of contradiction as the substance of life lived in the rational and the actual ... In the middle of imposed and negated identities and truths, in the uncertainty about who we are and what we should do, Gillian commends that we comprehend the brokenness of the middle as the education of our natural and philosophical consciousness. She commends us to work with these contradictions, with the roaring and the roasting of the broken middle, and to know that it is 'I'. (Tubbs 1998, p.34)

Other writers (Levine 1997) see the imposition of a unity external to the particular psyche as dangerous because it replicates previous attempts, often made by parents, to impose an external (and probably repressive) order. The therapist must wait for the order to arise from inside the person. Heidegger calls this 'authentic care'. (In dealing with this he stresses the need for the therapist to have entered into their own chaos *before* attempting to do this for others. This resembles the need for the shaman to have descended into the Underworld.) Notions of identity based on unity in the work of Derrida and Adorno (see Chapter Two) have been associated with a repressive imperial force. Psychologists like Michael Fordham (1986) have challenged the notions of unity that underpinned Jung's concept of integration. Fordham 'suggests that the process of de-integration and reintegration is an archetypal one, not belonging to myths as such, but instead being "much more primitive"' (Jennings 1999, p.45).

Joseph Redfearn (1992) explores in some detail the way in which Freud and Jung handled diversity within their own selves and in their theories, concluding with his own position:

Freud uses the terms *ego*, *id* and *superego* for the basic structural units of personality; Jung uses the terms *archetypes* and *complexes* for those various selves within ourselves. I use the term *subpersonality* for the structural unit of the personality because it begs no theoretical questions and it is not only an empirical finding of everyday life – we all readily recognise and describe each other's main subpersonalities – but also the main working unit of analysis and psychotherapy ... Although the subpersonalities are not complete human beings, they behave like persons in so far as they behave like characters in a story or on the stage, or like mythological or religious characters, or embodiments (personifications) of virtues, vices and instincts etc. ... They are indeed primarily units of the observed behaviour of the person, enacting themselves smoothly and unconsciously as behaviour in the normal state of affairs, only reaching awareness when blocked or in conflict with other predispositions in oneself. (p.59)

The concept of subpersonalities is very helpful in dealing with multiplicity in the self and will be used in Chapter Two to explain the psychological roots of composition in the classical tradition. This theory links happily with the theories of creativity:

The images of the opposites combining creatively is associated with images of new life ... If the energy cannot be contained, the images of the new creation take the corresponding negative form ... Rubbish and *prima material* can be converted into valuable things, intrapsychically speaking. (Redfearn 1992, pp.171–172)

Other writers in this area would see the necessity to de-integrate in order to re-integrate and see the crisis as an opportunity. However, the presenting symptoms of people entering therapy often seem like meaningless disintegration. In times of deep pain and suffering there is an *uncomfortable* sense of disunity, of fragmentation, of a loss of a central self that is seen as necessary for the personality to cohere. Such moments can be looked at in two ways: one is that the loss of an old persona is the prelude to new growth, a growth that leads to a greater and better unity; the other is that the process is one of the acceptance of another persona and the encompassing of greater diversity (Levine 1997). Here Levine retains the notion that the ultimate goal is unity.

In an article that resembles poetry more than academic text, Elaine Barkin (1994), writing about composer Pauline Oliveros, describes this process of remaking vividly. In it the notion of unity is far less clear:

On the way to becoming we most of us try others on. Not whole bodies. Those parts whose fit might still enable pores to breathe. Ultra tight fits unintentionally wanted by some constrain, intentionally put upon also constrain. The longer the wear the less the bind feels. Wanting fitness at first is all. Itself gets used to. Until. The want to become again revives. We cast off second hands exposing our remaining rawness, selfness. Ourselves becoming again consolidated. Refit. Until. Awareness momentarily that stupefies may become our real thing. Fitness is not all. When unawareness of prosthetic appliance environs us we are not us. Then to divest to unbecome to become. And invest ourselves with discards of now our own former moulting. Or refashion from some scratch never wholly unloosed of old fits. Or invent new starts. Or even as it were to unbecomingly flounder. And reimage ourselves barely unjointedly as we reimagine fitting ourselves out. Conjoining our unbound first hands. Until. (p.203)

Another psychologist, James Hillman, proposes a polytheistic psychology, seeing personal identity more as a 'multi-dimensional play of imaginative realities' (Levine 1997, p.19). This has been part of the thinking of post-modern philosophers such as Rosi Braidotti (1994):

The nomadic subject is a myth, that is to say, a political fiction, that allows me to think through and move across established categories and levels of experience: blurring boundaries without burning bridges. Implicit in my choice is the belief in the potency and relevance of the imagination, of myth-making, as a way to step out of the political and intellectual stasis of these post-modern times ... It entails a total dissolution of the notion of a centre and consequently of originary sites or authentic identities of *any* kind ... It is *as if* some experiences were reminiscent or evocative of others; this ability to flow from one set of experiences to another is a quality of interconnectedness that I value highly... Nomadic becoming is neither reproduction nor just imitation but rather emphatic proximity, intensive interconnectedness. Some states or experiences can merge simply because they share certain attributes.

Nomadic shifts designate therefore a creative sort of becoming; a performative metaphor that allows for otherwise unlikely encounters and unsuspected sources of interaction of experience and of knowledge... It is a retrospective map of places I have been...the practice of 'as if' is a technique of strategic re-location in order to rescue what we need of the past in order to trace paths of transformation of our lives here and now... I prefer to approach 'the philosophy of "as if"'...as the affirmation of fluid boundaries... I am committing myself to addressing issues of repetition, difference, and the subversion of dominant codes... [It] is a politically empowering sort of repetition, because it addresses simultaneously issues of identity, identifications, and political subjecthood... The nomadic subject as a performative image allows me to weave together different levels of my experience... There is a strong aesthetic dimension in the quest for alternative figurations. (pp.4–8)

She draws on Deleuze to elaborate her image, explaining his image of a rhizome to represent the connections:

What Deleuze aims at is the affirmation of difference in terms of a multiplicity of possible differences; difference as the positivity of differences. In turn, this leads him to redefine consciousness in terms of a multiplicity of layers of experiences that does not privilege rationality as the organising principle... The notion of 'rhizome'...points to a redefinition of the activity of philosophy as the quest for new images of thought, better suited to a nomadic, disjuncted self. (Braidotti 1994, pp.100–101)

Calvin Schraig (1997) links it with post-modern views when he describes the self as: 'A unity that is progeny of a transversal play of viewpoints ... Such is the dynamics of transversality, striving for convergence without coincidence' (pp.131–132).

In the plurality of modern society it is possible to take on a number of different musical traditions. These can be seen as expressive of difference within the personality. Initially most people will probably be immersed in the culture of one tradition to some depth. Having examined the strengths and weakness of that tradition it is then possible to explore other traditions and so explore different parts of the personality.

The process of re-forming the person, the acceptance of the more hidden aspects of the personality, leads to a 're-membering' of the personality. The newly accessed areas are now reintegrated to form new patterns, more reflective of the re-formed person. The new experience is of relationships of respect within the personality. Music has certain characteristics that enable it to play a real part in the processes of integration and de-integration. It uses motifs and ideas arranged in a whole which may have a greater or lesser degree of coherence. Beethoven's sketchbooks show us the process of refining and combining musical ideas into works and a willingness to abandon those which will not fit but may be used in another piece. So in these precious personal diaries we have a record of Beethoven wrestling with the process of 're-membering' himself.

The process of listening can enable the listener to participate in this process. Listeners are called to enter into the processes of the performer and composer. The listener tunes into, becomes 'in sync' with, the composer/performer. The listener shares the journey and is reassured by the fact that another person has been into that chaotic place that they are experiencing. They also become part of the journey and learn some of the strategies of the composer/performer. This has echoes in shamanic practices.

Most musical forms allow for a degree of repetition and contrast. This is a reflection of unity and diversity. Music allows for juxtaposition and simultaneous combination; it therefore can accommodate difference and differing degrees of unity. It allows for things to stay separate or to be recombined into new ideas. It allows for the existence of chaos in certain sections (especially in freer improvised structures) and more ordered sections at other times. As such it provides a mirror of a mature person happy with order and acknowledging the presence of chaos.

I have tried to bring various traditions together authentically in some of my pieces, which has enabled me to bring some musical integration to intercultural elements within my thinking. A piece entitled *The Call of the Ancestors* (1998a) used a large four-part choir and brass quintet in Western classical style, and Thai piphat (an instrument including circles of gongs and xylophones), Kenyan drums and a rock group. I decided to arrange the sections sequentially and only have the groups play together at the end; I felt that the integrity of the traditions would be compromised by merging the sections more than that. So it is in the personality. Certain things can be combined but certain others may always remain separate.

This often involves the exploration of the unconscious, subconscious or some personal Underworld. Thus it is part of the process of de-integration described above. Indeed, listening to challenging pieces can trigger this process. Through composing, performing or listening we can contact areas of the unconscious or subconscious of which we were unaware. Accounts of the creative process always involve some descent into chaos. These challenge the Western Enlightenment notion of progress which sees truth as being approached by means of logical steps that can be carefully charted. The ability to enter that chaos, with tools for handling it, would seem to be what differentiates the experienced composer from the less experienced musician.

What we need is to fumble around in the darkness because that's where our lives (not necessarily all the time, but at least some of the time, and particularly when life gets problematical for us) take place; in the darkness, or, as they say in Christianity, 'the dark night of the soul'. It is in these situations that Art must act and then it won't be judged Art but will be useful to our lives. (Cage, quoted in Ross 1978, p.10)

Anthony Kemp (1996), drawing on Jung, sees the gifted person as one with a profound need for this process to be accepted both by their peers and the wider society. He discusses this in relation to the education of the gifted. The process of education may be seen as the inculcation of the dominant value system; this makes the gifted person, who often has a high intuitive sense, very vulnerable. He draws on Pruett (1990), who writes:

> [Teachers have a responsibility to] encourage the very gifted to avoid the sense of the asymmetric, misshapen or unfinished life and self... The most enduring artistic achievements involve the whole person and his careful understanding and intimate expression of his imagination's light *and* dark components, not just his facile fingerings. (p.322)

Kemp goes on to make the justified and sensible step of requiring our society to nurture such figures more carefully. We could take one further step and say that such gifted people can be encouraged to explore both the prevailing value systems of the society in which they find themselves and their own preferred value systems. Then they can act as 'musical prophets' calling their society to rebalance, by exploring a wider range of experiences through the medium of music. It is a view similar to that developed by such theoreticians as Attali and Adorno (see Chapter Two). It depends, however, on the ability to value and contain diversity within the personality.

The acceptance of multiplicity within the self as natural can be an experience of great freedom: 'The changes...are to do with this increasing sense of conflict and plurality in the I or collective we, coupled paradoxically, with the consciousness of greater freedom and choice in the range of possible behaviours and an increase in the room to manoeuvre available to the I' (Redfearn 1992, p.261).

Case study

Olu Taiwo was born in the 1960s in Clapham, London, to Yoruba parents, who had just come to the UK from Nigeria. He was educated in South London and then went to Exeter University to study Fine Art where he discovered drumming and dancing traditions. He describes (in an interview with me in 1999) the shock of meeting Western Enlightenment traditions at his grammar school and wondering how they could possibly fit with the Yoruba backgrounds of his parents. Olu sees his drumming and dancing as a way of exploring the relationship between Yoruba and Western culture.

Although initially he tried to bring them together, he now sees them as very different and is interested in finding ways in which they can exist side by side. He has chosen an improvisatory art form as he feels it mirrors life processes. He has developed a notion of the 'return beat', which underpins much of his thinking and embodies more cyclical approaches to time, rather than the digital clock time of Western culture. These appear to mirror Levi-Strauss's distinction between 'hot' and 'cold' societies (see p.36). When he lectures he is able to call on his two selves, even giving each a hat, a way of moving and a distinctive accent to illustrate their diversity. He is an example of a person working musically at the diversity within his self.

Summary – unity/diversity

The self needs to be able to accommodate diversity within a non-repressive unity. Music has been seen as a way of producing unity in diversity by integrating small motifs into a coherent whole. It is also a way of living with the chaos until such time as the self is ready to re-integrate. However, there are psychologists and philosophers who challenge the model of the unified self and value a greater measure of diversity. Dis-integration and de-integration need distinguishing. Models of the creative process include a descent into the chaos of a personal Underworld. This is also part of the training of a traditional shaman, although here the Underworld is located outside of the self. The experienced musician has ways of entering and leaving the chaos with a creative outcome. Listeners can participate in this journey and gain insight into their own unconscious. This could also be seen to be similar to certain shamanic practices.

Challenge/nurture

The process of reshaping the personality often results in a sense of empowerment. The previously unharnessed energies, which were once a threat, are now harnessed and channelled into the service of the personality. This can result in a great sense of strength and a feeling of being centred, of standing firm, of self-knowledge. It is associated with the heroic quest discussed above (pp.34–36).

The polarity of nurture is connected with vulnerability. It is a way of handling this. The skill of the therapist is in knowing how to hold the de-integrated parts until they are ready to re-form. In the stages of growth where dis- or de-integration is happening (see pp.47–51) there is the necessity for being held, for someone other than the patient to hold the pieces until they find their own re-ordering. In this process of holding, the patient's sense of self is restored, but in a new form. The concept of holding is well defined by Sara Ruddick (1989) in her concept of 'maternal thinking'. She writes: 'To hold means to minimise risk and to reconcile differences rather than to sharply accentuate them. Holding is a way of seeing with an eye towards maintaining minimum harmony, material resources and skills necessary for sustaining a child in safety' (p.79).

Music is a way of holding. I was told the story of a therapist who gave a distressed client her scarf as a way of showing that the client was held by her even when she was not physically with her. A song can fulfil this function well. It can also be a way for a group of people to hold some of its members. I used a repeated drumbeat very softly under a heated discussion which threatened to break up. The attitude of confrontation changed and the group was able to function again.

Many New Age pieces are designed to hold people. They are the adult equivalent of the lullaby. The lullaby can be sung without physically touching the person. The song transmits loving holding through the medium of music. A song is a vehicle of transmission of love (as evidenced by the serenader singing the lovesong outside the beloved's window). In an age where the sense of touch has for many people been abused so that it is difficult to use as a therapeutic tool, the role music can play in holding people in their vulnerable moments has real possibilities.

But we can also listen to music to be challenged and this has been part of the post-Enlightenment aesthetic in classical music. The master composer on his heroic journey challenges the listener to join him and so move forward him or herself (see Chapter Two). Classical tradition based on challenge through attentive listening has despised 'wallpaper' music designed for the more subtle process of holding or nurturing.

Music teaching regimes have set pupils a series of challenges of increasing difficulty, often in the shape of examinations and competitions of some kind. The 'good' teacher is paid to move pupils forward, not to encourage them to rest peacefully where they are.

However, if we take the rapidly developing world of New Age tapes and cassettes, we find music at the opposite pole, designed to relax, to affirm people where they are – to nurture them in the same way as a mother might feed a child. If we accept that music can do this, then music becomes a backdrop to other internal action within ourselves; it is no longer only something to be concentrated on. It can be used as a safe home or relationship is used, to revisit old and new areas of oneself for purposes of renewal and sustenance. This can be seen in the contemporary phenomenon of having music playing while working. It provides a security in which new ideas can be explored and new risks taken.

Another aspect of this is that music helps to order the mind and think more carefully: 'Music creates order out of chaos; for rhythm imposes unanimity upon the divergent; melody imposes continuity on the disjointed, and harmony imposes compatibility upon the incongruous' (Menuhin 1972, p.9). Listening to Mozart has been particularly cited in this area.

When well balanced, challenge and nurture together lead to empowerment and the two work in tandem, especially in person-centred models of learning. The learning of musical skills is often part of the challenge. Singing has been extremely important in the empowering of people both at an individual and a cultural level. Estelle Jorgensen (1996), in a powerful article which brings together Paolo Freire's *Pedagogy of Hope* (with its notion of empowerment through pedagogy) with the role of the artist in society and education in the arts, highlights the role of itinerant singing masters in empowering the poor and the women in eighteenth century society. These men delivered the only formal education open to groups of people from otherwise disenfranchised groups, especially women and girls who were excluded from much music-making in the churches and communities. Jorgensen claims that the nineteenth century political movements, which encouraged the inclusion of music in the school curriculum of the emerging state-supported schools, were inspired by the work of these singing schools. She concludes: 'Indeed, my reading of educational history generally suggests that wherever there have been concerted efforts to teach people to sing, there has been a concomitant, deepening regard for self-improvement and general education, and heightened desire for freedom. Each has fed the other' (p.42).

Case study

Liz Wilcock was a classical violinist who decided to train as a music therapist. She found the classical tradition too challenging and demanding for a mother with young children. She was attracted to seeing music as a nurturing force, having already discovered the healing power of her own hands, and has had to challenge many of the prejudices engendered by her classical training. She makes a real distinction between performing from notation and improvisation, especially in the area of being able to tailor-make the music to a particular situation and reach the heart of the feelings of group. She has had from childhood a sense of the emotional power of music which she would distinguish from its effect on the mind, body or spirit. The process of expression when it is accepted by someone is the process of re-integration. She now has real sense of nurturing through music which can be done by concerts or improvisation and is slightly worried about her role in triggering 'difficult' responses or touching 'difficult' areas in people's lives.

Summary – challenge/nurture

Notions of challenge have been part of the post-Enlightenment classical tradition linked with the notion of the heroic journey. Composers have embraced innovation and teachers of music have set pupils a number of hurdles to jump over. The notion of music as nurture has emerged in New Age music-making and Western music therapy. Balancing challenge and nurturing successfully leads to empowerment, and there are cultural examples of the teaching of singing skills to empower disenfranchised sections of society.

Excitement/relaxation

The human being needs to establish a rhythm between excitement and relaxation to maintain physical, mental and spiritual health. This differs with age, experience and general stress levels. We live in a society that offers a very stimulating environment for a great deal of the time. The development of multimedia forms of communication allows for unprecedented degrees of excitement. Anthony Storr (1992) terms excitement arousal as 'a condition of heightened alertness, awareness, interest, and excitement: a generally enhanced state of being... Arousal manifests itself in various physiological changes, many of which can be measured' (pp.24–25). These include an increase in pulse rate, a change in respiratory rate and an increase in blood pressure. (Some of these are documented in Harrer and Harrer 1977.)

Most cultures have used music to excite and relax people. Although linked with challenge/nurture above, these states are concerned more with effects of hearing different sorts of music. The effects are simpler and more transcultural, and the effects of loud music which gets faster as an energiser appear in some researches to be cross-cultural. Glenn Wilson (1994) refines a table from Eibl-Eibesfeld (1989) on *Human Ethology*, which suggests some cross-cultural features that characterise joyful, sad and exciting music. Here Wilson suggests that in the area of frequency, joy is suggested by high frequencies, sadness by low, and excitement by varied frequencies. Strong melodic variation is connected with joy, slight with sadness and strong also with excitement. To be joyful, the tonal course moves moderately, first up and then down, while sadness has a downward course, and an exciting melody moves strongly upward and then down. Joyful music contains many overtones, sad music fewer overtones, and music that causes excitement has barely any overtones. The tempo of joyful music is rapid, that of sadness is slow and that evoking excitement is of a medium tempo. Joyful music is loud, sad music soft, and music to cause excitement varied in volume. An irregular rhythm suggests joy, a regular rhythm sadness, and excitement is caused by an irregular rhythm (Wilson 1994).

In order to understand how this happens, it is necessary to return to the notion of entrainment dealt with under community/individualism above. The normal heart rate is between 70 and 80 beats per minute. Music slower than this will have the effect of slowing this down and will be perceived as calming. Faster music will stimulate us, causing excitement. This is caused by the process of entrainment. We shall see in Chapter Five how this effect has been used in pain reduction: 'Entrainment music has been found to be superior to other types of music in eliciting psychophysiological changes with chronic/disease patients' (Rider and Welin 1990, p.215). Others link soothing music with the mother's heartbeat:

> Music with a pulse similar to the mother's heartbeat (about 72 beats per minute) seems to have a soothing effect on babies. In fact, it does not have to be music... Even if reminiscence of our mother's heartbeat is not an essential feature, our own pulse may be a marker that determines the emotional intensity of a musical piece. (Wilson 1994, p.21)

David Epstein, conductor and professor of music at Massachusetts Institute of Technology links tempo with our neurological make-up:

> Finding the 'right' tempo (tempo giusto) is essential to successful music-making. The right tempo allows the body to express musical gestures and emotions. The wrong tempo creates a chain reaction — the gestures of musical phrases cannot be expressed and the intuitive 'feel' of the music is lost, together with the necessary technical control. (Robertson 1996, p.30)

Robertson goes on to link this with the interdependence of motion – 'the quintessential basis of all music' – and emotion, which come from a common Latin root – 'to move'. He explains how Epstein's research reveals that 80 per cent of all musical tempo relationships (in a sample taken from seven different non-Western cultures) conform to simple ratios like 1:2, 2:3 and 3:4 (Robertson 1996, p.30).

Calming music usually combines a slow pulse with soft sounds. Many people have learned to use music for calming effects and to establish a rhythm in their personal lives. They have music to suit their mood. Classic FM regularly produces sets of CDs for various moods and times of day. Used wisely, music can be used to replicate the effects of the more powerful and less discriminating drugs either from medical or less legal sources. Music lovers need to be aware of the potential effect of certain pieces (see the section on Guided Imagery to Music, Chapter Six). Many good listeners have worked out the effect of music on their own sense of well-being and know (often quite precisely) how to use music to bring about a rhythm in their lives. Chris Brewer (1996) describes the subtlety of this process, linking it with the isomorphic (iso) principle which means that the music needs at first to match the mood of the listener:

> The iso principle is one of the most natural and intuitive techniques for moving into a new rhythm. With the iso principle, a change in tempo and mood is accomplished by entraining to the present mood and slowly altering the pace into the desired direction…rather than a quick change to a fast or dynamic mood, the use of the iso principle moves the mood gradually, almost unnoticeably into a different state. (pp.14–15)

A piece of music designed to excite starts with a pulse rate similar to the normal heart rate and then gradually increases it. By the end of the piece people are generally more excited. It is clearest in traditional war drums and military bands; but it can also be seen in the 'happy clappy' religious traditions and the bands of the Salvation Army. It is part of the rave culture, where young people are often very discriminating as to their own state of excitement and know how to use the 'chill out' rooms with discrimination. This is essential in a culture which uses multimedia presentations as a means of achieving excitement.

Certain instruments also seem to have soothing or exciting qualities. The drums are great energisers; the jingles of the tambourine also excite. A music therapist once said to me: 'If they are excited put the tambourines at the back of the cupboard.'[5] Harps and bells seem to have a calming effect. When I introduced a rainmaker (a long tube with seeds inside it) into a class of five-year-olds, one child asked if she could take it home to get her to sleep.

Music has often used the process of entrainment described above to regulate a group of people working together. Sea shanties, road-building and stone-breaking songs are just some examples of this. This is an extension of the use of music with dance to keep a group of people together and regulate

---

5   Unpublished conversation with Auriel Warwick, May 1980.

the speed at which they move. A military band orders the steps of the army and this unanimity of approach reduces fatigue. Its use in this way was extended to include piped music in factories; not only were repetitive tasks better performed with musical accompaniment, but also morale was raised.

Anthony Storr (1992) links this with the physical:

> Music brings about similar physical responses in different people at the same time. This is why it is able to draw groups together and create a sense of unity. It does not matter that a dirge or funeral march may be appreciated in a different way by a musician and by an unsophisticated listener. They will certainly be sharing aspects of the same physical experience at the same moment, as well as sharing the emotions aroused by the funeral itself. (p.24)

Case study

Chris Southall is a drummer and musician working in New Age circles. He describes himself as coming from a background of engineering, craft and practical self-sufficiency. He is strongly committed to community living and works leading drumming and dance, sweatlodge and self-development through creativity. (Sweatlodge describes a ritual with healing intentions which takes place in a very small hut heated by hot rocks in a central pit. The participants sweat and pray, while singing and drumming.) He includes workshops in trance dance, and Gabrielle Roth's Drumming the Five Rhythms, which take people through a wave pattern of various speeds and emotional qualities (see Chapter Four). Chris said in an interview with me in 1999: 'I first encountered Trance Dance in the work of Leo Rutherford and as I learned about African and North American drum dance my own path opened as a shamanic drummer.'

Chris is a drum-maker. His practice is eclectic, drawing on traditions from North and South America and various parts of Africa: 'For me, [my work] involved physicality in some way; mask work, dance, ritual drama, were probably the most important things for me... For me, and other people around the place, [what we] see going on is a fusion of traditional knowledge and contemporary knowledge, and how you bring the two together' (1999 interview).

Chris's conceptual frame is built around the concept of a dynamic energy which moves and flows through the body and the world. The notion of the connection between human beings and the world is central to this. His task is to support through his music the flow of energy in others and this is how he views healing. There was a clear notion of transcendence especially in the shamanic journeying but always rooted in the body and without a belief in God.

Summary – excitement/relaxation

Human beings need to establish a rhythm of excitement and relaxation in their lives. Music has long been used for these purposes because it has physiological effects which appear to be transcultural. The process of entrainment enables music to start where people are and move them to a more excited or relaxed state. Loud and fast music induces arousal and slower, softer music, relaxation. Certain instruments have exciting or calming qualities. Experienced listeners know how to use music to establish this rhythm in their lives, and radio stations like Classic FM are encouraging this use of music by classifying pieces by mood.

Embodiment/transcendence

Western culture has inherited from Graeco-Roman ideas and Christianity dualistic notions of the mind and body. In the pursuit of the transcendent, Western Christianity has often lost its sense of the body; indeed in its most extreme ascetic forms it denied the body, encouraging excesses that resemble those of anorexics today. This dualism has resulted in a divorce in medical practices treating the body and the mind. Post-Christian Europe has often dismissed notions of spirituality as superstitious, in line with scientific, objective rationality. Practitioners in New Age traditions have worked to restore the relationship between the body, mind and spirit and treat in a more holistic way. Shamanic practices have always regarded the two as inextricably connected.

The notion of transcendence is sometimes associated with notions of self-fulfilment. Maslow (1967) concludes by seeing freedom as an important element in these peak experiences:

1. giving up the past;

2. giving up the future;

3. innocence (without shoulds and oughts);

4. a narrowing of consciousness (concentration);

5. loss of ego (self-forgetfulness);

6. inhibiting force of consciousness;

7. disappearance of fears;

8.   lessening of defences and inhibitions;

9.   strength and courage;

10. acceptance: the positive attitude (giving up selectivity);

11. trust versus trying, controlling striving;

12. taoistic receptivity (a yielding to the authority of the facts);

13. integration of B-cogniser (an act of the whole man [sic]);

14. permission to dip into primary processes;

15. aesthetic perceiving rather than abstracting;

16. fullest spontaneity;

17. fullest expressiveness;

18. fusion of person with the world. (pp.45–47)

At the top of Maslow's (1987) hierarchy of human needs, he includes the aesthetic – the need for beauty, order, symmetry. This is placed immediately below his pinnacle of self-actualisation – realising one's full potential.

Robert Assagioli (1994) in describing the bringing together of areas of the personality uses a language of transcendence:

> Because of the multiplicity of human nature, of the existence in us of various and often conflicting subpersonalities, joy at some level can coexist with suffering at other levels... A vivid anticipation of future willed achievement or satisfaction can give joy even when one feels pain... The realisation of the self, or more of *being a self*...gives a sense of freedom, of power, of mastery, which is profoundly joyous. The mystics of all times and places have realised and expressed the joy and bliss which are inherent in the union of the individual will and the Universal Will. (p.201)

Such experiences are examples of the resolution of Aristotle's first polarity – limited/unlimited (see earlier discussion on Aristotelian thought, p.24).

The presence of the body has often been hidden in Western classical traditions, although interest in this area increased in the late twentieth century, particularly in feminist musicology. A number of injuries have been identified as a result of prolonged playing in positions difficult for the body. These include violinist's neck which results from long hours of holding the instrument under the chin and cellist's back associated with sitting with limited movement for long periods (Fry 1986). The International Society for

Tension in Performance is increasing awareness in this area. The classical concert involves sitting still, often in uncomfortable seats, in order to appreciate music. Even young children are told to 'sit still and listen'.

Because of this marginalisation of the body by the dominant Western classical tradition, little connection has been seen between physical medicine and music, except in the development of motor skills. However, interest is growing in the area. Musical elements are being detected in normal bodily discourse: 'The body of the speaker dances in time with his speech. Further, the body of the listener dances in rhythm with that of the speaker' (Condon and Ogston 1966, p.338). Others see musical links with the immune system: 'It is possible that live entrainment music can not only elicit a maximised immune response, but also increase patient compliance with home imagery practice' (Rider and Welin 1990, p.215).

Anthony Storr (1992) uses physical factors in distinguishing feelings and emotion:

> The patterns of mathematics and the patterns of music both engage our feelings, but only music affects our emotions. Herein lies the difference in our response to each. Emotions involve the body; feelings do not... Music promotes order within ourselves in a way which mathematics cannot because of music's physical effects... Music is less abstract than mathematics because it causes physiological arousal and because the sounds from which it probably originated are emotional communications. It is both intellectual and emotional, restoring links between mind and body. (p.183)

Paul Robertson (1998) cites Manfred Clynes' work linking the movement of music with emotion through the body: 'Manfred Clynes has superbly shown the exact connection between the physiology of emotional experience and its precise musical counterparts in musical gesture' (p.21). Clynes has extended his work to the area of computers, which brings us into the whole new area of 'the virtual embodied self' offered by computers and the cyborg (a human being and machine acting as a unit). He has developed interactive software called 'Superconductor'. This enables a person with musical interests to change the emotional aspect of a computer performance at will. This enables them to explore the notion of the aesthetic in direct relation to their own emotional needs.

Another area that has opened up new aspects of the relationship between music and the body is the advancing technology that has made access to the activity of various areas of the brain possible. The use of PET (positron emission tomography) in association with performing musicians at the

University of Texas Health Science Centre in San Antonio has revealed interesting features. It reminds us that performing music is a bodily activity. Scans taken when a musician is playing scales show activity in areas of the brain associated with feelings of movement and in areas in the left hemisphere associated with auditory perception. However, when a musician is playing the third movement of Bach's *Italian Concerto*, areas in the right hemisphere involved in auditory perception were activated (Robertson 1996). Research into the interaction of the two hemispheres of the brain would imply that the performance of musical pieces does cause activity in both hemispheres and requires the two areas to co-operate in a unique way. This is clarified by work with people who have suffered brain damage. Robertson (1996) also tells the story of Stephen Wade, a multilingual telephonist and amateur composer, who suffered a massive stroke affecting the left hand side of the brain. This left him with no words and serious impairment to short-term memory. He is, however, still able to use his left hand to play the keyboard fluently and use a pen to write music, although he is unable to write words.

In other societies the close relationship of dance to music-making has meant that the bodily aspects of music-making are more self-evident. The ethnomusicologist John Blacking (1976) deals with this area in relation to the Venda people of South Africa, outlining the relationship in other societies:

> Many, if not all, of music's essential processes can be found in the constitution of the human body and in patterns of interaction of bodies in society...when I lived with the Venda, I began to understand how music can become an intricate part of the development of mind, body, and harmonious social relationships. (pp.vi–viii)

From his experience with the Venda people, Blacking found that the relationship between the body and music is often clearer in cultures other than the Western classical tradition. A student from a largely Western classical background after a concert of Africa drumming said to me, 'At first I hated it. I found it strange, different and fought the power of the drums. Eventually, I yielded to their power and I found my whole body taken over by the drums so that they seemed to play my body. Then I never wanted them to stop.'[6]

Transcendence in the sense of connection to the Divine or spiritual was present in the thinking of the earliest Western philosophers of music (see Chapter Two). The profound links within Christianity between music and

6   Unpublished conversation with an undergraduate at King Alfred's University College, Winchester, 1992.

the experience of God perpetuated the notion. In the hands of the philosophers of the Enlightenment the link between music and the spiritual became weakened and the search for the spiritual which had characterised the musical tradition for hundreds of years became an essentially human search.

The notion of the connection with the Divine now reappeared in the human sphere and music and the aesthetic came to be about the highest expression of human achievement. Although an element of the sublime remained in the thinking (see Chapter Two), the notion of the spiritual was lost. Music came to be associated exclusively with the human mind. The way was therefore prepared for the development of music therapy as an adjunct to psychotherapy.

The notion of transcendence as part of self-actualisation leads people to regard the musical experience as the last remaining place for the spiritual in Western society. Hills and Argyle (1998) studied subjects who were members of both a church group and also a music-making group like a choir. They reported greater intensities in music-making in the areas of 'joy/elation', 'excitement', 'feeling uplifted' and 'loss of sense of self'.

This would certainly seem to be indicated by the presence of many pieces of religious origin in the concert hall and on disc, now dissociated from their religious roots. There are also descriptions of a unitive experience as part of the musical experience that resembles that of the religious mystics. This often takes the form of a feeling of being united with the universe, other beings and the natural world. Music may be seen as the most ubiquitous example of the contemporary 'sacred site'.

Peter Hamel (1978) sees the increasing use of drugs in the twentieth century as a fulfilment of the human need for a widening of awareness. He offers the possibility of music fulfilling the same role: 'What drugs failed to achieve – the creation of a lasting intensification of awareness – becomes possible through this new experience and appreciation of music' (p.3). He links this with a call to experience the magical mystical powers of music not in the unconscious way of the 'far-Eastern culture, the magic rituals of Africa, Asia and South America,' but in a conscious way, 'So that they might become familiar to us, stand at our service, help us to become complete people, in the sense of having achieved an integrated Wholeness' (Hamel 1978, p.7).

The New Age has rediscovered the notion of the spiritual (see Chapter Four), which is described in a variety of ways that includes higher self, a higher power and spiritual beings like angels. This diversity reflects the variety of traditions that make up the cluster of belief systems that constitute the New Age. Here transcendence is arrived at through physical practices such as chanting or dancing.

Case study

Michael Deason Barrow has had a varied musical experience. He started as a cathedral chorister in the 1960s. In an interview with me in 1998 he described himself as a natural musician and a Wiltshire bumpkin who was shot very quickly into cathedral singing in which he developed a sense of the spiritual that was to last for a lifetime. He has a very spiritual view of healing and music rooted within the Steiner anthroposophical system (see Chapter Four), together with the Alexander Technique (developed to help actors and musicians deal with stress) and his own wide reading. He works with his partner Lorin Panny who is experienced in Steiner eurhythmy, a movement system designed to balance the energies. Community for him is sacred and reached by exploring archetypal processes musically.

He has developed a theory of two complementary elements in music. The balance between the streaming connected consciousness of *rhythmos* must always balance the more individual awake consciousness of *tonos*, a principle which he sees as out of balance both in Western classical and rock music. He sees signs of a reasserting of that balance in all areas of music but especially in the rediscovery in the West of world music traditions. He gives certain instruments certain characters linked with their materials, the phase of the development of the person and the season of the year. He has formed his own organisation – Tonalis – within which to work towards these goals.

His life illustrates a developed sense of the spiritual in music born in a cathedral choir and developed by syncretising elements of various religious traditions. This is embodied by the links with eurhythmy which means that instruments are often played with flowing movement associated with their character and a concern for the materials of the instruments. He concentrates on what he calls streaming sounds and roots these in the natural world by building his own instruments out of specially chosen materials. The link with eurhythmy and his concern about the nurture of the singing voice gives the embodied dimension to his work. In this context the sounds on the instruments are often produced by flowing movements in tune with their character.

Summary – embodiment / transcendence

The mind/body/spirit split that characterises Western Enlightenment culture has coloured how the relationship between transcendence and

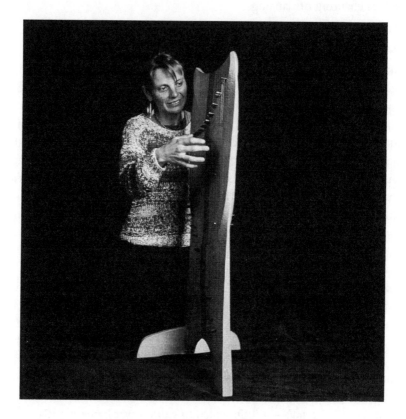

Figure 1.8 Streaming sounds: Lorin Panny plays a Tonalis instrument

embodiment is viewed and constructed in Western medicine. The influence of the mind/body dualism in Christianity has resulted in a disembodiment in Western classical traditions. This had led to lack of connection between physical medicine and music and the association of music with psychiatric medicine. There is currently a great deal of interest of the area drawing on traditions where the split has not occurred. The loss of a spiritual dimension in the Western suspicion of belief systems has led to the notion of transcendence being associated with aesthetic experience. This now is seen as having characteristics once associated with religious experience. The concert hall can be seen as a place of spiritual experience. New Age traditions have rediscovered notions of the sacred, and musical healing is set in this context. Here there are many versions of the spiritual and therefore diverse musical systems. Music can be seen as a way of rooting such experiences in the body. The achievement of the balancing of these polarities is regarded by many religious traditions as the ultimate wisdom.

Summary

This chapter has set out a model of looking at personhood as encompassing a variety of ways of knowing. Society chooses to value some of these and therefore implicitly to devalue others. As certain personalities favour different ways of knowing they will be in or out of tune with the prevailing value system. Those out of tune with it are more likely to be designated as 'sick', both because they are likely to undergo more stress and also because their chosen ways of knowing are more likely to be designated abnormal. There is evidence that people try to explore different ways of knowing in their leisure activities and that working situations can be 'improved' by validating a variety of ways of knowing. The value that Western society places on music reflects its own prevailing political and economic systems.

The self may be seen as dynamic and bringing into relationship a number of different polarities. These have been drawn from personal experience, sociologists, humanistic psychology and music education. Individuation has been approached differently by various musical traditions. The heroic journey myth has underpinned most Western models and has resulted in individualistic approaches to the musical self. Music can be a container for various powerful human emotions. Some traditions lay a greater value on structure or form than others; some include a greater degree of freedom, especially in terms of improvisation, than others. Music is a confidential medium whose meaning is not read in the same way as words. It is therefore both public and private simultaneously and is a way of expressing something of the self and gaining acceptance for it. Western philosophy and psychology have valued unity and integration but the process of growth and change involves the valuing of diversity both within the self and in the wider culture and including de-integration in the process of human development. This gives us the possibility of having multiple selves that can exist in harmony. Empowerment can be achieved musically with a right balance of challenge and nurture and different traditions have put varying degrees of importance on these two aspects of music-making. Music has been used to encourage the rhythm of relaxation and excitement in many different cultures, and notions of transcendence have been part of musical traditions geographically and historically separate. This is interpreted in different ways and within different spiritual systems. Some of these are related to bodily movement in some way and some traditions have stressed the embodied nature of the art while in others this element is not as clear.

These polarities need to be explored and balanced within the self and society. Music is seen as having a potential part to play in this process. The present book will examine how these polarities can be seen in various musical traditions – the Western classical, traditional societies involving shamans and spirit possession, Western music therapy and the cluster of practices designated the New Age. The final chapter will examine and compare the musical tools available and see how they might be used to inform the dominant health and education systems. Appendix I suggests some practical activities that can be used for this process. Appendix II lists the addresses of organisations mentioned in the text.

Above all we shall see how music is able to keep humankind rooted and centred in a balance that can delight in the exploration of the breadth of human experience. This book is designed to guide readers through a variety of musical traditions originating in different cultures using the model of the musical self as a map. I hope that it will encourage people, whether professional or amateur musicians, to explore their own constructs of musical healing. For each, in the end, will have to find their own way. I hope the map will provide some recognisable landmarks. We all need to feel both that we know where we are and that there is still somewhere to go and a treasure that may be found.

CHAPTER TWO

Of Philosophers and Thinkers

The myth of Orpheus

On the banks of the River Hebrus, long before the days of Homer, a son was born to Oeagrus, King of Thrace, and Calliope, muse of epic poetry. His name was Orpheus. He was a great man, a wise man and a maker of songs. As his fingers touched the strings of his golden lyre, given to him by the god Apollo, savage beasts were tamed and mountains and trees uprooted themselves and were moved to follow him. He could change the hearts and wills of both gods and mortals with his singing. In Hades all activity stopped when he made music; the torturers stopped their vicious tormenting, and the victims were soothed by the sweet sounds. The eternal turning of the wheel of Ixion was brought to rest; Sisyphus was freed because the stone which he was condemned to push uphill was stopped in its downward motion. He quenched the never-ending thirst of Tantalus with a melody and calmed the vultures who were attacking Tityus's liver. He played and the dreaded pursuance by the Furies of their appointed victims was halted. His melodies were able to save the Argonauts from being enchanted by the sweet songs of the Sirens which were almost as beautiful as his own. He loved the nymph Eurydice whom he followed to Hades when she died, and his song persuaded Pluto to release her. However, contrary to Pluto's conditions, he turned round to check that Eurydice was following and so lost her. After that he wandered howling in lonely places where animals and birds were still influenced by him. At his death at the hands of the Maenads, his severed head floated out to sea calling the name of his beloved Eurydice but his lyre was heard to be playing its amazing music still, so beautifully that Zeus, King of the Gods, took it and placed it for ever in the heavens as the constellation *Lyra*.

This chapter deals with the Western classical tradition, the dominant tradition in Western civilisation, despite the fact that of all the traditions to be discussed it has the least clear notions of healing associated with it. It is based on the work of musicologists, music historians, philosophers and mystics. Defining the term 'classical' is problematic since it has two meanings. The first is associated with music written between about 1750 and 1820. The second refers to notated European music from the foundation of the monasteries.

> 'Classical music', in this broader sense, is a conceptual product which, in Britain, has been formed since the eighteenth century, and at three moments in particular: the Industrial Revolution; the turn of the nineteenth and twentieth centuries, often called the 'English musical renaissance'; and the post 1945 reconstruction in education, broadcasting and state policy for the arts... Firstly then we have the emergence of the concert tradition, during the first industrial revolution... Through the eighteenth century, the rapidity of modernisation was paralleled by an increasing sense of the importance, the value, of established knowledges. There was an increasing urge to classify and compartmentalise, to order the world through category and hierarchy, and to establish standards of correctness in all fields of knowledge... This modernising epoch established, for the first time, the notion of a 'tradition' of music with its own repeatable and absolute values. Before this point, almost all music was 'contemporary'; however complex, scholarly and carefully constructed, music was written and performed for specific occasions and seldom revived, as with most music for film and television today. (Blake 1997, pp.26–28)

The theoreticians who constructed the tradition as understood today were often not practising musicians but theoreticians, intellectuals and critics. Musicians' accounts of their own practice often differ markedly from that of the theoreticians. This chapter will concentrate on the writings of theoreticians but will include some musicians writing about their work. Although in the second definition above, classical music starts from the advent of Christianity and the birth of the monastic traditions, the roots of the tradition lie in ancient Greek philosophy and it is here that this chapter starts. For the ancient Greeks, the gods of music, medicine and theology were brought together in several figures related to Hermes, the messenger of the gods. They believed in the healing power of music for both bodily and psychological illness. The Phrygian mode, for example, was thought to cure sciatica, while Pythagoras used songs to ease grief, calm anger and as an analgesic. From

Pythagoras onwards, the notion of the music of the spheres, which saw each planet circling with its own vibration influencing the earth's vibrations, runs like a thread through the history of Western music and Anthony Rooley (1990) charts a similar role for the myth of Orpheus.

Notions from ancient Greek philosophy like the music of the spheres became inextricably entwined with the Christian Church in Europe (Underwood 1999). James (1993) charts this in his book entitled *The Music of the Spheres: Music, Science and the Natural Order of the Universe*. The notion of God was central to medieval philosophies of music. Those who constructed these philosophies were often connected to the Church either as priests or religious or as musicians employed by the Church in some way. Within these systems there was no notion of 'music for its own sake'. Music was viewed as a vehicle for moral education or a reflection of the greater order of the cosmos. Technical aspects of music such as modes were examined as part of this wider order. Musical structures too were examined in the light of general cosmic or theological principles, not in relation to individual pieces of music. The music tradition was also a monophonic one – a single line of melody often closely associated with words. Gardner (1997) locates the loss of a healing dimension to mainstream European music to the advent of the harmonic texture and the associated loss of monophony. She ends by describing the chord as the corpse of the melody. This link between musical texture and healing is an individual interpretation, but it is true that notions of the healing power of music in the literature do decline as harmony became more central, from 1600 onwards. The Renaissance saw a revival of interest in Greek ideas. The work of Robert Fludd (1574–1637) shows this clearly as he likens the confluence of material and spiritual in music to 'sweet delight in contemplation' (Godwin 1987, p.146).

As the Church gradually lost its power, aesthetics became secularised. Notions of beauty replaced those of God based more on Plato's notion of 'the ideal' than his views on the moral and spiritual power of music. There have, however, always been religious notions on the margins of European aesthetic debate. In the Romantic period these tended to be drawn more from agnostic traditions than Christianity. In the twentieth century religious notions have been drawn from a greater variety of sources. Composers themselves have sometimes indicated their own spiritual and healing intentions, but these have not often been taken up by theorists, who have adopted a structuralist approach to music, concentrating on the analysis of the sounds (as revealed by the notated score). Composers like Scriabin, Stockhausen, Messiaen,

Pauline Oliveros and Terry Riley, to name but a few, have all included elements of spirituality in writing about their own works.

The origins of the idea of analytical tradition rooted in individual artworks is a product of the rise in scientific thinking after the Enlightenment. Such an approach emphasised objectivity, paralleling developments in the natural sciences. Individual works of art were examined in this period with regard to their content and their form. In the area of form this often meant fitting pieces (sometimes with difficulty) into existing musical proto-types, such as binary, ternary, rondo and sonata forms and so on. In general, this meant identifying the positioning of recurring themes within a particular piece. Content-based systems concentrated in general on harmonic analysis and developed various systems for chord identification. This involved an understanding of the Western construct of 'tonality'. The systems were often developed for the purpose of teaching composition to a wider group of people, but later they came to be used to help people in the process of what came to be called 'music appreciation'.

The roots of current musicological systems lie in these methodologies. They have been very much refined in the twentieth century. The more numerically based contemporary systems are called by Nicholas Cook (1987) 'formal approaches'. He summarises their characteristics as: 'Any kind of analysis that involves coding music into symbols and deducing musical structure from the pattern these symbols make' (p.116).

They include such approaches as pitch-set and semiotic analysis. The other set of approaches have sought to re-establish a greater link between human beings and music. Cook (1987) calls these psychological approaches and refers to work of Leonard Meyer (1956), who looked at how music communicates meaning to the audience, and Rudolph Reti (1961), who was not only interested in the role of motives in large-scale musical form but also in the psychological significance of these in the composer's creation of the music.

In the last quarter of the twentieth century, in keeping with the plurality associated with post-modernism, there has been increasing attention directed towards popular music (Frith 1987; Middleton 1990; Tagg 1982) and world music (Elliott 1995; Floyd 1995). In the hands of some theorists, this has raised a number of questions about the classical traditions (Cook 1998). Other theorists have attempted to establish a greater link between music and society (Shepherd 1991).

This is necessarily a very brief overview of the contexts in which philosophies about music have been developed, drawing on a literature that is perhaps more extensive than that associated with any other area in this book. From this it is easy to see that notions of the healing properties of music were deeply embedded in the Greek philosophies of music with its connection with the gods and moral education. Healing in the Middle Ages fell largely within the province of the Church and was set in the frame of the 'humours' – a medical system based on the balancing of natural forces within the body, mind and spirit. Musical philosophies were therefore conceived of in a cosmic frame and inextricably interlinked with theology. Under the influence of the Church with its dualistic division between body and spirit, the notion of physical healing through music became increasingly lost and healing was conceived more in the area of the spirit.

This prepared the way for the increasing relationship between the mind and music that characterised developments after the Enlightenment. Here the notion of healing became replaced by one more of personal enlightenment (which could be related to composer and/or performer and audience) or mental improvement. Although much music in Western civilisation would have been written for the purposes of entertainment, theoreticians have tended to stress notions of personal improvement. Music composed for entertainment is often seen as shallow. Aesthetic judgements came to be made according to notions of excellence based on the sensibilities of the educated classes; knowledge, understanding and music came to be inter-linked.

As theoreticians moved their attentions from global principles underpin-ning music as an art form to the examination of individual artworks in detail, a structural approach to music that saw it in a detached, 'objective' light developed. This necessarily had little place in it for notions of human con-nections such as healing. Modernism, with its inbuilt notion of progress, stressed notions such as self-expression and challenge and held notions like aesthetic excellence to be of supreme importance.

Post-modernism in the later twentieth century attempted to deconstruct the classical tradition (Subotnik 1996) and included a rebirth of more human-centred and contextualised approaches alongside the more formal approaches. Feminist theorists such as those of Kristeva (1989) and McClary (1991) have sought also to re-establish connections between music and the body. In this context, notions of the relationship of music to healing at an individual and a societal level have started to reappear.

So, notions of healing linked with music have, in general, diminished since the Enlightenment in the pursuit of objective and rational approaches to music theory. This chapter will chart the presence of the notions implicit in the polarities within the model of the self set out in Chapter One.

Community/individualism

Under this heading we will look at the development of the individualistic view of the composer out of a view of music that was more rooted in community, the relationship of the individual musician to the wider community, the nature of elitist views and debates about how the music itself can be related to social and political theory.

> In Ancient Greek philosophy music was related to a universal organising principle. The nineteen treatises attributed to Hermes Trismegistus (meaning 'Thrice greatest Hermes') in the early centuries AD drew on Egyptian mystery teaching in the context of Alexandrian philosophy. In one dialogue he draws a line between pure philosophy which leads to God and inferior sciences which only tell of the material cosmos. In this division lay the seeds of the elitism that was to develop in the European classical traditions. (Godwin 1987, p.16)

The notion of the central purpose of music as being to unite everything into a single order emanating from a divine source is also present in the Roman philosopher Boethius (c.480–524/25). His work is based firmly in Platonic principles and music is placed in the Quadrivium with Arithmetic, Geometry and Astronomy:

> Thus we can begin to understand that apt doctrine of Plato which holds that the soul of the universe is united by a musical concord. For when we compare that which is coherently and harmoniously joined together within our own being with that which is coherently and harmoniously joined together in sound – that is, that which gives us pleasure – so we come to recognise that we ourselves are united according to this same principle of similarity. For similarity is pleasing, whereas dissimilarity is unpleasant and contrary. (Boethius, quoted in Godwin 1987, p.45)

Within Christianity the origin of this unity was ascribed to a creator God. Hildegard of Bingen (1098–1179) writes:

> In music you can hear the sound of burning passion in a virgin's breast. You can hear a twig coming into bud. You can hear the brightness of the spiritual light shining from heaven. You can hear the depth of thought of the prophets. You can hear the wisdom of the apostles spreading across the world. You can hear the blood pouring from the wounds of the

martyrs. You can hear the innermost movements of a heart steeped in holiness. You can hear a young girl's joy at the beauty of God's earth. In music creation echoes back to its creator its joy and exultation; it offers thanks for its very existence. You can also hear in music the harmony between people who once were enemies and now are friends. Music expresses the unity of the world as God first made it, and the unity which is restored through repentance and reconciliation... (Hildegard quoted in Van der Weyer 1997, p.80)

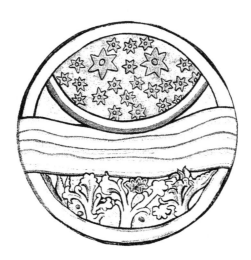

Figure 2.1 A contemporary depiction of Hildegard's vision. Taken from the cover of 'Singing the Mystery – Hildegard Revisited', composed by June Boyce-Tillman. Milton Keynes: British Music Label, 022

So in the Middle Ages music was seen as a representation of the Holy Spirit binding the natural world, God and human beings into a cosmic whole. Healing through music is the bringing of these three into a right relationship, the relationship intended by a creator God.

In the Renaissance, Greek views came into prominence again. There is an interesting discrepancy of opinion between the Renaissance teacher Ficino who believed that by communal singing human beings actually communicated with the deities and acquired some of their powers and his teacher Germistos Plethon who thought that the act of hymn singing simply moulded the minds of the singers so that they were more able to contemplate higher things (Rooley 1990). This represents a significant stage in the disembodiment of the tradition. The bodily act of singing in the second view is now disconnected from the pure act of mental contemplation. It is also the beginning of the loss of a schema in which the community was seen as being wider than human beings.

After the Enlightenment, notions of community were narrowed to be largely a human phenomenon. The elitism implicit in the Greek traditions gained prominence, with the result that philosophers of the Western classical traditions have been often more concerned about notions of excellence than notions of community.

The tradition increasingly became one of an elite group of initiated musicians. Within their hands the notion of a canon (described by Lydia Goehr as *The Imaginary Museum of Musical Works* in her 1992 book) developed. This created a group of masterworks from the past that was considered superior to the other works. The notion grew that somehow this was a 'natural' process – that historical processes somehow automatically make this selection on the grounds of excellence. This disguised the power structures that led to the creation of the canon. Cook (1998) reflects on this in the development of critical theory:

> [It] is in essence a theory of power; and it sees power largely in terms of the institutions through which it is channelled. Institutions, in other words, are crucial in naturalising power structures, in making it seem as if the unequal distributions of power we see across the world must be just 'the way things are'. (p.106)

He goes on to see the same process of selection now going on within rock music as it establishes itself in the Academy. Again certain works are being chosen and others rejected.

The development of this elitist view of music was supported by the development of a 'musical knowledge' based firmly on a grasp of musical notation. This ensured the centrality of the score to the notion of what constitutes a musical work. The opportunity to learn the skills of musical literacy has for most of this history been limited to a few – the gifted, rich, male and white. This has meant that the capacity to understand the notation has divided the musical world along the lines of who can and who can't understand the score. The understanding of Western classical notation formed the basis of music education at every level. In the second half of the twentieth century this was challenged and debates about the nature of 'the work' have included the notion of performance, aided by the development of the recording industry and the rediscovery by the dominant tradition of 'folk' and popular traditions.

Allied to this debate is that surrounding the construct of the musical genius. This saw the beginning of the alienation of the classical composer from his audience. Post-Enlightenment (or more particularly, post-Mozart and Beethoven), the construct has grown up as being male, isolated and rejected and only achieving fame after death. In this paradigm, well illustrated by the film *Amadeus*, it is essential that the composer follow his (and it was largely his) own destiny regardless of contemporary opinion. Rejection by the community of musicians made the likelihood of being perceived as a genius after death more likely. And yet, after death, the musical genius collected around him a great following – to which Mozart, Beethoven, Wagner, Mahler and many others bear witness. There are, however, degrees of rejection and some of these had around them a group of devotees in their lifetime. The notion of genius is deeply rooted in the notion of the classical hero pursuing his own destiny in the face of obstacles. In this climate it was possible to construct a musical canon from a collection of masterworks composed by master composers.

This notion sat uneasily with notions of shared community. It is a highly individualistic notion of pursuing one's own style regardless of what the 'world' thinks. It has dominated the classical tradition and persists today. Anthony Kemp, in dealing with *The Musical Temperament*, identifies that musicians have a certain 'boldness' arising from the quality of independence (Kemp 1996, p.66). However, he identifies the cost of individualistic notions in the training of musicians, particularly at special music schools:

> It appears ironic that, in an institution where pupils, and presumably teachers, will have so much in common from the point of view of interests and temperament, relationship problems seem likely to occur. These children appear to have deep, unarticulated personal needs, and yet, at the same time, emerge as jealous and arrogant. Nigel Kennedy, who attended a specialist music school, describes how at the age of seven he was required to practise for four hours a day on his own, and how lonely and depressed he became, seeking companionship by offering to share his Mars bar with other boys as a bribe.

What is interesting about the description developed above is how so many of these introverted and anxiety related traits reflect aspects of social skills or lack of them… The picture painted above is a worrying one because it suggests a psychologically unhealthy individualism that

may militate against the development of close relationships with other
fellow musicians in the special school... (Kemp 1996, p.248)

Such an individualistic climate based on elitism generated a suspicion of
notions of community. Doubt about the effect of social context on musical
discourse grew and characterised musicological debate. Only in the second
half of the twentieth century were there attempts to move from a view that
saw the masterworks of the canon standing freely on their own somehow
disconnected from the contemporary traditions in which they were
composed. This has caused a considerable debate among musicologists
(Meyer 1956). The work of Zuckerkandl (1956) and Shepherd (1991) has
attempted to tease out the distinctions between the experiential qualities of
sound and the cultural realities contained in these sounds. In summarising
the relationship between musical meaning and social issues, Shepherd and
Wicke (1997) write:

> As we have argued, music is capable of *evoking*, in a concrete and direct,
> yet *mediated and symbolic* fashion, the structures of the world and the states
> of being that flow from them and sustain them. In operating on people
> through a technology of articulation, we can now argue that the sounds
> of music serve as well to *create* those structures, and to create them in a
> dialectic of perception and action *consistent* with the quintessentially
> symbolic character of human worlds. (pp.138–139)

Michael Finnissy is quite clear about how music is inextricably bound up
with the values of the system that generated it:

> Musical metaphors also propagate the world-views of their particular
> era. From the beginning of a Handel piece, you can see how the people
> walked, you can see the clothes and you know what their attitude to the
> world was, at least the attitude that they wanted to have. But my world is
> not the same as Handel's. I don't even wish that it was. Other metaphors
> have to be found. (Finnissy, quoted in Brougham, Fox and Pace 1997,
> p.20)

Debates within and about modernism have swept political and sociological
discourse into the aesthetic debate. Notions developed of an elite who are
able to perceive a greater truth that they must articulate for the benefit of the
wider community. Within this the dangers of shared community are often to
the fore and the role of the artist is seen as over and against the 'egalitarian
commerce' (Rahn 1994a, p.6). An important role is ascribed by theorists to
the lone rebellious musician. He was often seen as representing the excluded

and the marginalised: 'Tolerance for the expression of singularities serves often as a safety valve for persistent injustice' (Rochlitz 1994, p.35).

This was an important aspect of the work of the significant theorist Theodore Adorno. Adorno is set apart from post-modernity by his efforts to save the concept of normativity and retain the possibility of the emancipatory power of reason, while rejecting the totalitarianism that it can spawn (Rochlitz 1994). Within this the theme of composer as saviour is developed. Jacques Attali (1985), in his significant work *Noise: The Political Economy of Music*, postulates the origin of this aesthetic phenomenon in ritual murder. In his essay *The Natural History of the Theatre*, he compares aspects of contemporary theatre and public music to violent archaic ritual (Collins 1994).

At the moment when the murderous rage threatens to tear a group apart an 'emissary victim' is chosen as a scapegoat who is accused quite falsely of being responsible for the dysfuntionalising violence (Rahn 1994b). After an expulsion or death which is seen to rid the society of its problems, this creature then assumes the role of the most sacred of humans. The French cultural theorist Renée Girard links the notion with the sacrifice of Christ in Christianity (Rahn 1994b).

These ideas relate to those of Nietzsche (1994 edition), who also recalled the power of the Greek tragedy to heal as a type of ritual sacrifice. In the contemporary absence of such pacifying rituals, Rahn (1994b) sees society as struggling to find a way to resolve its violent conflicts. Attali (1985) builds on this idea putting forward a theory of music to build a non-violent society. He sets up a hypothesis of four stages in the history of Western music. In his schema noise is a weapon and music the formation and ritualisation of the weapon, functioning as a simulacrum (change) of ritual murder. The first stage, characterised by Gregorian chant, is entitled 'sacrificial ritual'. This absorbs power and wipes away the possibility of violence. The second stage, emerging in the eighteenth century, which he called 'representation', is linked with the decline in feudal society and the birth of capitalism. Here music becomes a commodity with an exchange value. Music is freed from its regulations and rituals, and hence its discipline. The third stage he calls 'repetition' and dates from the invention of recording techniques in the late nineteenth century which made possible the: 'individualised stockpiling of music possible on a huge scale' (Attali 1985, p.32). He sees this as a crisis in which music 'no longer constructs differences. *It is trapped in identity and will dissolve into noise*', and leads 'to a society of repetition' (*ibid.*, p.45). In his pessimism that 'accessibility has replaced the festival' (p.109) he sees violence prevailing and shattering all codes (p.45).

He entitles a final Utopian stage 'composition': 'Music would be performed for the musician's own enjoyment, as self-communication, with no other goal than his [sic] own pleasure, as something fundamentally outside all communication, as self-transcendence, a solitary, egotistical non-commercial act' (Attali 1985, p.32).

Attali ends with some notion of a new community (which links with ideas present in New Age groups reviewed in Chapter Four) where music is produced for pleasure 'outside of meaning, usage and exchange' (p.137).

Other theorists have developed the theme of the artist as the challenger of prevailing values that would seek to normalise and stultify. Collins (1994) draws on the sociologist Cornelius Castoriadis to express the tension involved in this theme. In this thinking the single composer is seen as the heroic champion of different (perhaps higher) value systems which go against the values shared by the majority community. Notions of elitism and the heroic journey combine to produce this position. Michael Finnissy develops the theme of music and ritual in a different way:

> Music to me has always been more than simply the technical mechanisms; there also needs to be a spiritual and aesthetic apparatus in place... Spiritual activity for me also covers what other people would call tribal or ritual activity. Those are all under the same umbrella for me – ritualised and collective music-making: hymn singing and the Mass in parts of Western Europe. (Finnissy, quoted in Brougham *et al.* 1997, p.22)

Other composers have reacted against the sounds and individualism of modernism and attempted to return to more ancient value systems:

> My own feeling is that music of 'New Complexity', however powerful, dramatic and wonderfully constructed, represents a reflection of the hideous and complex world within which we live. Music, for me, is not about these things; rather it should be an attempt to depict a vision of the world we would like to see, and the musical language and idioms chosen should be ones which speak with passion and directness to the hearts, minds and souls of large numbers of people, enough indeed that the effect can have a wide ranging influence... In order for me to release my creativity, I have to abandon, for the period of creation, any sense of my own significance in society... I need to feel that my separate egotistical identity has been replaced by a sense of belonging to one wholesome organism, and that my function is to serve and enrich that organism... It

may seem odd that in order to be truly original one has, in some way, to deny one's individuality, but it is surely true that much of the world's most beautiful music has been created by people who are happy to remain anonymous. In Europe, Gregorian chant and much folk music fall into this category, as does most of the music from the remainder of the world. (Downes 1998)

As musicologists address a wider variety of musics different social functions for music become apparent. Nicholas Cook (1998) challenges the traditional view of classical aesthetics that 'music lies outside society'. He illustrates it with a description of the development of the classical orchestra:

> Consider the classical orchestra. It consists of a team of specialists (violinists, oboists and so on) all working to a pre-existing blueprint or master plan (the score). Where there are several specialists in the same area, there are identifiable hierarchies and management lines (first and second violins, the leader). Throughout the eighteenth century one of the team members (normally a violinist or the harpsichordist) had overall control of the operation, but early in the nineteenth century this managerial role developed into a specialist career (the conductor). Not held accountable for the success or failure of the entire operation, the manager acquired an executive status, quite distinct from that of the other team members, with a remuneration package to match... I might say that the classical orchestra and its evolution reproduces the organisational structures of contemporary society... I am not suggesting that it is the role of music to provide a kind of early warning system for society (though such a suggestion has been made), any more than that it is its role to reflect society. The point is simply that, as I said, it is *part* of society...
> (pp.79–80)

Cook (1998) then pursues this line of thinking into the area of world musics thinking about the political significance of *Nkosi Sikel' iAfrica*, the hymn which has become associated with the anti-Apartheid struggle in South Africa:

> It has a meaning that emerges from the act of performing it. Like all choral performance, from singing a hymn to chanting at a football match, it involves communal participation and interaction. Everyone has to listen to everyone else and move forward together. It doesn't just symbolise unity; it *enacts* it. And there is more. Through its block-like harmonic construction and regular phrasing, *Nkosi Sikel' iAfrica* creates a sense of stability and mutual dependence, with no one vocal part domi-

nating over the others... Again, it lies audibly at the interface between European traditions of 'common-practice' harmony and African traditions of communal singing, which gives it an inclusive quality entirely appropriate to the aspirations of the new South Africa. Enlisting music's ability to shape personal identity, *Nkosi Sikel' iAfrica* actively contributes to the construction of the community that is the new South Africa. In this sense, singing is a political act. (pp.80–81)

In this way singing together can shape a social identity in the same way that it can shape personal identity, as we shall see below.

Anthony Rooley (1990) also draws on the different cultures to challenge the prevailing individualism of the classical tradition. He challenges the notion of the lone 'master musician' by having a more tradition-based view of music based in gratitude to the 'musical ancestors'. He addresses the necessity for performers to relate to the audience, encouraging them to 'encircle the audience in your vision' (p.50).

Popular music criticism has always had a greater sense of context. This is partly because the background of the theorists is often in cultural theory. Andrew Blake (1997) starts a discussion of British popular music post-1950 by listing bands and groups such as Special AKA, UB40 and the Thompson Twins and then proceeding, not just to an analysis of the music, but to an analysis of the context:

> Both musical style and ethnic identity are in this mix, in a configuration of the city as a culturally interactive space which has affected people and their musics from all over the world. Apache Indian, raised in the Handsworth suburb of Birmingham, uses English, Punjabi and Jamaican patois interchangeably, rapping across language and dialect on the back of rhythm tracks which owe more to dance hall reggae than to Indi-pop, for all their use of dhol and tabla drums... Partly because of its continuing use of lyrics in Punjabi, Bhangra has a whole political economy. (p.117)

Writing about pop brings together the surrounding culture with musical analysis and sees the two inextricably related. The sleeve notes of the CDs and the publicity machines of the stars are inseparable from the music itself.

Summary – community/individualism

From notions of a higher and greater unity in the cosmos of which music plays a significant part, the classical tradition has moved towards one of isolated masterworks by composers isolated from the wider community.

These are supported by notions of truth connected with an elite. Post-modern theoreticians, in widening the musical styles that are addressed by a musicological debate, have enabled a move to examine again the relationship between music and the wider culture.

Containment/freedom

In this section I shall be examining the significance of musical form in the tradition and how improvisation, in particular, has been part of it. Nietzsche (1994 edition), in examining the roots of Western culture, identified the two poles which he termed as Apollonian and Dionysian. He saw the non-artistic visions of the modern world as Apollonian (Apollo was god of the sun and of justice, who controls the laws of the city) in its pursuit of the scientific concept of reason with its notions of order, coherence and clarity and separation from the body. An artistic society would be Dionysian (Dionysus was god of the vine, ecstasy, drunkenness and disorder, valuing community in which there is a sense of the loss of self), valuing the senses, community and belongingness to the earth. He saw the Enlightenment as crucial in the loss of the Dionysian but he did not advocate a Dionysian culture. He saw the answer in the transformation of Dionysian power by Apollonian clarity. This conjunction would produce living form.

Anthony Rooley (1990) develops a notion of balance of these extremes by exploring the idea of performance in a manual on courtly love by the Italian Platonic poet Pietro Bembo, written in 1528. This combines the idea of *decoro*, which 'embodies all that is understood by tradition, the laws and rules which hold right conduct in place' (p.11), with that of *sprezzatura* – 'a lightning-like energy which carries courage, boldness, even rashness, and excitement…a delighting in the moment, a love of improvisation, a kind of calculated carelessness' (pp.11–12). The task is to bring *decoro* and *sprezzatura* into balance. However, to these is added the idea of *grazia* which 'is not quite the same as the Christian concept of grace – it is that, but with a touch of pagan magic about it as well. It is a quality from the Divine, uncontainable, unknowable, unownable, without limit, belonging to no one' (p.13).

It is not clear whether Rooley regards this as the balancing point of these two ideas. Drawing on such notions, he later develops the notion of the 'per-former' whose true task is 'to bring into our sensual world those things (powers, energy, inspiration) which already exist in an un-formed stage – literally to "bring into form"' (p.25).

Post-Enlightenment, because of the centrality of rationality to the development of Western civilisation, debates in musical circles have far more often been about the formal structures of music rather than the freedom that might lead to the chaos, so feared and guarded against by rationalists. The notion of composer as craftsman has often meant that the well-crafted piece of music has occupied a more esteemed place than the feeling-ful piece with a looser structure. The music analysis of the Western system has been largely about containment and courses in musical composition have concentrated for a long time on the teaching of musical form, even to the extent of recommending that students for exams produce empty shells with no content (empty shells fulfilling the requirements of an academically constructed musical form but with no expressive content). From a textbook entitled *The Examination Fugue* comes the following vignette: 'The writer remembers asking a fellow-candidate for D.Mus. [Doctor of Music] what kind of plan he used for the fugue. The answer was: "Oh, I don't have a plan. I just write as I feel." He failed to complete his fugue; he also failed the examination' (Lovelock 1952, p.4).

The development of notation was central to the development of this construct musical form. John Sloboda (1985) writes of the significance of notation which he calls 'a cultural force':

Many world cultures are, or have recently been, essentially non-literate (or oral). That is, they have not used visual notational means of recording details of human transactions. There are many contrasts to be made between literate and oral cultures. I wish to concentrate on four broad proposals about the effects of the availability of notation:

1. The existence of written notation allows lengthy verbatim recall of complex meaningful material.

2. Notation allows proliferation and migration of material so that it exceeds the capacity of any one individual to know it all.

3. Notation encourages the separation of the content of an utterance from its context, and makes it easier for an utterance to be treated as a 'thing in itself'.

4. Notation selects certain aspects of sound for preservation, and, in doing so, both embodies current theory and also tends to restrict the future development of music in certain ways. (p.242)

His comments present an interesting collection of the freedoms provided by musical notation as well as the limiting power of notation in containing the notes of a particular piece and thus restricting improvisation. Containment (order) expressed in the classical tradition by producing a score in notated form sets the high art tradition apart from more popular traditions. John Rahn in 'What is valuable in art?' (1994b) sets out this philosophy very clearly and rates it highly above the non-notated traditions.

Popular musical criticism, however, has drawn attention to the presence of freer passages in the context of pieces controlled by a tight rhythmic structure to show how freedom and containment are held together in a single piece:

> Heavy metal revolves around identification with power, intensity of experience, freedom, and community. Musically, dialectic is often set up between the potentially oppressive power of bass, drums, and rhythm guitar, and the liberating, empowering vehicle of the guitar solo or the resistance of the voice. The feeling of freedom created by the freedom of motion of the guitar solos and fills can be at various times supported, defended, or threatened by the physical power of the bass and the violence of the drums. The latter rigidly organise and control time; the guitar escapes with flashy runs and other arhythmic gestures. The solo positions the listener: he or she can identify with the controlling power without feeling threatened because the solo can transcend anything. (p.54)

The notion of musical form as a container for the freedom of imagination on the part of the listener is well developed in the classical literature. Adorno saw a freedom from the everyday in the very nature of music. This is very like some of the ideas in developing notions of creativity in the twentieth century. Rochlitz (1994), summarising Adorno, writes: 'Art is not in the order of the everyday, even though it seeks epiphanies in the most ordinary life; it can take the liberty – and this is in fact what one expects from it – of ignoring the intersubjective demands which constitute the daily life in society' (p.31).

This is a strand in the thinking of Sartre who says that on leaving a concert he must return to 'the nauseating disgust that characterises the consciousness of reality' (Sartre, quoted in Cook 1990, p.152).

Nicholas Cook (1990), in the Introduction to his book *Music, Imagination and Culture*, develops the idea by seeing the formal structure of the music as a container in which the imagination of the listener can flow free. He stresses the importance, in this context, of the perception of repetition, contrast and permutations of material. So the music itself becomes like a ritual within which the listener is free to experience meaning. Without the container of musical form the work would be experienced as meaningless or just sound.

Cook (1990) goes on to explore the dilemma of Schoenberg who developed the use of serialism[1] as a means of defining musical form in an age when the power of tonality had been eroded. Paradoxically, Schoenberg himself favoured free fantasising in inspiration.

The debate has raged for a long time about how much one needs to be able to hear and recognise the appearances of the row or series in order to understand Schoenberg's work and how far Schoenberg himself required this of his listeners. What is clear in this debate is that there is a tension in the thinking about how far the form – of which the composer is necessarily aware in constructing the work – needs to be perceived *in the same terms* by the listener or whether it is simply a 'holding form', giving listeners freedom to impart their own meaning to the work. Cook (1990) attacks the elitist views on these evident in the work of critics like Roger Scruton (e.g. 1983). In the end, Cook links the process of listening to psychoanalysis: 'The psychoanalyst helps his patient come to terms with his predicament through rationalising it in terms of his past experiences; the music analyst renders a new work intelligible by interpreting it in terms of familiar structural prototypes. In both cases understanding results…from comparing the unfamiliar with the familiar' (p.242). He goes on to liken music to myth. Although such a definition presents a problem in a time of rapid movements of music across cultures, the linking of the meaning of music to myth which can be reinterpreted by each listener is a useful one.

The degree of control exercised by the notated score increased over a period of time in the West. Initially it was sometimes an aide-mémoire for the composer or a structure that allowed for some improvisation on the part of the performer. Right through the Classical period (1750–1830) there had been space for improvisation on the part of the performer. The score produced by the composer still had elements of sketch that to a certain extent and within well-defined cultural limits needed filling out by the performer. This is clearest in the moment of the cadenza in the concerto where the performer was free to improvise, but happened in other areas like the realisation of the ornaments written in the score. The late Romantic period, in the second part of the nineteenth century, saw an increasing control by the classical composer over every aspect of performance with less and less freedom for performers and an increasing level of demands placed on them. For example, the scores of the late Romantic symphonists like Mahler

---

1   Serialism is a system of generating music from a series (or 'row') of notes decided by the composer at the beginning of the process of composition.

include gradations of dynamic level that include a range of *pppp* to *ffff* and sometimes beyond. It is a short step from such demands for refinement to the abandonment of human fallibility. Electronic composition which results in a 'once for all' performance technologically on a tape is perhaps the most 'contained' and controlled form of composition that the West has known.

However, halfway through the twentieth century, this move towards absolute control, which could be regarded as the absolute negation of freedom in performance, was followed by a rise in aleatoric or chance/choice techniques. This led to the development of minimalism with its use of minimal resources, including much repetition and some improvisation. One of the most prominent figures here was Terry Riley who writes of his abandonment of classical techniques:

> In the last ten years I have given up the traditional role of the composer in favour of self-interpretative improvisation...the composed portions remain unaltered, but the musician is quite free to spin them out within the limits of his imagination. The mode used (tone row) and the accompanying melodic figures establish the mood and atmosphere in which the improvisation is carried out. (Riley 1974)[2]

Some of the chance techniques used by such composers as Riley involved the use of dice to decide on which direction the music should take next. But some, more significantly for my purpose, saw the handing over of the role of choice to the performers. In chance/choice music we also see a move to a greater communal ownership of the music; for the performer and composer together now have a more equal part in the piece. This allows greater freedom to both.

The notion of closure has been central to the development of Western form. The container must close at the end in the same key in which it began and with a real sense of 'coming home' or back to its starting point. In the twentieth century this has been challenged by feminist theorists like Susan McClary (1991). The contemporary British composer Michael Finnissy develops this idea further. He describes a dynamic and optimistic view of musical form:

> I try to make form active, conspiratorial, mobile, disturbing – but above all, audible. You're not supposed to have worked it out before the end... I prefer to just close the door, as if the music is still going on behind that

---

2   From the programme of the Meta-Music Festival, Berlin.

door… I'm presenting an optimistic view. Life must go on and beyond a piece there is life. It's false to tell the audience 'This is the end'. It isn't, they go home on the bus after the concert. (Finnissy, quoted in Brougham *et al.* 1997, p.20)

Summary – containment/freedom

The High Art traditions of the West have been increasingly contained by the development of a notation system (which has been extended in the twentieth century to include a greater variety of symbols). Although up to 1800 this included some measure of improvisation, which gave the performer a certain freedom to contribute to the process of composition, this was increasingly eroded in the nineteenth century in which Romantic composers sought to control every aspect of their work. In the twentieth century improvisation re-appeared to a certain extent but the notion of masterworks has been firmly rooted in a notated score. The stress on formal issues in the classical tradition has sometimes been seen as necessary to contain the free flights of fantasy that characterise the listening experience or the perception of musical meaning.

Expression/confidentiality

Under this heading we shall primarily look at the 'meaning' of music and how this is constructed theoretically and culturally. In ancient Greece the notion of the Muses which possessed the artist placed the origin of the expressive elements of music in the area of the Divine. Pre-Enlightenment theories would ascribe the process of musical creation to God and have human beings simply as channels of divine creativity. This is seen very clearly in Hildegard's notion of her music coming straight from God as part of her visions. It is present in an apocryphal letter ascribed to Mozart (printed in Vernon 1970) where he describes hearing a piece *tout ensemble* and then transcribing it as if from a divine source. However, post-Enlightenment, since the break of music away from the Church, such writing is less common and inspiration becomes more human-centred. As the centrality of human impulses started to hold sway after the Enlightenment, the notion of self-expression became paramount. It is often ascribed to the composer's unconscious or subconscious. The notion that the composer must express himself or sometimes herself, regardless of how it is received by the surrounding community, is deep within the notion of the Western construct of genius.

Debates about musical meaning have raged throughout the history of Western music. Its very impenetrability makes it an attractive form of expression for the introverts that Anthony Kemp (1996) identifies as numerous among classical musicians: 'Sensitivity features within a wider cluster of personality traits for which Cattell has adopted the term, "pathemia"... Taken together, this research suggests that pathemia, intuition, and feeling converge in identifying a fundamental quality of musicians' personalities' (pp.83–85). Here he highlights how people capable of handling complexity of aesthetic meaning and those having a desire for a certain form of privacy are drawn to music as a form of expression which allows for these qualities.

There has been a remoteness from human lives about the traditional musicological discussions:

> Methods of analysing affect and meaning in music have hardly kept pace with the increased diversity and currency of musical genres in every day life... Musicology has frequently avoided questions of affect and meaning altogether, claiming that its proper purpose is the establishing of the facts about music and history. When, however, it has considered questions of affect and meaning – either implicitly or explicitly – it has tended to do so in manner which isolates musical processes from their embeddedness in social and cultural processes and the everyday lives of people. (Shepherd and Wicke 1997, p.7)

Psychologists have been more likely to address these problems than musicologists. John Sloboda (1985) starts his book on *The Musical Mind* by linking the aesthetic and the emotional:

> Music is capable of arousing in us deep and significant emotions. These emotions can range from the 'pure' aesthetic delight in a sound construction, through emotions like joy and sorrow, which music sometimes evokes or enhances, to the simple relief from monotony, boredom or depression which everyday musical experiences can provide. (p.1)

It is the notion that people intuitively feel music to be connected to human emotions which they designate as being 'universal' that leads to the notion of music being a 'universal' language (Cook 1998).

However, how far it can stand alone and how far it needs the 'mediation' of words is a subject for debate. Andrew Blake (1997) claims that the words are needed to give music 'meaning', moving it from the realm of physiological response:

> We all approach music through speech and writing. Concert programmes, CD sleeve notes, reviews of gigs and albums; writing about music is everywhere. There are dedicated magazines: for followers of particular genres (e.g. *Folk Roots*), or particular forms of listening (*Hi-Fi News*), or users of specific musical instruments (*Guitarist*) and recording devices (*Sound on Sound*)...[taken] from the 'natural' physicality of sound to the 'cultural' state of sound endowed with human meaning. (p.7)

The correspondence between the leading figures in German Romantic music in the nineteenth century (like Robert Schumann and Johannes Brahms) about 'absolute' or 'programme' music is but one example of a debate about words and music that has been increasingly refined by musicologists throughout the twentieth century. The question being discussed concerns how far musical meaning rests in the interplay of the sounds themselves and how far these sounds can be related to a narrative structure 'outside' of the sounds themselves. Composers and musicologists have contributed to the debate.

Theorists from a variety of backgrounds favour the notion that musical meaning is to be found in an intense intersubjective relationship. It is produced, not by the composer who channels it via the performer to the listener but is, in essence, a relationship between musicians and listener. The real meaning is in the relationship constructed through the music. John Rahn (1994a) sees the creative act and its relationship to the hearers as being 'more complete than any normal social interaction could provide' (p.2). Rochlitz, dealing with Adorno, denies the possibility of putting this meaning into words: 'In truth, the stakes of art are for him foreign to signification; art is a kind of "non-signifying language"... Art – especially modern art – is thus a language, but a language charged with intense energy and which denies communication' (pp.28–30).

Later he makes a clear distinction between art and psychotherapy:

> The demand for aesthetic validity which characterises an intensified proposal of meaning calls for a symmetry between the 'voice' emanating from the work and that of the receiving subject; so long as it is a 'proposal of meaning', the work is not a psychoanalytical 'case' which one studies, and this symmetry is the basis of aesthetic rationality. (Rochlitz 1994, p.32)

So it can be seen that these debates give the lie to a simplistic notion of musical meaning in which the composer encodes a meaning in his work which is then decoded by the listener.

Once the listener is included in the construction of the meaning of music the way is open for more functionalist approaches to music. John Rahn (1994b) distinguishes between what music is valuable *for* from what is valuable *in* music. His writing is from an essentially high art position and so he downplays the functionalist view of music. In attempting to define a pure aesthetic value, he defines what the aesthetic is not:

Functionalism also underlies less sophisticated views on these questions. The married couple who value Our Song because of its personal associations with a period in their history illustrate the phenomenon of *induced aesthetic value*; they have learned to love the song, beyond their initial aesthetic reaction to it, as the great personal-historic value they use the song to contain spills over to the aesthetic domain. The immigrant, or exile, living in a foreign land, may use the native or folk music of his homeland to focus and contain his nostalgia, his *Heimweh*, to keep his feelings about his native country alive while sequestering them from his day-to-day activities. The powerful and deep emotions evoked may well spill over into the aesthetic domain, investing the music with a beauty of a kind not pertinent to it in the old country. (p.55)

Lucy Green's books *Music on Deaf Ears: Musical Meaning, Ideology and Education* (1988) and *Music, Gender, Education* (1997) make a very useful contribution to the debate in defining two different meanings within the music itself. The first she calls *inherent*. This operates 'in terms of the interrelationships of musical *materials* or, to put it simply, in terms of the sounds of music' (1997, p.6). The other she calls *delineated*. This conveys 'the idea that music metaphorically sketches, or delineates, a plethora of contextualising, symbolic factors' (1997, p.7). She describes how the two meanings interact with special reference to gender issues in delineated meaning. Important in her debate is the discussion around 'alienated' experiences of listening. She outlines her argument thus:

The listeners do not feel at one with the delineations, and are dissatisfied with the inherent meanings. At the opposite extreme, listeners find themselves 'celebrated' through a positive relationship to the delineations, and a fulfilling response to the inherent meanings. Clearly, there may often arise situations in which a listener's responses to inherent and delineated meanings do not necessarily tally. (1997, pp.133–134)

The resulting ambiguity occurs in two ways, as shown in Figure 2.2.

First (ambiguity B), a person may respond positively to the inherent meanings of, say Mozart's operatic music, on the basis of a lifetime's listening experience; but he or she may at the same time feel negative about the delineations of the libretto, or about the social milieux in which the operas are perceived to circulate. Secondly, vice versa (ambiguity A), a person may be dissatisfied with the inherent meanings, unfamiliarity with which produces difficulties in distinguishing salient elements; but he or she might nonetheless feel entirely positive about the narrative contained in the libretto, or about the social function of going out to the opera. In ambiguous musical experience, there is then a contradiction between the quality of experience in relation to the two virtual aspects of musical meaning. (Green 1997, p.134)

This table is helpful, for it explains ambiguities in our relationships to certain music. I have encountered this particularly strongly as I have encountered more music by women. In some of this I have felt myself in a relationship to the music that I had not experienced in the male tradition in which I was brought up.

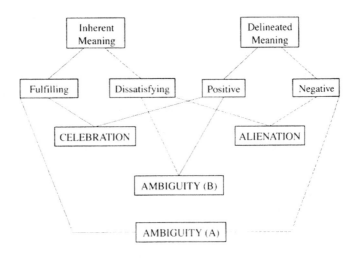

Figure 2.2 Lucy's table (adapted from Green 1988, p.138) With kind permission.

The inclusion of a wider variety of musics in those subjected to musicological scrutiny has meant that social meanings are more likely to be taken into account in contemporary debates. Nicholas Cook (1998) talks of the meaning of advertising music:

> You could think of television commercials as a massive experiment in musical meaning. Advertising uses music to communicate meanings that would take too long to put into words, or that would carry no conviction in them. The Prudential commercial [which features a young man who wants to be a musician] uses music as a powerful symbol for aspiration, self-fulfilment, the desire to 'be what you want to be' as the voice-over says. More than that, it uses a particular sort of music – rock music – to target a particular segment of society, the twenty- or maybe thirty-somethings. [The commercial is advertising pension plans that you can take with you from one job to another.] (p.3)

The whole area of the use of music in the media where it is allied with visual images and words, especially in advertising contexts, has increased the multiplicity of music's possible meanings.

The application within theories of music of ideas from feminists like Kristeva has resulted in the inclusion of the body in musical meaning. In this debate the 'signifier' is the music itself and the 'signified' is any meaning that may be ascribed to it by interpretation. Barthes (1985a), drawing on Kristeva's work, requires us to 'immerse ourselves in the signifier, plunging far away from the signified into the matter of the text' (p.125). He seeks to break the link between the signified and the signifier. Interpreting him, Engh (1993) writes that 'the move to the field of the signifier is not be understood…as valorisation of nonmeaning against meaning', concluding that Barthes 'wants to loosen the fixity of meaning, to pluralize it' (Barthes 1985a, p.71). Barthes concludes that music is 'a field of *signifying* and not a system of signs, the referent is the body. The body passes into music without any relay but the signifier' (1985b, p.308).

To understand this, he says that we need 'a second semiology, that of the body in a state of music' (1985b, p.312). In this writing the way is open for the physiological response to music being a meaning in its own right. By drawing the body into the debate about musical meaning it is possible to see music's meaning as closer to the world of action than to that of signs (which constitute the world of language). There is inevitably a sense of movement within musical discourse. This brings music closer to the world of processes (Middleton 1990). In this debate we are drawn back to the thinking under individualism/community where:

> All media of human expression and communication are capable of several
> levels of signification, none of which is free of the influence and media-
> tion of others. In the case of music, meaning and ideology have to be rec-
> onciled with the non-denotative and asemantic modes of articulation
> that are fully formal and structural in character. (Shepherd and Wicke
> 1997, p.203)

Shepherd and Wicke go on to ask for the development of a new semiology
taking into account '[t]he *total* set of dialectic relations obtaining between
music, language, society, the body, cognition and affect' (1997, p.203).

The notion of a plurality of meanings developing around a single piece is
developed by Rainer Rochlitz (1994). He teases out the plurality of musical
meanings that can be ascribed to an individual work:

> The elaboration of this language 'for one' transforms it into a language
> 'for all', made virtually universal by dint of its intelligibility, which neces-
> sitates a deciphering... Aesthetic comprehension – and criticism – is
> thus an art of translation which causes the apparent singularity of the
> work (and of the experience which constitutes it) to attain a virtually uni-
> versal signification, but which is for its own part a function of a particular
> actualisation. The unity of aesthetic 'validity' does not in any way reduce
> the diversity of the 'non-significant eloquence' particular to each work,
> nor the plurality of interpretations of which each can become the object,
> precisely to the extent that it is successful. (p.31)

This somewhat complex and dense writing shows how the individual event
for the composer is changed in the process of being 'musicked'. The acceptance of the work as a language 'for all' leads to it acquiring a plurality of
meanings. These mask the original event that gave it its original life. Rochlitz
(1994) deals with the risk involved in this: 'The work is "proposal" of
meaning at the risk of failure: of a meaning which can remain private or of
limited interest' (p.32). Rochlitz is here dealing with the establishment of
works of art in our society. There is a notion that the putting out of a work of
art is a risk, for it is now in the hands of forces out of the control of the
composer who may ascribe a variety of meanings to the work or, perhaps
worst of all, see it as 'meaningless'. John Rahn (1994a) echoes this when he
writes: 'The dimensions of the creative act are at once intimately personal –
this is *me* out there – and intensely, inevitably involved with ideologies,
religions, metaphysics, politics, matters that constitute a dangerous arena in
which to present oneself naked' (p.2). This is the closest that the literature
gets to the notion of the importance of the acceptance of the composer's

piece as an expression of him or herself. Much of the classical literature concentrates on the need of the composer to express himself, regardless of how it might be received.

Summary – expression / confidentiality

Whereas the Greeks and the Christian philosophers of the Middle Ages saw music as an expression of the Divine which flowed through a human source, the notion of self-expression became prominent post-Enlightenment. Although there is a strand that would see music as a universal language, some views have sought to define musical meaning in ways that separate it from human responses to music. Some stress the need for words in the process of giving music meaning and debates about programme music raged in the nineteenth century. Some differentiate between aesthetic and personally constructed meaning. Some stress the intersubjectivity of meaning; others involve the body in the notion. However, it is clear that the meaning of music is not easily decoded and resists simplistic notions of understanding. There is a notion that the act of composition puts something of oneself into the public domain and this can be a risk and implicit in this is the need for acceptance. However, debates about the meaning of music stress its plurality – how audience and composer/performer interact in the establishing of meaning.

Unity/diversity

This section will examine the creative process in music and its relation to the personality of the musician. The pursuit of integration has coloured much of the Western tradition. The establishment of 'harmonia' was deep in the Greek notion that 'beauty heals'. The development of classical musical forms is often seen as that of integration between different elements, growing out of a

> personal need to create order and wholeness. Musical works reveal how the composer's craft largely comprises the synthesis and analysis of fragmentary musical ideas. In adopting these contrasting and complementary processes composers bring creative order to chaos, ambiguities, and conflicts within them. In this way they may maintain an equilibrium in their levels of neuroticism and stress... Composers' works frequently reveal considerable insights about their personalities and perceptual styles, and can open up windows on their internal worlds and psychological needs. (Kemp 1996, p.216)

Anthony Rooley (1990) expresses similar aims on the part of the performer and listener. These are linked with Greek ideals. The three desires in a performer are:

A desire to sing the song

A desire for aspiration

A desire for unity. (p.122)

These are linked in the listener with three longings:

A longing for peace

A longing for uplift

A longing for unity.

> In every breast is a degree of turbulence, creating a longing for peace, closely followed by a longing to be raised to a higher state of awareness. Out of this is revealed, deepest of all, a longing to be reunited. With Orpheus' song, channelling divine frenzy, Euridice's longings are assuaged. (Rooley 1990, p.123)

The process of finding the appropriate shape for a piece may be linked to the process of re-shaping the personality. The search for a unifying principle is particularly clear in the work of certain composers, particularly those who have left sketchbooks or writing about their music. If we relate Beethoven's sketchbooks to notions in Jungian psychoanalysis, what is happening is the integration of various aspects of the personality. We could also relate them to the 'subpersonalities' of psychosynthesis which need to be brought into relationship (see Chapter One). Caldwell (1972) deals with this in some detail in his discussion of Beethoven's String Quartet no.6 in B flat, opus 18. The movement consists of sections of alternating moods including slow, melancholic and even quite playful sections. The opening he relates to a struggle to keep going despite inhibiting depression. The following fast theme is full of a restless energy. Suddenly the depressed mood returns. The swings appear more and more frequently. Caldwell sees these as Beethoven's attempt to depict manic-depressive swings. He does not suggest that Beethoven was a manic-depressive but says that it indicates how Beethoven was able to use these aspects of his understanding of human personality (perhaps drawing on the contemporary philosophy of *Sturm und Drang* – Storm and Stress – which in music was reflected by sudden changes of mood) to shape his creativity.

Paul Robertson (1996) links Mozart's *Dissonance Quartet* with the two hemispheres of the brain. It opens with a passage of clashing discords that have even been rewritten by a musicologist who thought it was an error of judgement. Robertson draws attention to the fact that the piece was written to impress his mentor Haydn and that, uncharacteristically for a very intuitive composer, he spent a long time labouring over it. Such intellectual effort would, according to Robertson, bring into play the more intellectual hemisphere of the brain. The quartet then can be seen as a bringing together of the contrasting characteristics of the brain.

Another composer with a psychological make-up within which he was even able to name two contrasted personalities was Robert Schumann. He was a man of extreme moods. Sometimes he wrote separate pieces to express the diverse aspects within himself. Liszt saw his dilemma as trying 'to reconcile his romantic personality, torn between joy and pain…with the modalities of classical form…this struggle against his true nature must have caused him great suffering' (Liszt, quoted in Jamison 1993, p.207). We shall see below how Schumann struggled with the construct of the classical tradition. It is interesting to speculate that if the stress on integration had not been so high within the classical tradition and there had been a greater tolerance of diversity, both within the personality and within the individual piece, then he would have been able to manage his own changing temperament more easily.

In line with notions of the heroic journey, we can see in such stories that the journey of the composer is now apparent in the form of his work, which is able to contain its diversity within a single structure. Insofar as the composer achieves a balance within himself of diverse elements within the piece, the piece itself will have the power to take its audience through a similar journey towards integration. The composer becomes a therapist or indeed a shaman who takes the listener on his or her own internal journey by 'singing his or her song'. This idea will be explored further.

Anthony Rooley (1990) describes the role of the performer in this process: 'The performer takes the audience's attention with his own to the heart of the matter, and there through the medium of the work contemplates the nature of inspiration as it flows through the composition' (p.26).

The progress to enlightenment is deliberately set out in Mozart's opera *The Magic Flute*, heavily influenced as it is by ideas taken from Mozart's experience in Freemasonry. Peter Hamel (1978) links this with the descent into the Underworld of the mystery-initiation rites. Bruno Walter links it with Mozart's preoccupation with death at the time: 'Since death, properly regarded as the ultimate purpose of this life of ours, I have over the past few years made myself so familiar with this true, best friend of man that its mere portrayal no longer holds any terrors for me, but does contain for me much that is soothing and consoling' (Walter, quoted in Hamel 1978, p.20). Through the process of listening to *The Magic Flute*, listeners follow a similar journey and undergo similar initiation rites themselves. Many contemporary composers (in both jazz and classical traditions) have entered the world of their own unconscious or subconscious quite deliberately.

The theory that this opens up a similar journey for their listeners is set out particularly clearly in Stenhammer's letter to Sibelius after hearing his Second Symphony;

> You are in my thoughts daily since I heard your symphony…it is indeed a large catch of marvels that you have brought up out of the depths of the unconscious and the inexpressible… Give humanity hope, give us the drama!… all the many who turn away from a riddle they cannot solve, they require it… (Stenhammer, quoted in Ekman 1946, p.173)

Here he sees the composer as solving his own problems and in so doing helping his listeners in their problems. Anthony Rooley (1990) gives an account of a similar nature when he describes the cathartic effect of performances of Dowland's *The Songs of Mourning*:

> Emma [Kirkby] and I have performed the work on a number of occasions and have had the chance to observe in some detail the means of transformation, for that, essentially, is what happens to everyone witnessing the unfolding of the cycle in the twenty-five minutes it takes. It is a guided meditation – guided because the route for the mind is plotted out in very great detail, every stage of the meditational journey is pre-set… As each phase of the cycle concludes, the listener, in the silence between sections, is brought to join, more consciously, his own, still, observation point beyond words, character, mask, and in this manner transformation appropriate to each person's own standing is effected, the whole experience is a controlled, ritualised journey of such rare beauty, that we are brought to a different point in ourselves. (pp.98–99)

This account has more of a sense of meditation about it and in it each person takes those parts of the journey that are appropriate for them.

The French theorist Paul Ricoeur develops a theory (Rahn 1994b) of mimesis as refiguration of reality through the configuration of the artwork itself, and I would agree with this from my own experience. If the classical composer configures his or her own reality, what effect does this have on the audience's reality? Can listening to music be a reconfiguration of reality? John Rahn (1994b) deals with this:

> It is possible to refer to the value of expression to a kind of Aristotelian catharsis, and a distancing of emotion that allows us to get a perspective on it. The intricacies of musical development within a piece work through a kind of analogy to the structure of world, of ourselves experiencing not only the world but our emotional and intellectual concomitants to the world as part of the world... In this view, the value of expression in music would partly lie in its providing a kind of jungle-gym on which to exercise our capacity for dealing with reality, increasing our survivability and teaching us wisdom. The pleasure we gain from this aspect of the musical experience would derive from the same sources as the pleasure of learning, of satisfying curiosity, of increasing our abilities. (p.57)

So, in this view, the experience of a piece of music gives us an opportunity to look again at our own processes and exercise our own creativity in dealing with our circumstances.

The stress of the dominant traditions of Western culture has been on the uniting power of the elements of musical form. However, it could also be seen as a way of handling diversity through the bringing together of divergent elements into relationship in some way. There was not necessarily a thematic relationship, for example, between the movements of a baroque suite or a classical symphony. Composers put together movements from different works to form new works and debates have existed about the nature of a relationship between different movements of a symphony which have no overt thematic or harmonic links. The development of the aleatoric traditions in the twentieth century (where performers have a choice of a number of motifs) has a clear notion of diversity encapsulated within a structure.

In the work of individual composers we do see sometimes shifts to a more fragmented style. It is seen very clearly in the contemporary Norwegian composer Per Norgard's engrossment with a schizophrenic character called Adolf Wölfli: 'It was as though the cries and phantasms of a lonely person, afflicted for decades, suddenly demanded entry into Per Norgard's music and thereby brought about a sudden interruption in a grand scheme of making the world cohere musically' (Jensen, quoted in Beyer 1996, p.9). Before this period Norgard had been taken up with systems of establishing unity within music and with the environment – techniques based in the natural overtone series and golden-section rhythms[3] through which he had explored the infinity series (the notion of infinity):

> This composer who, in the 1970's, perseveringly and systematically had established a more and more widely branched balance in music, and who had opened horizon after horizon...almost passionately, his music now focused, not on continuity and wide horizons, but on the cup that is full to overflowing, the intensity of the moment, abrupt changes and drastic alterations. (Jensen, quoted in Beyer 1996, p.9)

Smetana's (1824–1884) first two quartets are musical autobiography. The first entitled *From My Life* describes his early life and loves. The finale is a joyful celebration of Czech music but it is dramatically interrupted by a tremolo and a high E which represents the onset of tinnitus, an early symptom of tertiary syphilis. The second quartet was written in the asylum where he experienced terrifying symptoms while various areas of his brain were destroyed. This took the form of tormenting voices. The effect on the music is that dislocated musical gestures without a sense of any 'home' key. Paul Robertson (1996) writes: 'It is a moving testimony to the power of music that this quartet simultaneously records the nature and destruction of the composer's persona and brain neurology, whilst remaining a fine and effective musical composition' (pp.40–41).

Such ideas can be linked to an autobiographical approach to the process of composition. Here the Underworld is sometimes identified with childhood experiences. In an interview I conducted in 1998 the contemporary composer Jennifer Fowler relates some of her own inspiration to a childhood dream which was frightening. She sees herself as reworking this in her adult life in her compositions. Writers concerned with psychological roots have concerned themselves with the way in which music makes use of childhood experiences. Anthony Kemp (1996) in writing on *The Musical Temperament* relates his own attraction to music to his experience of the loss of his father at the age of two. He goes on to cite Jacqueline du Pré's choice of the cello. She relates that, at a critical moment before her fifth birthday, she heard the sound of the cello on the wireless. This is described as a 'crystallising experience' by Walters and Gardner (1992) which they locate within Gardner's theory of multiple intelligences. They describe such experi-

---

3   The golden section is based on the mathematical sequence known as the Fibonacci series – 1, 1, 2, 3, 5, 8, 13, 21, etc.

ences as '[a]n overt reaction of an individual to some quality or feature of a domain: the reaction yields an immediate but long-term change in the individual's concept of the domain, his performance in it, and his view of himself' (p.137). John Sloboda (1985) also claims that many musicians can point to a single experience that is seminal in forming a lifelong engagement with an instrument. He claims that this is often in the context of an enjoyable family situation or as part of a good experience with friends:

> The outcome often takes the form of an obsession relationship with an instrument from which the child finds it difficult to be separated. The instrument becomes endowed with a personality of its own; significant characteristics are projected on to it, and these may or may not be associated with a particular music, or a specific musical style. (Kemp 1996, p.141)

Kemp (1996) sees Jacqueline du Pré's choice of the cello sound as filling a void. Easton, in her biography of du Pré (1989), identifies her relationship to William Pleeth, her 'cello daddy', as closer than that with her real father. In such stories we have the possibilities of exploring the needs of our unconscious by means of a relationship within the tone colour of a particular instrument and the choice being linked with an extra-musical event or need.

Summary – unity/diversity

The stress on unity that has characterised the Greek notion of harmonia and Christian notions of a single God have led to a concentration of the uniting aspects of musical form. This is sometimes linked with notions of self-integration on the part of the composer. However, the classical stress on structure could be seen as a way of containing diversity and keeping diverse elements in relationship. Contemporary composers, especially those using aleatoric techniques, have embraced unexpected elements more readily. It is also possible to see in the development of some composers periods of greater fragmentation, which are embraced as part of the creative development of their life. The process of listening takes listeners on a journey into their own subconscious with the possibility of reshaping themselves with the help of the composer who becomes a musical guide or therapist.

Challenge/nurture

This section will deal with the roles classical music is perceived as playing by composers, performers, listeners and theorists. There was strong sense of moral education implicit in Greek views of music. These became subsumed in thinking about the journey of the soul and its needs on that journey in medieval Christian thinking. Music could nurture the soul on that journey. In post-Enlightenment traditions there has been increasing stress on the notion of challenge. This was seen above in the debates about individualism and community, especially in the notion of the individual who is impelled to challenge prevailing norms.

It enters also as part of the ongoing debate about art as entertainment and art as an aesthetic experience. Here it may be linked with social issues around the employment of musicians. Before the French Revolution, art was produced to 'entertain the guests of the nobility' and composers were paid to fulfil this task, however they might view their own activity. High art critics have, however, largely favoured aesthetic value systems. This is particularly true from the Romantic period onwards when patronage was in decline. The argument about the challenging nature of the art through which one is empowered is linked with the Western idea of 'progress'. This has coloured the structuring of Western history and, therefore, Western music history and musicology.

The notion of progress combined with the heroic journey encouraged notions of challenge. The individual composer was pursuing his own heroic journey and a composition is a chance for others to join. This may result in a challenge to the audience. This was clearly seen in the first performance of Stravinsky's *Rite of Spring* when the challenged audience walked out. But such behaviour is not common in classical audiences; we could, however, see the declining audiences for the avant-garde in the classical tradition as an example of audiences voting with their feet. The role of challenge is central to Leonard Meyer's (1956) theory of musical meaning. The degree of information communicated to the audience was related to the element of 'surprise' in the audience: 'The inhibition of a tendency to respond or, on the conscious level, the frustration of expectation was found to be the basis of the affective and intellectual aesthetic response to music' (p.43).

Mireille Besson, at the Cognitive Neuroscience Laboratory in Marseilles, researched what she called event-related activity. She highlights how the brain anticipates events and how a regular pattern becomes established as an anticipated event. Her research shows that both professional musicians and non-musicians are sensitive to musical incongruity. Paul Robertson (1996) summarises:

> The real significance of these studies seems to be that we are all wired to be 'musical' in the sense that we all of us implicitly understand the clichés

of familiar tonal melodies... Music relies on inherent neurological responses that we all have... One curious observation is that, unlike language, which provokes a negative electrical response, music elicits a positive electrical response. To the best of my knowledge nobody understands the significance of this or why it should be so. (p.10)

Later Robertson illustrates this with reference to Hindemith's (1895–1963) work for string quartet entitled *Minimax*. Here Hindemith pokes fun at the precision of a military band marching by introducing the odd wrong note into the texture.

So, as outlined in the debate about musical meaning, the nature of musical meaning as interrelationship between composer, performer and audience becomes clarified. The audience's attention is held by the right degree of contrast or surprise. Cultural factors are clearly very important here:

This analysis of communication emphasises the absolute necessity of a common universe of discourse in art. For without a set of gestures common to the social group, and without common habit responses to those gestures, no communication whatsoever is possible. Communication depends upon, presupposes, and arises out of the universe of discourse which in the aesthetics of music is called style. (Meyer 1956, p.42)

It is a position that presents problems for a world of wider interchange between cultures than the one in which Meyer was working.

The role of challenge now underpins the training of the classical musician who is expected to surmount a number of hurdles in order to enter his or her chosen profession. These include the competitions and examinations that are increasingly defining the musical world. It is questioned by Anthony Kemp (1996) in his work on *The Musical Temperament*:

A key aspect of special music schools, emphasised by the Calouste Gulbenkian Foundation report (1978) into the training of musicians, was 'the stimulus of competition' within a boarding school environment. One wonders how unhealthy this might be should it get out of hand in a community where, in a sense, all the pupils are in competition with each other, and where, at each level, there are winners and losers, and no escape... Most children, however precocious they are, like to have friends of their own age and, what is more, to feel accepted by them. The interpersonal dynamics created by an unruly competitive environment may result in destroying the possibility of pupils developing genuinely close and nurturing relationships. (p.249)

His book shows how the challenging competitive situations characterise the world of classical music. He sees real dangers in the competitive nature of the music world: 'The personal investment that musicians make in music, which is inimical to feelings of personal esteem, appears to be intertwined with the manifestation of competition at every level' (Kemp 1996, p.102). Kemp cites members of the Vienna Symphony Orchestra who reported problems in relationships within the orchestra and believed that envy is an integral part of the musical profession. Back-stabbing and personal competition was described by a researcher into two London symphony orchestras and was even higher in a London conservatoire. All of this sets out a profession based on the notion of challenge at every level.

And yet there is a strand in post-modernity that challenges notions of progress and therefore leaves the door open, theoretically, for more 'nurturing' notions of art. The development of Classic FM has shown how the familiar is now seen as nurturing and that pieces that were challenging in their own time are now perceived as nurturing. In an article entitled 'Art and entertainment' Eric Gans (1994a) points out that the roots of the word 'entertainment' are in the French verb *entretenir,* 'to nourish'. He castigates the Romantic notion of an art divorced from notions of entertainment, and draws heavily on French philosophers of art, especially Mallarmé, Valéry and Artaud, in his exposition, defining a position where there is no longer a distinction between two audiences – one, the un-self-conscious masses who regard art as entertainment and the other, the self-conscious elite who regard it as art for its own sake (aesthetic) and separate it from entertainment. These two attitudes reflect the nurturing and challenging aspects of music. Gans expounds how art is linked to the religious experience of contemplation and also how art is consumed like food, and sets out a theory in which art is the satisfaction of desire. In this theory he links them together: '...to think of art as separate from satisfaction of desire is to externalise the originary moment of contemplation, to cut it off from the appetitive satisfaction that ritual has always preserved, in however attenuated a form' (p.48).

His article is dense and complex but contains fascinating reflections on how to resolve the theoretical dichotomy between the individual, challenging nature of the lone artists and the desire for entertainment of a consumer society. He makes the interesting point that what is consumed turns into the culture itself:

> Culture arises as a reflection on what has already been consumed. If that is true then in sociopsychological terms when we look to the culture of the past already consumed we in effect return to our ancestors or at least

our grandparents as a source of nurture; when we strike out to explore new avenues and challenges we move away, forming our own path with the more adventurous explorers of our culture. (Gans 1994a, p.49)

He refuses to condemn the 'entertainment' function in a way that classical theorists have traditionally done, linking it with the needs generated by a consumer society:

The 'alimentary' nature of entertainment no longer implies a necessary complicity with the anonymous violence of the periphery. Instead, there is an exploration of the surface of experience which, by offering easy solutions to insoluble problems, permits us to defer the necessity of finding such solutions... Entertainment provides solace from the anxieties of the market on which these [social] differences are bought and sold. The stock exchange on which we are obliged, for well or ill, to spend our lives. (Gans 1994a, pp.52–53)

Andrew Blake (1997) in addressing the jazz revival in Britain in the 1980s sees it too caught in the dilemma of entertainment and art:

Jazz has attracted more of its fair share of the fantasy of opposition, the individualised, implicitly male, 'heroism' of the great artist working in defiance of social norms... Jazz also has a shadow existence as an entertainment form, as good music to dance to, converse to, chat up to. The tension between art and entertainment has dogged jazz (as it has other forms such as opera) throughout its history. Many moments of public interest in jazz have enthused on its danceablity – the rhythm or groove, rather than the technical ability of the soloists so revered by musicians. (p.113)

There are isolated examples in post-Enlightenment European music when composers have included healing in their intentions for their works. The most famous example is the *Cavatina* from Beethoven's (1776–1830) late quartets. In these it is generally accepted that Beethoven reached elevated states of being and touched on the world of the transcendentally sublime. He wrote that he was writing them for the nurture of future generations. Robertson (1996) describes its power in this way:

Each fragment of the Cavatina is somehow invested with a significance that transcends its apparent content. The seemingly simple phrases develop and extend in a miraculously tender fashion and the middle section, *beklamt* ('heavy of heart, desolate'), transports us by means of a few notes into a rootless and hopeless netherworld of the human psyche.

Such explorations of the psyche's dark side are not to inflict pain but rather to act as a catharsis. As Beethoven said, 'I leave my music to heal the world.' (p.42)

Contemporary composers like Terry Riley have been vilified for the creation of 'function music' because they produce music of a more nurturing nature in a tradition which is more at ease with notions of challenge. Ideas from other cultures finding their way into the classical tradition have produced sleeve notes of composers in a way more reminiscent of the New Age (see Chapter Four) and of a more nurturing feel. They indicate more spiritual intentions to the music. For example, Lawrence Ball's *Meditational Music Number One*, issued in 1982, contains the following description:

Meditational Music-Philosophy. In sensitive music, something is experienced expressing itself like a second music over and beyond physical sound. This image is ancient, occurring in Indian music treatises as the 'Unstruck Sound' (i.e. not blown, plucked or struck)... In my musical composition, improvisation and performances, I am concerned that audiences become conscious of this second level directly, otherwise the music is failing. (Ball 1982)

Summary – challenge/nurture

Although the nurturing function of music was prominent in Greek and early Christian thought, notions of challenge have been prominent in the construction of the notion of the master musician, although the entertainment function was present in the age of patronage. As individualism progressed, the tradition became more competitive. It was inevitable that the development of the public concert had to give its audience a degree of challenge: the audience is expected to pay its full attention to the music for the duration of the concert. More nurturing music is often condemned as 'wallpaper' music, regarded as boring by the elite. The centrality of the public is central to an understanding of this development. People are unlikely to pay to be sent to sleep! The general growth of the entertainment industry in the late twentieth century has fuelled the debate about nurturing and challenging functions of music. Many theorists are still uncomfortable with notions of nurture although some are asking for a bringing together of the two polarities.

Excitement/relaxation

This section will examine the perceived effects of listening to music. Classical literature is filled with stories embodying the potential power of music as enshrined in the Orpheus myth. Jamie James (1993) in *The Music of the Spheres: Music, Science and the Natural Order of the Universe* cites the following story from the biography of Pythagoras by Iamblichus:

> A young man from Taormina had been up all night partying with friends and listening to songs in the Phrygian mode, a key well known for its ability to incite violence. When the aggravated lad saw the girl he loved sneaking away in the wee hours of the morning from the home of his rival, he determined to go and burn her house down. Pythagoras happened to be out late himself, stargazing, and he walked in on this violent scene. He convinced the piper to change his tune from the Phrygian mode to a song in spondees a tranquillising metre. The young man's madness instantly cooled, and he was restored to reason... The Pythagoreans, when they retired for the night, cleansed their minds of 'the noises and perturbations to which they had been exposed during the day by certain odes and hymns which produced tranquil sleep and few, but good, dreams.' When they woke up in the morning, they got the day off to a proper start by playing songs that dispersed the torpor of sleep. Iamblichus concludes: 'Sometimes the passions of the soul and certain diseases were, as they said, genuinely lured by enchantments, by musical sounds alone, without words. This is indeed probably the origin of the general word *epode,* or enchantment.' (p.32)

The sixth century theorist Boethius had similar ideas:

> From this same principle radical changes in one's character also occur. A lascivious mind takes pleasure in the more lascivious modes or is often softened and moved upon hearing them. On the other hand, a more violent mind finds pleasure in the more exciting modes or will become excited when it hears them. This is the reason that the musical modes were named after certain peoples, such as the 'Lydian' mode, and the 'Phrygian' mode; for the modes are named after the people that find pleasure in them. A people will find pleasure in a mode resembling its own character, and thus a sensitive people cannot be united by or find pleasure in a severe mode, nor a severe people in a sensitive mode. But, as has been said, similarity causes love and pleasure. Thus Plato held that we should be extremely cautious in this matter, lest some change in music of good moral character should occur. He also said that there is no greater ruin for the morals of a community than the gradual perversion of a

prudent and modest music. For the minds of those hearing the perverted music immediately submit to it, little by little depart from their character, and retain no vestige of justice or honesty. This will occur if either the lascivious modes bring something immodest into the minds of the people or if the more violent modes implant something warlike and savage.

For there is no greater path whereby instruction comes to the mind than through the ear. Therefore when rhythms and modes enter the mind by this path, there can be no doubt that they affect and remould the mind into their own character. (Boethius, quoted in Godwin 1987, p.45)

In this description we see the necessity for a match between the music and the characteristics of the people or person – the notion that the effect of music cannot be reduced to simple cause and effect equations.

In the twelfth century, Hildegard of Bingen saw music as having a softening function:

Just as the power of God extends everywhere, surrounding all things and encountering no resistance, so too the sound of human voices singing God's praise can spread everywhere, surrounding all things and encountering no resistance. It can rouse the soul lost in apathy, and soften the soul hardened by pride. (Hildegard, quoted in Van der Weyer 1997, p.79)

Such writing is less common as Western music history progresses and the classical composer becomes more separate from his audience and less concerned with its reaction. Most musical forms that have developed in the classical tradition do, however, contain a balance between faster and slower sections (although the balance between these have differed in different periods). The balance between exciting and more relaxing sections formed the cornerstone of forms like the baroque suite and the classical symphony and sonata.

The pursuit of discord in the twentieth century has led to a greater stress on energising rather than relaxing. Paul Robertson links this with sexual energy in the work of Leos Janacek (1854–1928). He called his first string quartet, written in 1923, the *Kreutzer Sonata*. It was based on an overtly sexual Tolstoy story in which an obsessively jealous husband who hates music murders his music-loving wife. All of Janacek's late music was coloured by his obsession for Kamilla Staeslava, 25 years younger than him: 'The increased levels of neurological arousal and hormone releases associated with sexual love certainly change our subjective experience of the world. Are we right in suggesting that the supremely exciting frenetic *ostinatos* (short repeated phrases) of the first string quartet relate to the composer's aroused state?' (Robertson 1996, p.39.)

The advent in the UK of radio stations such as Classic FM has clearly highlighted the effects of listening to music of the classical repertoire, perhaps more clearly than ever before. Pieces of music are now classified as relaxing, uplifting, exciting and so on and clustered together to form CDs of a particular mood. These are designed for listeners who are aware of their own responses to music and wish music to help maintain a rhythm in their lives. The classical canon is now perceived as relaxing, more so than the avant-garde tradition.

Summary – excitement/relaxation

The ancient Greeks had a sense of the relationship of music to the human condition. Music was used by them and also by the Church in the Middle Ages to influence people in certain ways. Although the classical forms include a balance of faster and slower movements and sections, this dimension does figure highly in contemporary theorists' work. However, the advent of radio stations like Classic FM have developed an awareness of this dimension as a way of marketing collections of music for different moods.

Embodiment/transcendence

This section will look at how far the process of music-making contains notions of the body or of the Divine and how far these concepts are interrelated. Music and religion, or the concept of the Divine, have been inextricably bound together for much of Western history. The relationship of the Muses and the gods of classical tradition were moved across into the Christian traditions within the notion of a single creator god. For much of Western history, the Church has been the main patron of the classical tradition.

In the ancient Greek culture, Pythagoras saw a resolution of the perceived division between body, mind and spirit in his notion of three sorts of music. In the words of James (1993):

To use modern nomenclature of a later era, *musica instrumentalis*, the ordinary music made by plucking the lyre, blowing the pipe, and so forth; *musica humana*, the continuous but unheard music made by each human organism, especially the harmonious (or inharmonious) resonance between the soul and the body; and *musica mundana, the music made by the cosmos itself, which would come to be known as the music of the spheres.*

To a modern person, the most salient observation to be made about these three classes of music is their enormous discrepancy in scale. Yet for the Pythagoreans, again, there existed among them an essential identity: a piper and the cosmos might sound the same note. That is because to Pythagoras it was purely a matter of mathematics. There was no more of a difference among these three classes of music than there was among a triangle traced in the palm of the hand, a triangle formed by the walls of a building, and a triangle described by three stars: 'triangleness' is an eternal idea, and all expressions of it are essentially the same. (p.31)

In the Middle Ages the notion of God was central to music theory. Hildegard writes: 'Music is the echo of the glory and beauty of heaven. And in echoing that glory and beauty, it carries human praise back to heaven' (Hildegard, quoted in Van der Weyer 1997, p.79). Later she attempts to reconcile the duality that had developed in Christianity between spirit and body by means of music: 'The words of a hymn represent the body, while the melody represents the soul. Words represent humanity, and melody represents divinity. Thus in a beautiful hymn, in which words and melody are perfectly matched, body and soul, humanity and divinity, are brought into unity' (Hildegard, quoted in Van der Weyer 1997, p.79).

In the Renaissance the revival of Greek ideas led to writing like this fine description of an improvised performance by the lutenist Francesco di Milano:

The tables being cleared, he chose one, and as if tuning his strings, sat on the end of a table seeking out a fantasia. He had barely disturbed the air with three strummed chords when he interrupted the conversation which had started among the guests. Having constrained them to face him he continued with such a ravishing skill that little by little, making the strings languish under his fingers in his sublime way, he transported all those listening into so pleasurable a melancholy that – one leaning his head on his hand supported by his elbow, and another sprawling with his limbs in careless deportment, with gaping mouth and half-closed eyes…they remained deprived of all senses save that of hearing, as if the spirit, having abandoned all the seats of the sense, had retired to the ears in order to enjoy more at its ease so ravishing a harmony; and I believe (said M. de Ventimille) that we would be there still, had not he himself – I know not how – changing his style of playing with a gentle force, returned the spirit and the senses to the place from which he had stolen them, not without leaving as much as astonishment in each of us as if he had been elevated by an ecstatic transport of some divine frenzy. (quoted in Rooley 1990, p.8)

The notion of the soul leaving the body transported by music underpins such Renaissance thinking linked with the ancient Greek ideas. The notion of the music of the spheres occupied many philosophers of the Renaissance. A letter from the philosopher Marsilio Ficino, who sang the hymns of Orpheus regularly as spiritual exercise, illustrates the tension between soul and body that characterises the tradition in which Greek ideas are combined with Christian notions of God:

> According to the followers of Plato, divine music is twofold. One kind, they say, exists entirely in the mind of God. The second is the motions and order of the heavens, by which the heavenly spheres and their orbits make a marvellous harmony. In both of these our soul took part before it was imprisoned in our bodies. But it uses the ears as messengers, as though they were chinks in this darkness. By the ears, as I have already said, the soul receives the echoes of that incomparable music, by which it is led back to the deep and silent memory of the harmony which it previously enjoyed. The whole soul then kindles with desire to fly back to its rightful home, so that it may enjoy that true music again. (Ficino, quoted in Rooley 1990, pp.13–14)

The emphasis on the Divine as an aspect of music declined as the influence of the Church declined. In Romantic philosophy it reappeared in the concept of truth. Martin Heidegger (1886–1976) refines this in his thinking, as Nielsen explains:

> Heidegger approaches a work of art from two angles. On the one hand he asks what can make a human being see the world in a new light: on the other, he asks what the role of art actually is. The two questions turn out to be related. Heidegger's aim is to show how the work of art *still* – as in the aesthetics of the Romantics – is concerned with truth. Indeed it emerges that the work of art is one of the few things that can seriously open our eyes to the world in which we live… Unlike previous philosophical schools, Heidegger does not associate truth with 'the world' as it is 'in reality' nor does truth have anything to do with measuring whether something is 'correct' or 'incorrect'. No, the true is what we human beings sense, purely and simply… Heidegger was a phenomenologist. The main point of phenomenology is that we consider objects as they appear. We should not worry about how they are constituted 'in reality', independent of human beings. For a phenomenologist it is only

meaningful to ask about 'the world' as it manifests itself to the human being. The world of phenomenology is always the world of man. (Nielsen, quoted in Beyer 1996, p.174)

Heidegger describes how art makes truth happen:

A work of architecture, a Greek temple, is not an image of anything. It simply stands there in its rocky cleft. The building rests on the rocky ground. Its state of rest draws the hidden...bearing quality out of the rock. As it stands there, the building holds its ground against the storm that rages against it, and then and only then shows the might of the storm. Apparently only there by the grace of the sun, it is the lustre and gleam of the stones which make the light of day, the expanse of the heavens and the dark of the night shine forth. The assured towering of the temple makes the invisible space of the air visible. (Heidegger, quoted in Beyer 1996, p.179)

Nevertheless, notions of the sacred still struggled to find a place in contemporary aesthetics. Georges Sorel (1945) argues that the sublime died with the triumph of the bourgeoisie but Jules Monnerot writes: 'The sublime is an element which western societies cannot afford to do without' (Monnerot, quoted in Rahn 1994b, p.17). However, Rainer Rochlitz concludes: 'As for works of post-avant-gardist modernity which content themselves with seeking a "secular illumination" in the frame of a world which is neither the worst or the best, their critical force will be all the greater as their normative reference is no longer an inverse image of redemption, but rather a meaning which is conceivable ere below, here and now' (p.35).

Cook (1990) describes a concert as being a transcendent experience. The act itself is characterised by a loss of boundaries. He quotes Sartre when saying that the listener has to return 'always to a reality from which we had been drawn away by the image building process... The significance of this process lies in the fact that image building eliminates the subject–object division essential for all perception, so that when we "awaken" to the real world, this division seems all the more accentuated' (Sartre, quoted in Cook 1990, pp.152–153).

The linking of this freedom in listening with images and fantasy (seen under containment/freedom, pp.83–88) can be traced back to ancient Greek notions as filtered through Renaissance philosophers. The teacher Ficino, for example, saw the soul as being refreshed by seven conditions: sleep, syncope (fainting), melancholy, aloneness, reverie, chastity of mind, devotion to God (Rooley 1990). Notions of transcendence linked with reverie still colour the aesthetic writing. The notion of transcendence occurs even when the sense of the divine is absent. Adorno states that 'the novelty of avant garde art is its incessant transcendence of negativity' (quoted in Rahn 1994b, p.25). Gans (1994b) in a challenging article entitled 'The beginning and end of aesthetic form', parallels the activity of contemplation with the reception of a work of art. This echoes W. B. Yeats who in *Ideas of Good and Evil* writes:

> The purpose of rhythm, it has always seemed to me, is to prolong the moment of contemplation, the moment when we are both asleep and awake, which is the one moment of creation, by hushing us with alluring monotony, while it holds us waking by variety, to keep us in that state of perhaps real trance, in which the mind liberated by the will is unfolded in symbols. (Yeats, quoted in Hadfield 1960, p.237)

Notions of the mystical are more likely to be found in composers' own accounts of their processes than in those of musicologists. Clara Schumann's account of Robert Schumann's madness provides an interesting case study here:

> From the night of Friday the 10th February, 1854 until Saturday the 11th, Robert suffered from so violent an affection of the hearing that he did not close his eyes all night. He kept on hearing the same note over and over again, and at times also another interval. By day it was covered up by other sounds...

> [Written in April, 1854] The aural hallucinations increased markedly from the 10th to the 17th of February. We consulted another doctor, Regimental Physician Dr Boger, and Hasenclever also came daily, but only an advising friend.

> On the night of Friday the 17th, after we had been in bed for some time, Robert suddenly got up and wrote down a theme, which, as he said, an angel had sung to him. When he had finished it he lay down again and all night long he was picturing things to himself, gazing towards heaven with wide-open eyes; he was firmly convinced that angels hovered round him revealing glories to him in wonderful music. They bade us welcome, and before a year had passed we should be united and with them ... Morning came and with it a terrible change. The angel voices turned to those of demons and in hideous music they told him he was a sinner and they would cast him into hell. In short, his condition increased to an actual nervous paroxysm; he cried out with pain (for as he said to me afterwards, they pounced on him in the forms of tigers and hyenas, to seize him, and two doctors, who luckily came quickly enough, could

scarcely hold him. I will never forget this sight, I actually suffered the pains of torture in it...

On the 20th, Robert spent the whole day at his writing desk, with pen and ink before him, and listened to the angel-voices...[he] would often write a few words, but very little, and then listen again. He had a look full of rapture that I can never forget; yet this unnatural rapture wounded my heart as much as when he was suffering from the evil spirits. Ah! all this filled my heart with the most dreadful worry about how it would end; I saw his mind ever more unsettled, yet had no idea of what still awaited him and me...

During the days that followed, things remained much the same. He felt himself surrounded alternately by good and evil spirits, but no longer did he hear them only in music, often they spoke. At the same time his mind was so clear that he wrote touching, peaceful variations on the wonderfully peaceful, holy theme which he had written down on the night of the 10th; ... On Sunday, the 26th, he felt a little better...he ate a large supper very hastily. Then suddenly, at 9:30, he stood up and said he must have his clothes... 'It will not be for long. I shall soon come back, cured.' (Schumann, quoted in Godwin 1987, pp.234–236)

This account of his madness shows clearly how processes that had served him well in composition are now out of control. The passage reads not unlike a shamanic journey (see Chapter Three). It is interesting to reflect that if the notion of the divine and the mystical had been more part of the Western tradition, Schumann might have developed ways of handling the 'other world' in which lay both the roots of his creativity and the roots of his madness.

Leading contemporary composers have absorbed ideas from other cultures, sometimes located in particular phases in their lives. These have provided conceptual ways of linking the transcendent and the physical. Karlheinz Stockhausen wrote widely on religion and music, drawing heavily on Eastern traditions. Here he uses the notion of the chakras (see Chapter Four) to explain his ideas on music and healing:

Each of us is...a person with many levels ... I have a sexual center, three vital centers, two mental centers and a suprapersonal center. If I can perceive that, I have come far enough to have awoken seven different centers in myself. And with different things I can bring each center into vibration...

There is also music that goes through all the centers: hence there are moments in which you are addressed in a purely sacred, a purely religious way; and other moments in which you are addressed purely sensually, purely erotically. That is pretty reckless music. One must be very strong to be able to experience that completely. Above all, this music must be exceptionally well balanced, fantastically composed. If it is not, then there are overloadings, and when one hears it one is overexcited in a certain way, and brought out of equilibrium. Hence it is naturally better if one hears music that draws one up higher than one is by nature. We are mostly pretty physical sacks, are we not – all of us? (Stockhausen, quoted in Godwin 1987, pp.288–289)

We can see here how he struggles to bring the embodiment of the Eastern tradition together with the more transcendent Western tradition; in the middle we can see how he rates the physical as 'lower' than the spiritual. His work *Aus den Sieben Tagen* required of its performers that they fast and meditate for seven days before playing it. Its instructions read more like a manual of meditation than a musical score:

A note lives, like YOU, like ME, like THEM, like IT.
Moves, stretches and contracts.
Metamorphoses, gives birth, procreates, dies, is reborn.
Seeks, stops seeking, finds, loses, marries,
Loves, tarries, hurries, comes and goes. (Stockhausen 1968)

Stockhausen's work influenced the growth of free improvisation groups using aleatoric principles (see p.87) like those run by the American composer Pauline Oliveros (see Chapter One) and Terry Riley.

More composers explored such ideas as the twentieth century progressed. In the first quarter of the century Scriabin developed a mystical scale, while Erik Satie was a member of the French Rosicrucian Order, a sect devoted to the exploration of the esoteric. Schoenberg was immersed in the mysticism of Swedenborg while Paul Hindemith concerned himself at the end of his life with 'The Harmony of the World', exploring the secret tradition of Pythagoras in his final works. John Cage was heavily influenced in the 1940s by the Japanese Zen master D.T. Suzuki in such works as *Silence* and *Empty Words*.

The German composer and music educator Carl Orff had notions of ecology underpinning his musical philosophy and used it to bring the physical as a significant element in the musical experience:

Elemental Music is never just music. It is bound up with movement, dance and speech, and so it is a form of music in which one must participate, in which one is involved not as a listener but as a co-performer. It is pre-rational, has no over-all form, no architectonics, involves no set sequences, ostinati or minor rondo-forms. Elemental Music is earthy, natural, physical, capable of being learnt and experienced by anybody, child's play... Elemental Music, word and movement, play, every-thing that awakens and develops the powers of the soul builds up the humus of the soul, the humus without which we face spiritual soil-erosion. When does soil-erosion arise in nature? When the land is cultivated in an unbalanced way, when the natural hydrological cycle is disturbed by over-cultivation, when forest and hedge are sacrificed on utilitarian grounds to the drawing-board mentality – in short, when the balance of nature is undermined by one-sided encroachment. And in the same way we face spiritual soil-erosion when man estranges himself from the ele-mental and loses his balance. (Orff, quoted in Hamel 1978, p.18)

The French composer Olivier Messiaen (1908–1992) made his own synthesis of Christian/Gnostic mysticism with Hindu belief systems. This underpinned many of his works, many of which had religious themes. Minimalism was also associated with meditative techniques and ideas from the East. Both Terry Riley and La Monte Young studied with Prandit Pran Nath of the singing school of Kirana in northern India. The work of Steve Reich and Philip Glass bear the marks of similar influences. The contempo-rary Danish composer Per Norgard is pictured on the front of a book on his music in a position in which he 'listens for the deep "shadow tune" of the ocean surf' (Beyer 1996, p.17).

Other composers have developed meditative techniques to aid the process of composition. Andrew Downes (1998) writes:

For me, prayer and meditation...lead to the ability to calm one's mind and focus one's thoughts in the context of an inner personal environment of peace and tranquillity, however stressful life has become. In this way I an able to practise my art whatever the circumstances, whereas previ-ously, any kind of personal stress or problem was liable to stem the creative flow.

For a composer such techniques are invaluable. Indeed, I would say that they are essential. Focusing logically and entirely on the sound of music is incredibly difficult in a world filled with words, unharmonious noise, deadlines and stress...

The contemporary lutenist Anthony Rooley (1990) writes in similar style when he sets out the sense of sacred space that a performer needs to create:

As audience and performer become more attuned to this simple truth, the more the performing space is filled with awe and wonder. In the beginning...there is utter rest, utter silence...from which the performance begins to manifest. In the symbolic beginning of creation as represented by the beginning of the performance we need some simple techniques to exercise ourselves with... Like taking a breath... The simple technique for beginning a performance clearly is not always easy to do when several hundred people are watching your every quiver. (p.49)

Although the transcendent figures in much of this writing it is only occasionally linked with the body. To find the theme of the body in contemporary aesthetic theory one must turn more to the work of feminist musicologists or those dealing with the injuries inflicted on the body by prolonged playing in the classical tradition. Criticisms of modernity also focus on the demands made on performers by composers. Singers, for example, have often been asked to explore the very limits of their capabilities. Some critics have regarded this as an example of dualistic elements within modernism where the body must be persecuted in the service of the mind.

The advent of the inclusion of different musical styles within the scope of musicological enterprise has also brought notions of the body back into critical discourse:

One of the importances of Afro-American music lies in the fact that often the voice seems to be treated more as an 'instrument' (the body using its own resources to make sound) ... From work-song grunts through 1930s jazz styles (Louis Armstrong singing 'like a trumpet'; Billie Holiday 'like a sax') to the short phrases of funk and scratch textures (used like percussion, bass or synthesiser), we hear vocal personality receding as the voice is integrated into the processes of the articulating human body. Of course, at the same time, instruments in this tradition often sound like voices. But the often noted importance of 'vocalised tone' is only part of a wider development in which 'instrumental' and 'vocal' modes meet on some intermediate ground: while it is true that the instrument-as-machine (technological extension of the body) becomes a gesturing body (the 'voice' of the limb), at the same time the voice-as-a-person becomes a vocal body (the body vocalising). (Middleton 1990, p.264)

From here it is possible to see music again as an essentially embodied art. The notion of being controlled by a force beyond in the act of music-making fills this passage from the ethnomusicologist John Blacking (1977):

If there are forms intrinsic to music and dance that are not modelled on language, we may look beyond the 'language' of dancing, for instance, to the dances of language and thought. As conscious movement is in our thinking, so thinking may come from movement, and especially shared, or conceptual, thought from communal movement. And just as the ultimate aim of dancing is to be able to move *without* thinking, to *be* danced, so the ultimate achievement in thinking is to be moved to think, to be thought…essentially it is a form of unconscious cerebration, a movement of the body. We are moved into thinking. Body and mind are one. (pp.22–23).

Summary – embodiment / transcendence

The Western classical traditions have inherited the division of body, mind and spirit implicit in ancient Greek traditions and carried over into Christianity. As beliefs in the Divine declined, the notion of the transcendent was subsumed in notions of beauty and truth. In the twentieth century, composers have explored other belief systems and musics from other traditions that include various ways of bringing body and spirit together. There is still a greater sense of valuing and searching for the experience of the transcendent, in whatever tradition this is perceived as happening, than of valuing the relationship of the music to the body. Feminist theoreticians, in particular, have been concerned with re-embodying the tradition.

Summary

The roots of Western classical traditions lie within ancient Greek philosophy which was revived in the Renaissance. The notion of music for divine purpose or moral education and healing were present but weakened post-Enlightenment. Connections with society were stressed by an overarching scheme for the cosmos. However, individualism gained sway post-Enlightenment with development of notions of master composers and master works. These were often seen challenging the prevailing culture and calling people to a higher notion of art. This elitist construct has been maintained by the guardians of the tradition in the academy who have created the notion of the canon of masterworks. Although challenged by post-modernism, musicology has been somewhat resistant to ideas that link social theory and music too tightly together. The power base created by the development of an elitist theory has served to keep the tradition contained by a written notation and a concentration on musical form. This has limited improvisation within the tradition. Freedom, however, has been seen within the area of 'music appreciation' when the listener is freed from everyday concerns in flights of fancy. As the concentration on masterworks became the centre of the tradition, links with human expression weakened until more psychological approaches to musical form were developed in the later twentieth century. The 'confidential' nature of music has been explored in depth in debates about musical meaning. This has established that the meanings are plural and often negotiated between musician and audience. Notions of the body are increasingly part of the debate, thus redressing the concentration on mind (and to a lesser extent the emotions). Post-Enlightenment notions of challenge dominated the thinking of the relationship of the master composer to society. More nurturing traditions tended to be despised as mere entertainment or wallpaper music. The development of the public concert for which people paid played a significant part in this. However, the development of Classic FM has linked the notion of nurture with that of the canon and highlighted awareness of the emotional effect of various pieces of music. This notion has replaced the notion of moral education that filled pre-Enlightenment treatises. Notions of transcendence have taken different forms. Starting with Greek gods it moved towards the Christian God. Notions of beauty or the sublime or truth replaced this. However, in composer's accounts, notions of the divine are often present. Ideas drawn from a variety of religious traditions have been part of the journey of many musicians in the twentieth century.

CHAPTER THREE

Of Shamans and Healers

A woman healer

Nisa is an !Kung woman in Botswana. This account of her healing was collected by Marjorie Shostak in 1970 and 1971 (see Shostak 1983; see Young 1993 for an anthology). Nisa describes the 'n/um' – the power to heal – as a very good thing, and says it is like Western medicine because it is strong. The ability to heal with n/um is linked with trance, as Nisa explains:

> ...because it is in trance that the healing power sitting inside the healer's body – the n/um – starts to work. Both men and women learn how to cure with it, but not everyone wants to. Trance-medicine really hurts! As you begin to trance, the n/um slowly heats inside you and pulls at you. It rises until it grabs your insides and takes your thoughts away. Your mind and senses leave and you don't think clearly. Things become strange and start to change. You can't listen to people or understand what they say. You look at them and they suddenly become very tiny. You think, 'What's happening? Is God doing this?' All that is inside you is the n/um; that is all you can feel. (Young 1993, p.248)

Nisa describes how she touches people, lays her hands on them to cure them through touch. She tells how, in this process, she is in an altered state of consciousness: 'When you finish, other people hold you and blow around your head and your face. Suddenly your senses go "Phah!" and come back to you. You think, "Eh hey, there are people here," and you see again as you usually do' (Young 1993, pp.248–249). She sees the origin of her power in her father's ability to cure people with 'gemsbok-song trance medicine'. These are trance songs named after certain animals, like gemsbok, eland and giraffe. They were given long ago, by God, to her people to sing and to work with. The work is part of the fabric of their lives and is very important, good work.

Nisa describes God as the power who made people:

He is like a person, with a person's body and covered with beautiful clothes. He has a horse on which he puts people who are just learning to trance and become healers. God will have the person in trance ride to where he is, so God can see the new healer and talk to him. There are two different ways of learning how to trance and of becoming a healer. Some people learn to trance and heal only to drum-medicine songs. My mother knew how to trance to these, although she never learned to heal. There are other people who know how to trance and to heal to drum-medicine songs as well as to ceremony-dance songs. The n/um is the same in both. If a person is lying down, close to death, and someone beats out drum-medicine songs, a healer will enter a trance and cure the sick person until he is better. Both men and women have n/um, and their power is equal. Just as a man brings a sick person back to health, so does a woman bring a sick person back to health. (Young 1993, p.249)

It is difficult to use the power of n/um; it is very powerful but tricky, sometimes effective and sometimes not. This is because, sometimes, God doesn't want the sick person to be cured as Nisa explains:

Sometimes he tells a healer in trance, 'Today I want this sick person. Tomorrow, too. But the next day, if you try to cure her, than I will help you. I will let you have her for a while.' God watches the sick person, and the healer trances her. Finally God says, 'All right, I have only made her slightly sick. Now, she can get up.' When she feels better, she thinks, 'Oh, if this healer hadn't been here, I would surely have died. He's given me my life back again.'
That's n/um – a very helpful thing! (Young 1993, p.249)

Nisa's mother taught her about drum-medicine when she felt she was becoming a young woman. As part of the training, Nisa was given a root to help her learn to trance. It was put it in a little leather pouch where she had to keep for a few days. Then her mother took it and pounded it together with some bulbs and some beans. They were then all cooked together. The taste of it was horrible – it made her mouth feel foul, and made her vomit. Pounding it up with the other foods made it more possible for the stomach to accept it – if it had all been vomited up, it wouldn't have been effective. She had to drink it many times and she threw up again and again. At the end she started to tremble. Her mother, Peiole, rubbed her body as the effect got stronger and stronger. As her body shook harder, she started to cry. They were many people touching her and helping her while all this was happening.

In the end she learned how to break out of herself and trance. She started this when she heard the drum-medicine songs. At that time people would decorate her hair with beads and copper rings, as she describes:

> As I began to trance, the women would say, 'She's started to trance, now, so watch her carefully. Don't let her fall.' They would take care of me, touching me and helping. If another woman was also in trance, she laid on hands and helped me. They rubbed oil on my face, and I stood there – a lovely young woman, trembling in trance – until I was finished. (Young 1993, p.249)

Nisa enjoyed curing people with the drum-medicine songs. She was taught by an elderly uncle, for her mother had never learned the art. She says that he struck her 'with spiritual medicine arrows', which is how everyone starts. Now when she hears the drum sound, she is grabbed by her n/um. This is the time when she has the power to cure people. However, she says that she has become afraid of the pain involved in the process, so she hasn't wanted to cure anyone even though they have asked her. She is afraid of the way it pulls at her 'insides, over and over, pulling deep within' (Young 1993, p.249).

She describes herself as a master at trancing to drum-medicine songs with many successes in curing people with her hands:

> I know how to trick God from wanting to kill someone and how to have God give the person back to me. But I, myself, have never spoken directly to God nor have I seen or gone to where he lives. I am still very small when it comes to healing and I haven't made these trips. Others have, but young healers like myself haven't. Because I don't heal very often, only once in a while. I am a woman, and women don't do most of the healing. They fear the pain, the pain of the medicine inside them because it really hurts! I don't really know why women don't do more of it. Men just fear it less. It's really funny – women don't fear childbirth, but they really fear medicine! (Young 1993, p.250)

Within this account are many of the strands that characterise writings about shamanic cultures: the communal basis of the training and the healing, the use of trance, sometimes associated with herbs of some kind and the connections with natural phenomena such as animals. There is also the reluctance to be a shaman and pain involved in the calling. The cultural context also offers a very different worldview from the major religions of the Western world.

There is an acknowledgement of another world, often entered through trance, which is different from ordinary consciousness. This is a given, not a matter for debate. In some cultures this other world is regarded as more real than that experienced with ordinary consciousness. The world of spirits has been termed a 'separate reality' (Castaneda 1971). For many of the cultures in which trance is used, spirits and their doings are in many ways part of daily life. It is not only in times of crisis that belief in spirits and their power is activated. People have regular dealings with them as they go about their daily business of growing crops or fishing. Because spirits are everywhere, it would be impossible to ignore them, and because of their amoral and capricious nature, it is difficult always to know how to avoid offending them. They thus provide an important reservoir of explanations for afflictions of various kinds, as well as a theory of care (Caplan 1997).

The dimensions and belief systems that make up that world differ from culture to culture and music is an important component part in within these systems:

> There is something paradoxical about music and possession... Music occurs as one of the component parts of those systems, and the role it plays varies with the models upon which those systems are structured. But, since music is itself a system, its relations with each model is equally determined by its own organisation, thus accounting for their protean character. How can we try to grasp such a constantly shifting reality? (Rouget 1985, p.31)

Shamanism cannot exist in a culture that disputes the existence of such an 'other' dimension, because it relies on this 'other' realm for its practices and procedures. This other is intimately connected with the natural world and inextricably connected with the process of human living:

> It is clear that possession cannot be understood unless it is set in the system of representations of the society concerned. These representations, in their turn, must then be brought into relation with the way in which they are experienced in daily life, outside any form of ceremony. The least one can say is that we are very ill informed about this last kind of experience. What we do know however, is that in societies having preserved an archaic way of life, which are precisely those in which possession cults are frequently found, the individual lives in constant sensorial contact with nature. He lives in perpetual intimacy with the elements, plants and animals. For him [sic], the frontier between the animate and inanimate worlds is extremely vague. Men [sic], beasts, plants, and things

all have souls or are receptacles of souls. Every phenomenon is interpreted as resulting from the action or presence of a soul. The visible is constantly animated by the invisible. (Rouget 1985, p.123)

This chapter is based on a number of different sources from ethnomusicologists and anthropologists, recorded both in aural and written form. Certain phenomena occur as part of the role of music in the healing and these need to be distinguished at the outset. First there is the nature of the trance experience. Rouget (1985) in his definitive text on *Music and Trance* emphasises that trance is made up of two components. One of these is psychophysiological, the other is cultural. The trance is different from that used for everyday routine and is often associated with music. There is an important distinction to be made in the way in which music and trance are related. In this context Rouget (1985) coins two very significant terms: the 'musicant' and 'musicated'. The musicant is the person who makes the music and the musicated is the one for whom the music is made. Trance can be 'conducted', in which case the person makes the music for him or herself; that is, he or she is the musicant. It can also be 'induced'. In this case, the subject is led by music made by others – he or she is musicated.

This has close links with another distinction that needs to be made – that between shamanism and possession – which many writers regard as crucial (Eliade 1951; Rouget 1985). The use of the term 'shaman' was taken in the seventeenth century from a people in Siberia and originally limited to that region. However, ethnological writings have gradually expanded its usage to include central, northern and south east Asia, Melanesia and the Americas. Spirit possession is found largely in Africa. The distinction is in the direction of the flow of the communication between the two worlds. In shamanism the soul of the shaman leaves the body to journey in the other world; in possession, the spirits, the dead or the gods leave the other world and visit the one possessed, the possessee. The shaman may be accompanied by his spirit guides or may transform himself into an animal in order to undertake the journey, but he or she is essentially in control of the process. In possession cults, the possessee is controlled by the spirit and the process is involuntary:

It could be expressed by a series of three oppositions: journey to the spirits/visit by the spirits; control over the spirits/submission to the spirits; voluntary trance/involuntary trance. This triple opposition could be further condensed into only one: acting/undergoing. Shamanism appeared to be, if one may say so, essentially *acted*, possession as *undergone.* (Rouget 1985, p.132)

The distinction can be refined by many shadings and nuances and possession states are found in many cultures including shamanic ones. Indeed, the onset of a shamanic vocation may be discerned in a disturbance caused by possession. From this start the shaman learns to master the spirits that tormented him or her and use them as auxiliaries to accompany him or her on their journey. Cultures identify some possession as helpful to their society, as noted among the Vodun people in the People's Republic of Benin; in others possession states are rejected and the possessee is seen as being in need of exorcism. This latter term is a very difficult one, for its use within the cultures that practise spirit possession has often been coloured by the proximity of a monotheistic religion which is politically more powerful. What is clear, however, is that music is used in possession ceremonies in cultures which welcome the intrusion of the divinity in the form of possession.

Exorcism does not use music. Schéhérazade Qassim Hassan in her work in Iraq distinguishes between 'non-musical ceremonies' that 'exorcise the spirits of Evil' and 'musical ceremonies' that 'invoke beneficent spirits.' (Hassan 1975).[1]

This chapter will concern itself with cultures that use both shamanism and possession in alliance with music in the process of healing. There will also be some discussion of the wider use of singing in these societies and its role in maintaining group and individual balance.

Community/individualism

In this section we will look at the relationship of the individual shaman or healer and the individual sick person with the surrounding community. It has already been acknowledged that the notion of community in these societies will include the natural world. It will also include the ancestors through an a-temporal view of time. We have seen in Chapter One how Levi-Strauss (1970) divided societies into 'hot' societies who favour the construct of historical time which underpins their development, like Western cultures, and 'cold' societies where the relationship between past and present is conceived as parallel and the view of time is more circular. The view of time in 'cold' societies enables the concept of a close relationship with the ancestors.

---

1   It is interesting to compare this with the philosophy of Hildegard of Bingen
     (1098–1179) (see Chapter Two) who saw music as a way of connecting with the
     Divine, and portrays the Devil in her morality play with music Ordo Virtutum as only
     speaking and therefore lacking a connection with the Divine.

What is central to practice in societies using possession or shamanism to heal is that it is in the context of a society with a shared belief system that supports the practice. Roger Bastide (1972) identifies the following characteristics of possession as a religious phenomenon in which such shared belief systems are vital:

1.   There is a certain relationship between a deity and certain believers, that may cause these believers to become possessed by the divinity.

2.   Possession is socialised behaviour characterised by a change of personality, when the unusual personality is replaced by that of the deity who now controls certain behaviours, the person being in a state of trance.

3.   This creates an alliance with the divinity, who can now be asked to use their power in favour of the possessed person or group (like protecting them from evil or curing an illness or revealing the future) or else to stop using their power against them. (Bastide 1972, p.84).

Although the shaman and the 'sick' person are central to the ritual, the event usually involves the whole community and can include social as well as healing elements. In this North American ceremony from the Yurok people recorded in the first half of the twentieth century there are 'light' songs and 'heavy' songs:

The Brush Dance brings people together in a ceremony to heal a sick child. The medicine woman makes medicine to uplift the spirit of the child so that it will live a good life. About thirty-five men and unmarried women dance in a counterclockwise circle, with the medicine women and the child sitting in the centre facing east. The dancing lasts from until dawn for two or three nights depending on the area.

The singers perform both heavy and light songs. The heavy songs, which must be sung first, are more religious (heavy with prayer) than the light songs. The heavy, slower songs bring in the spirit, after which the medicine woman prays and all the people focus their attention on her and the child. If everyone is there for the right reasons and has the right thoughts, it brings good to the child.

The light songs inspire the dancers to move more vigorously... Shouting precedes and accompanies this strenuous activity of the men...

Although the Brush Dance is a curing ceremony, it has some social aspects. The words in Yurok songs frequently deal with nonmedicinal and nonreligious themes. Songs are still being composed today and sometimes have very modern themes...

The music of the Brush Dance features a complex leader–chorus relationship. In each song the leader begins the strophe, followed by the chorus singing a softer ostinato pattern. Toward the middle of each strophe the volume of the chorus increases, almost overpowering the leader... The only instrumental accompaniment is the rhythmic sound of the shells sewn on the girls' dance dresses... The Brush dance is performed nowadays primarily on social occasions. The joking and encouragement heard in this performance is indicative of the social interaction of the group (Figueroa 1977).

Contemporary native American healers use songs and drumming as part of their healing prayers in the sweatlodge (see p.59). Spirit possession may be seen as maintaining the unity of a community and correcting imbalances:

Spirit possession and similar states seem more closely related with social situations which regularly, though not necessarily, give rise to conflict, competition, tension, rivalry or jealousy between members of the *same* sex... Thus, although possession, and the forms of illness with which it is associated, may be psychological in nature, the important aspect for the anthropological viewpoint is that it is also a social phenomenon (i.e. it is public, sanctioned and ritualised) and this helps to confirm that we should look for tensions arising out of the relationship of socio-structural positions or statuses. (Wilson 1967, pp.366–367)

To support this view, Wilson refers to the likely possibility that a married woman whose husband is about to take a new wife will become possessed: 'I suggest that a woman whose marital status and prestige is threatened by the public action of her husband in taking a new wife is able, through possession, to re-affirm that status and prestige in public – especially her standing with respect to the new wife'. (Wilson 1967, p.371). These issues will be revisited under expression/confidentiality below (see pp.135–139).

Spirit possession ceremonies fulfil a range of important social functions: 'Spirit possession is obviously a multi-faceted phenomenon which plays a major role in individual therapy and healing, which provides entertainment...and even employment' (Wilson 1967, p.376). In its entertainment aspect it has been likened to the cathartic effect of drama (Beattie and Middleton 1969). Others have likened it to psychodrama (Lewis 1966). The rituals certainly provide a great deal of spectacle for their audiences. Kirby (1975) sees shamanic rituals (in which he includes spirit possession) as 'the antecedent of established theatre forms'. He makes an important distinction, as follows:

> shamanic performance may be considered the ur-theatre or prototheatre implies a very important distinction. Shamanistic ritual is unlike rites-of-passage or other forms of what may be called ceremonial ritual in that it depends upon the immediate and direct manifestation to the audience of supernatural presence, rather than its symbolisation. All ritual and ceremony can be theatrical, but the theatricality of shamanistic ritual is related to its function in a particular way. In order to effect a cure of a patient, belief in what is happening must be held, reinforced and intensified, not only in the patient, but in the audience as well, for their experience contributes directly to the effect. The audience actively reinforces the experience of the patient, and its own belief in a particular worldview or cosmology is in turn reinforced by direct experience of it. Shamanistic theatre, founded upon manifestation of supernatural presence, develops from a small curing séance which in effect needs only patient and shaman as participants, but actually depends upon the audience. (p.2)

He goes on to describe, using examples from the work of anthropologists, the staging and the 'magic illusionism' which he links with Western conjuring tricks: 'Dialogue, enactments, ventriloquism, incantations, music, dance, and song create a swirling stream of images drawn from a number of performance modes. The effect is literally hypnotic and hallucinatory' (p.5).

The active role of the audience in the ceremony is often stressed. The shaman and possessee can work together, surrounded by a group clapping or playing. Joseph Moore (1979) in his work 'Religious worship in Jamaica' looks particularly at the Cumina (sometimes referred to as African Dance) and revival cults ('a syncretistic group drawing on characteristics from western Christian and African beliefs and practices' – Moore 1979, p.293). Both of these traditions involve music and dance in rituals that involve possession by the ancestral zombie spirits (in Cumina) and saints and ancestral spirits (in revival cults). Moore comments on the training (especially physical) of the musicians and dancers and the careful planning in the engaging of the musicians, the food preparations, the invitations, the costumes. He draws attention to the fact that the ritual is both an individual and community expression:

The audience is both observer and participant... Participation...helps to make life tolerable and brings its followers a sense of security... To an observer, an art form brings stimulation and, perhaps, a deepening insight, but to a participant it is a vehicle for self-expression and a release of inner tensions. This psychic outpouring restores vitality and refreshes the whole person... The completed event had a psychological effect on all present and there was a prevailing sense of deep satisfaction. (p.308)

This is a view shared by Nketia (1957) in his work based on spirit possession rituals in the Gold Coast. He describes possession dances as a 'religious dance drama purposely organised for impersonating the gods' (p.4). He sees the drama as existing not only as something done because of the requirements of the belief system but also as having aesthetic merits for the communities in which it is staged. He distinguishes between the feelings of the believers who receive 'an assurance of fellowship and the protection of the gods' and the general company who go home 'with thoughts of a day well spent' (p.7).

Lorna Marshall (1969), writing about the !Kung bushmen's 'Medicine dance' of the Kalahari in South Africa, concludes: 'In their singing, clapping their hands, and dancing, the people are united, people unite and dance together whatever the state of their feelings. [Even if they are abusive in the course of the dance]...the next moment, the people become a unit, singing, clapping, moving together' (p.380). Feng (1973) in a study of songs of the Dinka tribe talks about song as a way of solving disputes:

'Fighting with songs', as one might put it, is, however, institutionalised, and goes beyond therapeutic singing. Apart from war songs which are presented in dancing, with mimed battle, there are age-set and insult songs. Young men competing over girls fight with songs sung to others but not face to face... The very idea of songs implies non-violent competition... The idea of pacification also applies to sub-age-sets and even to the warring territorial units, which compete in war songs... War songs are more dramatic because they are presented in public dances in which the opposing groups may take part. (p.79)

There are many societies where music plays an important part of rituals designed to resolve disputes, to heal the community. This can be linked with conservatism on the part of the elders who use the rituals as a way of containing rebellion (Floyd 1998). The notion of the reinforcement of a community and its values is one that enables traditional healing rituals to exist alongside Western allopathic medicine. People will return to traditional healers when they feel their links with their own community are weakened. They will use it as a type of cultural healing.

However, in the training of a shaman, in particular, the concept of the individual journey is marked with characteristics similar to that of the heroic journey. As seen in the opening account in this chapter, there is the powerful notion of a call. Mercia Eliade (1989) describes practice among the Yakut of Siberia: 'One destined for shamanship begins by becoming frenzied, then suddenly loses consciousness, withdraws to the forests, feeds on tree bark, flings himself into the water and fire, wounds himself with knives' (p.16). This is a call from conventional limits characterised by an 'illness' of some kind. After this he or she undertakes a period of training with a teacher, including techniques such as fasting and meditation and learning the myths around the art including those of solitude and wilderness. The training often involves a lonely journey into the other realm; but this is always guided (as seen in Nisa's story at the opening of this chapter) by members of the community who understand the herbs used and the experiences. It is usually regarded as very dangerous to undertake such experiences alone and unsupported. The last stage is characterised by some sense of death and rebirth, when the 'old' self is left behind and the shaman realises his or her healing energy.

Summary – community/individualism

The societies in which healing through shamanism and spirit possession occur have a strong sense of the importance of community and have a number of systems including music for maintaining it. Healing ceremonies will take place in the context of communal gatherings and will be conceived of in relation to the natural world and the world of spirits and other spiritual beings including the ancestors. There will often be social elements in them. A shared belief system is an essential part of the healing process. The rituals are also ways of resolving disputes and including people who might feel marginalised. However, within the journey of the individual healer there is a sense of a heroic quest that ends in finding his or her healing power.

Containment/freedom

The cultures dealt with in this chapter have not developed a written musical notation. The notion of containment is seen more in the traditions and training of potential healers. Because of the tightly knit nature of the societies in which shamanism is practised there is a great stress on the traditions and the practice of the elders. These are handed on from one generation to another, as seen in the opening story of this chapter. The societies are aware of the power of the ceremonies, so the tradition is contained by the society.

The experienced priests, shamans or mediums are used for the public ceremonies. Nketia (1957) in his work in the Gold Coast describes how the underlying belief is that the gods can posses anyone, but how, at public worship, there are official representatives or media of the gods:

> These media are people who have been previously possessed by the particular gods being worshipped and who have chosen to remain in this type of ritual connection with them.
>
> In Akan society the duty of impersonating a particular god falls on the priest, who may be assisted by a few priestesses attached to the particular shrine. The Akan priest goes through a long period of apprenticeship during which he learns the secrets of the profession, masters the music and dancing of the particular cult and the dramatic art of possession. A priest is expected to be a good artist and a convincing representative of his god during public performances. In Ga society, the office of medium and that of priest are separated for effectiveness of action. The media of the gods are mostly women, who also undergo special training in the dramatic art of possession as well as in the forms and symbolism of the cult dances. (pp.5–6)

Although the notion of self-expression is very different from that of Western cultures (see pp. 88–95) there is a notion that the sickness of the patient is 'contained' by the music of the ritual. In a BBC radio programme (1992), Janet Topp-Fargion talks about the role of trance in African societies and gives an example from South Africa of the curing of a pregnant woman. The repeated patterns being played by the community behind this can be seen as a container in which the pregnant woman is able to shake off her illness. The training of the initiates or shamans often involves the learning of the musical motifs associated with a particular spirit – this can be regarded as the 'holding form' of the spirit.

However, the notion of another world entered by trance gives the possibility of an escape from everyday consciousness. The shamanic 'flight' has elements of freedom about it. The calling of the traditional shaman (see above, p.130), Black Elk (a Sioux who was part of the Wounded Knee massacre in 1890) has the quality of a vision of another place beyond the ordinary:

For Black Elk the call to shamanism came early in life. When he was five he had a spontaneous shamanic experience and as he said himself: 'This was not a dream, it happened.' As he looked up at the sky, two human figures seemed to descend from the clouds: They sang a sacred song and the thunder was like drumming ... The song and the drumming went like this:

'Behold, a sacred voice is calling you;
All over the sky a sacred voice is calling.'

'I sat there gazing at them,' Black Elk told Neihardt, 'and they were coming from the place where the giant lives [north]. But when they were very close to me, they wheeled about toward where the sun goes down, and suddenly they were geese. Then they were gone, and the rain came, with a big wind and a roaring. I did not tell this vision to anyone. I liked to think about it, but I was afraid to tell it.' (Drury 1989, p.64)

The series of flights that Black Elk now embarks on has similar visionary qualities. He moves through the heavens, where he sees dramatic scenes of violence and renewal. He passes through four 'ascents', which he interprets as representing the future of the American Indians of the planet. The first and most beautiful ascent included a holy tree (the characteristic world tree of the shaman) surrounded by a green and fertile land. The other ascents portrayed incipient disaster. In the second he saw people transformed into animals of the hunt growing more afraid. The leaves of the holy tree started to fall. In the third ascent the animals went berserk and the winds and wild beasts of the universe were fighting. The holy tree appeared to be dying. In the fourth ascent the animals were transformed again into starving. The holy tree had completely disappeared. The world was filled with lamentation. In these visions he was given a song of power while riding a stallion:

'I sang it there in the midst of the terrible place ...

A good nation I will make live.
This the nation above has said.
They have given me the power to make over...

The virgins danced, and all the circled horses. The leaves on the trees, the grass on the hills and in the valleys, the waters in the creek and in the rivers and the lakes, the four-legged and two-legged and the wings of the air – all danced together to the music of the stallion's song.

And when I looked down upon my people yonder, the cloud passed over, blessing them with friendly rain, and stood in the east with a flaming rainbow over it.' (Drury 1989, p.67)

What is interesting in this account is how this visionary experience is allied for Black Elk with concepts of freeing his own people from their problems.

The healer regularly goes into the other world in order to find a healing song. This is often given in dreams, as in this example from the Temiars who live in the Malaysian rainforest, which was recorded in 1982. Here the healer works on the patient while a woman provides the percussive accompaniment with a pair of bamboo stampers beaten against a log drum:

> When a medium sings the song he or she has received in a dream, the medium becomes imbued with the long-range vision and knowledge of the spirit who gave the song. Thus empowered the medium becomes a healer. For Temiars illnesses come from the animated spirits of the land-scape; to counteract these illness agents, they call upon those animated spirits with whom they have entered into benevolent relationships, as spiritguides. When a medium sings, his voice and vision are those of a spiritguide who can see and extract illness agents from a patient's body.
>
> In this healing ceremony two mediums work as a team. While chorus and other community members converse on the sidelines; the first medium (nicknamed... 'Old Man Bitterness' for his biting humour) blows through his fist onto the patient's body, then intones a chant taught to him by his spirit guides, ordering the illness agent to depart. He yelps to frighten the illness into running away. Blowing, sucking, working over the patient's body, he draws the illness out, then claps his hands to send it back out beyond the community. A chorus member complains, 'O you sent it in my direction!' Another onlooker replies, 'No, he released it up into the ceremonial leaf ornaments hanging from the rafters!'
>
> For Temiars, the head-soul travels with the voice; thus, during healings, the curative head-soul of a spiritguide flows through the medium's vocalisations into the patient. (Smithsonian Folkways 1982)

In this account we see the range of sounds used by the healers. These include 'yelping, breathing, blowing and sucking'. The range of sounds used includes a wider or different range than that validated by Western society. The songs, in general, are monophonic. If there is an accompaniment it is often provided by percussion instruments of some kind, although simple bowed string instruments are found in some traditions such as the Boori cult in West Africa. The structure of the songs will use the traditions of the surrounding culture.

This means that they are often traditional pentatonic or heptatonic scales. The traditional native American songs often start high and end low signifying the descent to earth.

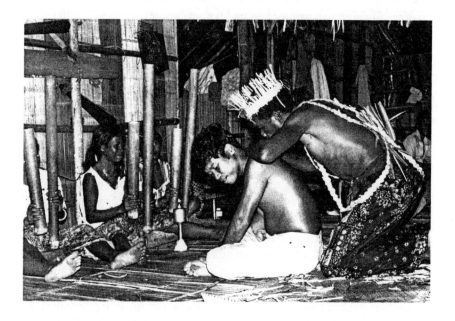

Figure 3.1 Malaysian healing treatment. Reproduced courtesy of the Ralph Rinzler Folklife Archives and Collections Centre for Folklife and Cultural Heritage, Smithsonian Institute.

Many of the traditions will be allied to movement of some kind. Sue Jennings' (1985) work with the Temiars highlights the disordered movements of the dance which contrasts with their ideal of an ordered society. She describes the trance dances, 'which appear to be a response to a level of tension in the village' (p.3). The singing shaman controls the sessions. The cosmology of the Temiars sees them as living in a hostile universe with a powerful tension between violence and non-violence. Jennings says it is possible to see trance dance as a mechanism for releasing the 'head-soul' to cathartic effect, but she concludes:

> In this way, Temiar society, which cultivates belief in tiger and thunder, also provides the mechanism by which fears of cosmic threat are assuaged. If one is led to accept a theory of 'tension release' as the most

logical explanation of Temiar dance, then this should be coupled with an understanding that this operates at the level of the group rather than the individual, and serves at the same time to reinforce those beliefs which together form the Temiar cosmos. (p.10)

Summary – containment/freedom

These traditions believe in the power of music to 'contain' the illness in some way. The rituals are controlled by tradition and practice. Within the call and training of healers there is an important place for the freedom of the experiences in other worlds. These can empower the healer to work in the everyday world. In healing rituals there is a role for the community in providing a secure supportive environment – a 'container' in which the healer can work.

Expression/confidentiality

The notion of what is being expressed here is different from Western culture. The sounds are conceived of as coming from the wider universe, not from the personality of the healer. One profound difference here is that usually patients do not make their own music. This is clear in the account above from the Temiars, where the patient is passive while the shaman works musically, constructing the music for the patient. The concept of patients making up their own song to 'express' their problem is not found. In general, it is the healer who finds the right song for the patient and this is often done apart from the patient in dreams or trance states. If the sickness is deemed at all to have come from the person's 'experience', it is not regarded as necessary that this is expressed in words. Although the body may express it in dance or in movement of some kind, the essence of the healing does not lie here; there is a sense in which the sickness 'is not that person' and needs to be taken away. The way this is done is not by it 'being expressed' but by it being counteracted by a song or drumming pattern that will withdraw the sickness. In this way the business of confidentiality is not so much of a problem. The 'events' that may have caused the sickness are never expressed in any form, so confidentiality is maintained and the healing can be carried out in a communal context without such issues arising.

The notion of the Western self is often alien to the world concepts that characterise the shamanic culture. There is a greater sense of interconnectedness between selves or souls, which makes the Western notion of 'self-expression' more like 'soul expression'. The healing sounds are magical sounds designed to produce a consciousness of a wider cosmos. Various techniques were developed for this:

> The shamans of Mongolia listened very carefully to the sound of the singing bow. As they bowed or plucked it, they listened particularly – more so than any other ancient culture – to the melody of the single note: the harmonics, the tone colour melody. Thus the Mongolian was from the earliest times in a position to appreciate the secret of music, the physical basis of sound-production, and learnt to realise vocally this original, archaic phenomenon of the 'monotone'. A whole singing technique was developed for it – xoömij, which means pharynx or throat.
>
> With this technique the individual Mongolian is able to sing in two voices at once. He hums or sings nasally a note of medium pitch and alters the volume of his mouth cavity by opening and closing his mouth, thus varying the harmonic spectrum of this single, long-drawn-out note. (Hamel 1978, p.80)

Hamel goes on to link other 'unnatural' sounds with this notion of the evocation of the mystical (see Chapter Four). He refers to the call of muezzin in Islam with its use of the high falsetto voice and Sufi chanting of the Scriptures where in ecstatic moments 'the singer brings off a kind of hiccup or very rapid yodel which, as with an overblown flute, switches the voice to a higher harmonic pitch' (p.81). He summarises his findings as follows: 'It is above all the Gnostic schools and sects with their shamanistic cult elements who have undertaken the journey into the collective unconscious via the world of sound' (p.81).

If we take the Western sociological view of spirit possession given above, the notion of expression of one's own experience through the medium of being possessed by a spirit does make it a form of expression (albeit vicarious). It becomes much closer to Western ideas of the role of mental illness in a patient's life circumstances and the part music might play in expressing this (see Chapter Five). Wilson's (1967) position, that it is a way for women to express their low status and acquire individual therapy and healing in the context of the group, opens up possibilities for the use of music more publicly. By being possessed by a spirit (a non-self), feelings of low status can safely be expressed, particularly in societies where such expression is ritualised. It becomes another expression of the link between individual 'illness' and cultural injustice (see Chapter One). Indeed, the link here is clearer than in the concepts of psychiatric illness in the West, particularly with regard to attitudes to women.

Lewis (1966) makes this point very powerfully when he sets out to chart an 'epidemiology of possession' (p.308). He points out how much literature has concentrated on the 'expressive' aspects of spirit possession, the drama, music and bizarre and exotic exercises, but that little attention has been given to the 'social roles and statuses of the chronically possessed – whether these are identified as mediums, shamans, or prophets...[Such research] views the prominent role of women in spirit possession as a compensation for their exclusion and lack of authority in other spheres' (Lewis 1966, p.310).

He draws clear examples of this from Somali society, dominated by a very 'male dominated and highly puritanical' Islamic culture. He shows how spirit possession is associated with jilted women, deprived and frustrated young herdsmen, women struggling to bring up a family with little support or attention from their husband and men who are over-stressed. He emphasises the common themes of 'deprivation and confinement' in these instances.[2]

Levi-Strauss (1960) wrestles with this dilemma of whether the phenomenon is a psychopathological one or a sociological one when he writes:

> The contradiction that I have spelled out can be resolved in two ways. Either the forms of behaviour described by the terms 'trance' and 'possession' have nothing to do with those that we, in our society, call psychopathological; or one may regard them as being of the same type, in which case it is the connection with pathological states that must be regarded as contingent, and as resulting from a condition particular to the society in which we live. In the latter case we would be faced by a further choice of alternatives: either so-called mental illnesses, in reality outside the realm of medicine, must be regarded as sociological events affecting the behaviour of individuals who have been dissociated from the group in a particular way by their personal histories and constitutions, or we must recognise in these sick people the presence of a state that is truly pathological but of physiological origin, a state that tends to create a terrain favourable, or, if you wish, 'sensitising', to certain symbolic forms of behaviour that still fall solely within the realm of sociological interpretation. (Levi-Strauss, quoted in Rouget 1985, p.16)

Lewis (1966) also makes a link with psychoanalysis, including parallels between the shaman and the analyst. These are similar to those made in Chapter Two between the role of the composer and the shaman. Lewis

2   It is very interesting to compare this with Western figures such as Hildegard of Bingen who found authority and freedom in the mystical experience through music and have linked this with work with justice issues in the wider society.

acknowledges the interest in these phenomena in the closing years of the nineteenth century. He adds, however:

> Although...spirit possession in its traditional guise is, with other marginal mystical practices, by no means defunct today... [The decline in interest in it] seems to coincide fairly closely with rise of modern psychology and psychoanalysis... And no one, I fancy, will question that many of the symptoms associated with spiritualism in our own past as well as in traditional societies are today treated on the psychologist's couch... For at least in psychoanalysis, not only is the mode of entry to the profession similar to that of the shaman's spiritual travail and apprenticeship, but the treatment situation of the patent is implicitly and increasingly explicitly psychodramatic in its essential characteristics... I am not of course arguing that all psychological illnesses can be regarded as responses to deprivation, nor am I proposing that the whole of psychotherapy is a deprivation cult. The parallel seems to me best restricted to the incidence and treatment of the neurotic disorders and particularly to psychosomatic and hysterical afflictions. (p.325)

It could be added that psychiatric practice still struggles to make sense of such experiences because of the absence of a transcendent dimension in its constructs (see Chapter Five).

So spirit possession can be seen as allowing for a form of expression of elements that might otherwise not be socially acceptable. It provides for a community of carers around a patient (Janzen 1987) and it encourages the alleviation of stress (Obeyesekere 1970). It enables people to play with their identity (Bourgignon 1965), including their sexual identity (Crapanzo 1977).

Shamanic ceremonies are also part of other rituals associated with rites of passage. Here they express the feelings of the community as well as performing the ceremonial necessary to enable the rite of passage to be successfully accomplished. Death rituals, for example, involve both the expression of grief as well as dealing with the passage of the soul. The Ssikkimgut on the Korean island of Chindo shows how these elements are joined together. It is an all-night ceremony and the music is used to invoke the spirits as well as to bid them farewell, for which gongs are also used. Other music used includes local funeral songs sung by the group while the shaman performs the necessary ritual actions. The chief summoning instrument is a six-holed pipe. The songs are of three tones and involve the shaman assembling a set of stock musical motifs, part improvisatory, part responsive and part fixed (Lewis 1985).

Summary – expression/confidentiality

The notion of expression in these cultures is very different from that of the 'self' as constructed in Western culture. The music is made 'on behalf of' the patient, not 'by' the patient him or herself. It is related to other beings in the wider cosmos. This enables the ceremonies to be performed publicly and for the community to have a role. The function may be seen as enabling the suffering of marginalised persons to be legitimised and socialised. Rituals associated with rites of passage include the expression of community feeling like grief alongside more functional elements.

Unity/diversity

Within the frames of reference of healing involving shamanic and spirit possession there is a sense of diversity within the self. The shaman can take on the persona, for example, of power animals, while in the concept of spirit possession the person is inhabited by a spirit which is other than their everyday self. These enable diversity to be encompassed within a frame of 'normality' within that society. This is a central question in looking at other cultures, at people with symptoms that we would regard as pathological: how far is trance regarded as a pathological condition and in need of 'changing' and how far is it 'normal' within the culture? The notion of the co-existence of difference in the self is interestingly 'solved' by the notion of the possessing spirit who is 'not' the possessee and has a separate identity. Erlmann (1982) in his work with Hausa Trance and Music in Nigeria identifies how each spirit has a praise-song of its own and that its 'adepts' (people chosen to represent that spirit) must learn these small melodic and rhythmic fragments.[3]

> Trance may be seen as a technique through which the adept, in a voluntary, self-controlled, learned change of self-consciousness, introjects the persecution by a spirit and assumes his new role as worshipped spirit. Music, however, simply serves as a praise song in that it says to the adept who he should be and whom he should identify with. (Erlmann 1982, p.56)

---

3   It is interesting to compare these, for example, with small motifs used by Beethoven for composition. I have suggested in Chapter Two that these might represent 'subpersonalities' of psychosynthesis, which need to be integrated into some form of whole.

The training of a shaman involves his or her own ability to enter other worlds safely and there are parallels with the training of a psychoanalyst who has to enter his or her own Underworld in order to help others. The notion of death and rebirth is essential to it. Traditional shamans regarded this as an actual death with images of skin being stripped from bones and their own dismemberment as illustrated in this account of the initiation of an Australian medicine man, a karadji:

> The candidate goes to the mouth of a particular cave where he is 'noticed' by the spirits of the dreamtime. They throw an invisible lance at him which pierces his neck and tongue, and another which passes through his head from ear to ear. Dropping down 'dead', he is now carried by the spirits into the cave and his organs replaced with new ones... When he rejoins his people as a person 'reborn', he has a new status as a healer-shaman, although he will not normally perform as a karadji for a year or so. (Elkin 1977, p.66)

Such crises can be sudden and short or prolonged and may precipitate the entry into an apprenticeship or come at the end of the training. After them, the self is regarded as completely new, transformed. Grof with Bennett (1993) call it, in psychological terms, an 'ego death' which they describe as 'an experience of annihilation on all levels – physical, emotional, intellectual and spiritual' (p.74). Halifax (1979) adds: 'The shaman not only survives the ordeal...but also is healed in the process...and as a healed healer, only he or she can truly know the territory of disease and death' (pp.10–11).

To enter the chaos and be able to find a route through it is an essential part of the training. The initial crisis often occurs outside the ritual context and seldom involves music. The use of songs has an important part to play in finding this safe passage through this other world, for his or her later voluntary trances are seen to re-enact this crisis. The music is now a way of inducing onset of the trance, controlling its form, so that what was at first an unregulated phenomenon can now be turned to a useful purpose.

The anthropologist Arnold van Gennep saw parallel stages in any ritual. This he entitled 'severance, transition and return' (1908, quoted in Roose-Evans 1994, p.6). Severance he associated with leaving everyday life by means of ritual gestures like holding hands or lighting candles. In the transitional or liminal phase contact was made with the transpersonal; and this might take the form of a change of consciousness. The return phase signalled a coming back to earth and the beginning of a new life. Such phases can also be seen in Western rituals. What happens here is that a community is now taken on a similar journey to that of the individual one of the shaman. This is an area explored in Chapter Two with the notion of the public concert being a ritual act, with the composer acting as shaman.

There is in many spirit possession traditions the notion that at the end of the ceremony the adepts have to brush the spirits off. This is very different from the exorcism addressed at the beginning of this chapter. The spirits have been seen as helpful to the healing process, but the process of getting rid of them may prove difficult. A young Moroccan musician writes of an application of the concept in the context of Western culture: 'I believe in the liberating value of trance through music, as a means of exorcising not the spirits of evil, but, symbolically, the spirits of the twentieth century' (quoted in Rouget 1985, p.166). It is interesting to compare this with the Western performer 'winding down' at the end of a performance, losing the persona of the composer he or she has been playing and resuming his or her everyday persona.

The notion of transformation by such controlled interaction with the 'other' world is central to many practices. Gerhard Kadir Tucek's (1994) account of Oriental medicine makes an important distinction between Eastern and Western practice. Setting out a system that involves body movement and singing in combination he says: 'We want to remind you of the typical oriental idea of changing emotions by special impulses [here, music and gesture], rather than "Katharsis" [meaning exaggerating]' (p.31).

Tucek's work (1994) describes how the shamanic practices of the local Bakse were merged with Christian, Buddhist and Islamic elements in Central Asia. In this literature the idea of integrating body, mind and spirit appears, as in the following ninth/tenth century description of the power of music to strengthen:

> The body is sick when the soul is weakened and the body loses power when the soul is affected. This is why physical healing happens through spiritual healing, by re-establishing its powers and bringing its substance into the right order, by means of sounds that can do so and fit the purpose. (quoted in Tucek 1994, p.13)

The constructs of spirit possession cults are different from those of the shamanic cults in the area of transformation. In Wilson's (1967) thesis set out above (see p.127), spirit possession is a way of acknowledging a person's identity in a formal communal context. This change of self, therefore, becomes part of a new identity in society. The effect of the ritual is both personal and social. Through it the society can contain the diversity:

I wish to argue that sociologically the act and subsequent rites of spirit possession are a form of *rite de passage* whereby social identity is changed and social status defined. In societies where spirit possession is not professionally employed, spirit possession is confined to re-affirming marital and situational status or re-defines it. In societies where possession is institutionalised, where individuals are 'professionally' seized, the achievement of specific, formal social status – shaman or priest – is quite clear. (Wilson 1967, p.374)

Feng (1973) sees this as a function of Dinka songs, similarly linking the personal with the social:

In the interest not only of social harmony, but also of each person's inner harmony, songs are used as a means of turning experiences which are painful or otherwise undesirable into a subject of art which enhances one's inner pride and recognition by society. The indignities of prison life, traditionally unknown in Dinka society, the result of rejection by a girl, or of divorce imposed on a loving partner, and the misery of 'orphanage' (a condition which continues into adult life in the Dinka view) or of being without dependable relatives or friends are examples of themes which it is better to sing about than brood over.

Songs do more than to achieve honour and dignity for the singers. The use of the word dheeng for singing and dancing indicates that these sensuous skills, both in their words of exaltation and in singing and dancing, are seen as essentially arts of grandeur in which a person does not have to excel to be exalted. In addition, they are established means towards winning recognition and enhancing one's social position. (pp.79–80)

The musical structures used in the rituals vary from one geographical location to another. The pieces often involve a great deal of repetition – both melodic and rhythmic. Judith Vander (1986), working on the songs of the Shoshone Indians, sees them as characterised by inexact repetition, which is in contrast to other analyses of similar songs. She writes of the musical structure of the songs:

Repetition is the most important characteristic of Emily's Naraya songs. Not only is there repetition of the phrases or progressions within the song, but the song itself repeats several times... Repetition gives symmetry to these songs. At the same time, because the repetition is often 'inexact, imperfect' casting up slightly variant forms of itself – it is dynamic and lively. (p.17)

What is interesting in this account is how the minute variants are perceived by the ethnomusicologist as giving its dynamic quality. It is interesting to compare this with the ideas of Leonard Meyer, discussed in Chapter Two, where the interest of the audience is held by 'surprise' within the music. Witherspoon (1977) coins the term 'dynamic symmetry' which he relates to Navajo art which fuses the ideas of symmetry/asymmetry into a dynamic whole:

> Just as perfect symmetry in art is basically static, perfect equality and balance between two parts of a pair also produces a static result... Dynamic symmetry is based on ideas of similar and complementary but inexact, imperfect, and unequal pairing or balancing... Dynamic symmetry is more characteristic of the dynamic flow and flux found in nature and in the proportions of the human body and in the growing plant. (pp.197–200)

Frances Densmore (1943), working with the indigenous Americans, describes the irregularity of accent in the songs, which takes the form of interruptions to the rhythm. She describes this as necessary to impress the rhythm on the mind of the patient. The songs which are given to the healers in dreams are sung many times and often have a distinctive beginning and ending section. The songs will have been given to the doctor in a dream.

In the Voodoo traditions of Trinidad each of the gods – of wind, water, fire and war – have their own drum signal. These are very similar: 'The differences consist of minute rhythmic hesitations, short gaps and pauses between the beats and the minutest gradations of volume. These acoustic signs are detected not by the head – i.e. the intellect – but the belly, or rather in the human centre of consciousness' (Hamel 1978, p.77). So the musical forms reflect notions of unity and diversity formed out of minute variations in repetitive patterns.

Summary – unity/diversity

The notions underpinning shamanic and spirit possession cults have a way of explaining diversity within the self by reference to another world which interacts with the everyday world. This world is explored safely by musical means. The training of shamans involves the concept of a difficult journey into dangerous areas, which is where the healing songs are to be found. The rituals are a communal entering into similar territory guided by the experienced healers. Insofar as they result in a personal transformation on the part of the patient they represent a change on the part of an individual; insofar as that person through this process finds acceptance within the group the group is also encouraged to include a greater degree of diversity.

Challenge/nurture

The notion of challenging the evil is part of the notion of healing but there is also a strong sense of nurture for the patient. The challenge is, in general, undertaken by someone who is 'well' on behalf of the patient, who is in a role of being nurtured. This combination leads to a strong sense of empowerment. Within these cultures the power of music to challenge disease is undisputed. Often this is allied to dance as in this account by a Wind River Shoshone woman, Emily Hill:

> It's something like somebody knows something: measles or fever or some kind of disease coming. Flu or measles or scarlet fever... One person knows when he's asleep. He knows that it's coming. It's coming like a ball of those bees. He can see them at nights asleep. That bad stuff's coming to us. We better be dancing...sending it back... That's the way they dance it. It isn't just a dance... It's the same way with Sun Dance. The leader that's going to give the Sun Dance. He's going to dream that he's giving that dance, so everybody can live out the winter good. The children should grow up good. That's the way they dream things like that. (Emily Hill, quoted in Vander 1986, p.8)

This shows a clear sense of how cause and effect operates within this world. Emily, who was born in 1911, was a medicine woman using plants, songs, dances, prayers, touching and blood-letting in her healing practices. Judith Vander collected 17 songs from her between 1979 and 1982 connected with the Naraya (a Ghost Dance tradition). She sees the tradition as rooted in the 'cruel times' (1885–1905) – a time of privation, sickness and traumatic change. The renewal of the Sun Dance, combining old beliefs and Christian symbolism, she sees as a way of challenging the sicknesses of that time. It is a social and political challenge achieved through the revival of rituals involving music and dance. Many of the songs were concerned with water related to the dry sage country which is their territory. This is reflected in the structure of the songs, full of words for various states of water – running water, snow and fog. One song repeats the word for fog over and over again, stretching out over a long temporal space in the music. This reflects the stretching of the fog across the landscape and serves to concentrate the power of the song in the notion of the water:

Although Shoshones no longer perform the Naraya it is important to note that the religious matrix from which it sprang remains vital. Beliefs concerning water, power, health and nature which shaped the Naraya in the past still influence and inform religious ceremonies and personal lives today. For example, water, a prominent image and concern in Naraya belief, also plays a prominent role in the Sun Dance... Abstinence from water is central to the dancer's ordeal and acquisition of power. When power comes, it is often experienced in a vision involving water. The outer forms may come and go but not the currents of traditional Shoshone belief, a nourishing source which continues to run below the surface. (Vander 1986, p.69)

Animals are often seen as a source of strength for the shaman. These power animals can appear in the form of bears, wolves, stags and all kinds of birds (Eliade 1989). It can also be a natural phenomenon like the wind or 'a great water' or a mountain shaken with a 'mysterious power'. Densmore (1943) describes an affirmative Chippewa Midewiwin song said to have been given by a power animal: 'You will recover, you will walk again. It is I who say it. My power is great. Through our white shell... I will enable you to walk again' (p.3).

Various views about the source of the power of trance traditions have been expressed. Some anthropologists taking a more phenomenological position (Boddy 1990, 1994) suggest that the power lies in the cultural knowledge that provides a schema explaining human relationship to the world. The *causative* element in them makes them satisfying and comforting as well as making the cure more efficacious and helping to prevent disease (Janzen 1982; Turner 1968). The reinforcement of a belief system within which the sickness 'makes sense' has a nurturing or 'holding' feel to it; the fact that the 'holding' function of the repeated rhythms is often held by the audience as well as the musicians is also clear. There is much debate about whether the power of the music is purely symbolic, or psychic, imaginary or real, somatic or effective (Rouget 1985). The 'holding' function is very clear in the stress laid on support in the ceremonies. This is often done by the community holding a repeated rhythm while the shaman works.

Summary – challenge/nurture

These functions of challenging and nurturing are tightly interwoven in the literature to produce a sense of power. The power of the shaman or healer challenges the sickness. Through this act the patient is empowered. The community often has the function of holding the patient musically during the rituals.

Excitement/relaxation

The role of music in the creation of altered states of consciousness is much discussed. One of the main distinctions between the shamanic and the spirit possession cults is who makes the music. The possessee in the spirit possession cult seldom plays an active role in the music. As he or she moves from initiation to the role of officiant, his or her role becomes more active. In contrast the shaman generates his or her own music (that is, is a musicant) from the very beginning of training. The shaman enters the trance state by singing or drumming him or herself but the possessee is often responding to the music of others. The shaman's music may be taken over by an assistant later in the ceremony.

The role of the drum in the trance state is much debated and many experiments have been performed (often on Westerners outside of these cultures). These are dealt with in some detail by Sheila Walker (1972) in her chapter on 'The neurophysiology of possession'. Although Rouget (1985) rejects the idea of neurophysiological effects of music he does see an accelerando in tempo as a possible universal technique for generating trance. Erlmann (1982) qualifies this by saying that although this may be true of individual tunes, in ceremonies lasting two or more hours there are variations in tempo, especially in the third part when musicians do not want to overstress the dancers' ability. The adepts are covered in blankets during the induction of the trance and there is a slowing down of the tempo when the spirit appears. Erlmann (1982) sums up the usual conclusions of this debate:

> The technique [trance] itself may work on a physiological basis as far as drugs are concerned, and one cannot deny that 'auditory driving' [by repeated drum rhythms often getting gradually faster] and other factors, such as hyperventilation, may support it, once trance starts. However, trance is not generated physiologically by music. (p.56)

He draws attention to the fact that trance may occur without music and to involuntary trance on the part of uninitiated people. This is considered to be 'savage' trance and linked with incurable mental illness. He also locates music in the first stage of the ceremony but says that the second possession phase, which may last several days, is maintained without music. He agrees with Rouget's (1985) thesis that although percussion instruments are part of most ceremonies practically any instrument can be used. He highlights the fact that the Boori cult in Nigeria gives the power to the one stringed lute on which the tunes appropriate to each spirit are played. The Yuraks of Northern Europe also used a bowed instrument called a 'singing bow' which is a single stringed trance-inducing instrument. The shamans of Siberia use a stringed instrument called the kobuz. Here trance is produced by using the harmonic produced by a single note (Hamel 1978). There is little doubt that the power lies in the role assigned to the instruments by the belief system of the culture and not in the instruments themselves. Dancing or an emotional situation are also often needed and the power of the songs resides not only in the songs or the music but also in the ability of the healer to use them efficaciously. The use of such techniques as hyperventilation in warrior societies also accompanies war songs as an energising technique.

Michael Harner (1990), however, sets out the notion that the monotonous drum rhythms of a shamanic session activate theta patterns in the brain. These waves are associated with creative thought. They also simulate the rhythmic beating of the heart:

> There have been very few scientific studies so far on what happens to a shaman making the journey. We need much more of this kind of research. But in one research project that was done using electroencephalographic equipment to measure brain waves it was found that the shaman in just ten minutes of journeying achieved a state of consciousness, empirically, scientifically measured, that had only been duplicated once before and that was by Japanese Zen masters in deep meditation after six hours of work. So the effect of the drumming, as well as the shamanic methods, is very, very considerable. (Harner, quoted in Drury 1984, p.86)

The songs the shaman uses operate in various ways. Some summon the auxiliary spirits while others tell the story of his journey. They are designed to make the power of the shaman available to the community for healing. All have the form of incantations and their role is to bring to life the 'imaginary world of the invisible' (Rouget 1985, p.319). He also deals with the phenomenon of induced group trance. Discussing the Arab sama tradition, he outlines how the sung poetry is used to induce the trance, while it is maintained during the dancing by the rhythm.

Singing in particular is very much part of the general life of these societies and would be used outside of ritual to get people into the right mood for various tasks and situations:

> Songs constitute an important part and everyday aspect of life among the Dinka, and every Dinka sings both as an individual and as a member of a

> group... They may be composed by the owners themselves of for them by experts... During the season of cultivation, many people can be heard, each singing loudly in his own field. In the stillness of the night, a mother may be heard singing any song as a lullaby at the top of her voice. (Feng 1973, p.78)

When the shamanic tradition was synthesised in central Asia with Christianity and Islam, elements of the culture were retained. These included systems for relating music to various moods:

> From the ninth century El-Kindi connects the four strings of the lute with certain body humours, ages, mental states, special rhythms, types of melodies, certain times. He recommends certain tunes in the night to calm the sickness and slow its power. 'Because if the things that are similar in nature increase and come together, their action will become powerful and their effects come out to overthrow opposites.' (Tucek 1994, p.13)

Later in this tradition in 1486 Sultan Bayeazid II included in his beautifully decorated hospital in Edime a fountain. It was by this that the doctor and six or seven musicians worked (Tucek 1994). There was also the notion that various instruments could induce various states. Around 950, Hakim El-Farabi developed the instrument known as the Ud (a lute) especially for this. He was renowned for creating joy and deep sleep in his patients (Tucek 1994).

Summary – excitement / relaxation

To summarise, the role of trance in healing ceremonies is much discussed. This often takes place in societies where music is better established as a way of managing moods. There is much debate about the role of music, particularly in the creation of trance, which is usually part of a ritual involving many elements like hallucinogens and movement. Experiments on Westerners cannot reproduce the religious and social elements which are an important part of the phenomenon.

Embodiment/transcendence

This is a central theme to this subject for in most of the cultures dealt with here, there is no dualism in the belief systems.

Grimes (1982) suggests that ritual is not a discursive reflexive activity but a bodily way of knowing designed to move consciousness from the head to the body. He sees its efficacy as being rooted in the total bodily attitude, which is a combination of inner movement and external manifestation. Trance is a very clear example of this. In the first section of this chapter I referred to the state of trance as a state of consciousness distinguishable from that used in everyday living. Rouget (1985) lists the following characteristics: it is a temporary state and regarded as unusual; there is a change in the relationship of the person in trance to the surrounding world; there may be neurophysiological disturbances; the abilities of the subject may be increased either in imagination or in reality; and this increased ability can be seen in behavioural symptoms by others.

The word 'trance' is also used in the West and some would see it as a continuum that runs from daydreaming to the full trance practised in shamanic cultures (Topp-Fargion 1992). In American literature in particular the term 'altered states of consciousness' has become popular (of which trance is one among many). It occurs in writings from the human potential movement where there is no clear relation to music and is used in relation to hypnosis, and sometimes in relation to epilepsy, hysteria, sleepwalking and brainwashing. Ethnologists are concerned about defining 'trance' clearly in societies other than those dominated by Western value systems and would limit its use to that described at the opening of this chapter. In a religious context it is sometimes allied with the word 'ecstasy'. Rouget (1985) distinguishes between the two terms, associating ecstasy with immobility, silence, solitude, the absence of crisis, sensory deprivation, recollection and hallucination. Trance, on the other hand, is characterised by movement, noise, the presence of others, crisis, sensory overstimulation, amnesia and no hallucinations. But Rouget has to admit that the two are at opposite ends of a continuum and that any particular example of it may include a configuration of features from either list.[4]

Trance is central to the shamanic cultures. As we have seen, this is only partly caused by the music; but the corporeal nature of the combination of dance and music in a particular way makes the link between the body and the trance crucial. Rouget (1985) describes the trance of the Muslim dikhr and Christian sects like the Shakers as 'above all a corporeal technique' (p.317), for the dancer and the singer are merged into one person. He notes certain

4   It is interesting to compare Hildegard's visions with this model as an example of a particular configuration of these elements. For her they were often moments of crisis and had a musical component to them. Most of her music was received in visionary experiences.

techniques of auto-excitation, like breathing techniques and physical movements that may be seen as consuming or liberating energy. He sees changes
of speed as linked with emotional intensity and sees the repetition of the
words as important. But again he emphasises the role of the whole event in
the occurrence of trance and not just the musical or physical phenomena
alone. However, he concludes:

> To shamanize, in other words, to sing and dance, is as much a corporeal
> technique as a spiritual exercise. Insofar as he is at the same time singer,
> instrumentalist, and dancer, the shaman, among all practitioners of
> trance, should be seen as the one who by far makes the most complete use
> of music. (Rouget 1985, p.319)

Many writers draw attention to the spiritual significance of the drum:

> It is from the branch of this Tree [the World Tree], which the Lord causes
> to fall for this purpose, that the shaman makes the shell of his drum...
> Seen in this light, the drum can be assimilated to the shamanic tree with
> its notches up which the shaman symbolically climbs to the sky... The
> drum depicts a microcosm with its three zones – sky, earth, underworld –
> at the same time that it indicates the means by which the shaman accom-
> plishes a break-through from plane to plane and establishes communica-
> tion with the world above and the world below. (Eliade 1964, p.168)

> Since the drum is often the only instrument used in our sacred rites, I
> should perhaps tell you here why it is especially sacred and important to
> us. It is because the round form of the drum represents the whole
> universe, and its strong steady beat is the pulse, the heart, the throbbing
> centre of the universe. It is the voice of Wakan-Tankan [The Great Myste-
> rious/The Great Spirit/ The Absolute] and this sound stirs us and helps
> us to understand the mystery and power of all things. (Black Elk, quoted
> in Brown 1989, p.69)

The making of the drum is a sacred act and the shaman is guided to the right
tree by the spirits. He or she must trust the intuition, and the vision of 'right-
ness' may be given in a dream. A Siberian shaman describes his choice in this
way: 'Then the spirits led me to a young larch tree which was so high that it
reached right up into the sky. I heard voices saying: "It is ordained that you
should have a drum made from the branch of this tree"' (Vitebsky 1995,
p.81).

The link between embodiment and transcendence is clear in many
cultures where bodily movements and gestures are endowed with spiritual
significance and regarded as efficacious in some way. Lisha Li, examining the

use of mystical numbers in Manchu traditional music, outlines the way that the special mystical number three is applied to drumming:

1. 'Drumming on the high road'. The drum is beaten towards the sky and held higher than the player's head to contact the gods who live in the sky, using only the 'Old Three-accented Patterns'.

2. 'Drumming on the middle road'. The drum is held in front of the player's chest to contact the gods who have come to the ritual place to pass the gods' intention to the people. To contact the gods who have come to the ritual, the 'Old Three-accented Patterns' are also used and the player should respect the altar. To pass the gods' intention to the people, the 'Five-accented Patterns' should be used.

3. 'Drumming on the lower road'. The drum is held in a lower position and is beaten towards the ground to drive away demons, using the 'Seven-accented Patterns'. 'Drumming on the middle road', however, is the most common style in ceremonies. (Li 1993, p.113)

So the bodily positions reflect shamanic views of the cosmos. These are also reflected in the expressive style:

1. In singing the special kind of chanting songs involving the names of the gods, the shaman adopts a kneeling position in a secretive manner and sings very weakly to avoid the song being heard by others... 'It is disrespectful to read the sacred names of gods loudly. We should read them inside the heart.'

2. In singing songs which are especially for the gods living far away, such as the God of the Sky who lives in the sky and Goddess of the Earth who lives under the earth, the shaman adopts a very solemn manner...and sings very loudly to make sure that the gods can hear.

3. In singing the songs for the gods who have come to the altar, the shaman stands in front of the altar and sings with normal volume in a relaxed manner. (Li 1993, p.114)

This fascinating article shows in great detail how mystical odd numbers are seen to create and transmit messages across the different worlds and how they permeate all the musical forms and performance styles of the Manchu, especially those used in shamanic rituals (Li 1993).

In contemporary Africa the belief systems and practices associated with them co-exist with systems based on monotheistic traditions and allopathic medicine. Pat Caplan's (1997) book *African Voices, African Lives* illustrates clearly how the Swahili people living on the east coast of Africa now distinguish between the causes for various illnesses to decide which medication they will use. For this process they seek the help of a diviner who identifies the source of the sickness, including sorcery, the evil eye, ancestors and spells. Once a person is sick a group of relatives will decide on appropriate therapy and may well choose a range of possibilities which in the account of Mohammed (Caplan's source) may include herbal, Islamic, biomedical, cupping or spirit possession. The ceremony described had three stages, the first involving all-night dancing, with drums, hand-clapping and singing, during which people become possessed and need to be restrained. The next involves ritual slaughter of an animal, whose blood is consumed by the possessed. The third stage is divination, which may last into the early hours of the morning, when the sick consult the still-possessed shamans. (This is the term used by Caplan, but using the definitions at the beginning of this chapter, this is a spirit possession cult and not a shamanic one.) Mohammed, who was born in 1935, describes this ceremony thus:

> The initiate was ill after being taken by the spirit, so they said that if it left her alone and she got better, they would hold a *kitanga* [a spirit possession ritual] since the spirit wanted here to become its medium...

> WA was watching the ritual, and JM of Karibu village was possessed and took WA over to the bed [where the people who are possessed sit]. Mohammed told WA to sing the *mwingo* song 'It is finished, that foolishness'...so he called the singer who sang the song and WA [also] became possessed and danced on the bed. (Caplan 1997, p.187)

Here we see a number of characteristics that mark these cults, including the notion that 'sickness' may be a mark of being 'chosen' by the spirit.

These ceremonies take place in cultures where the distinction between the animate and the inanimate is very unclear. Human beings are in close contact always with the natural world and the gods are to be found within places, natural objects and humans; the invisible world is filled with the souls of the dead. Scott Cloud Lee (1995) summarises much of the thinking: 'We are Spirit and approach Spirit with our own voices singing. We are co-creators with Spirit and recognise ourselves as fit controlling powers... Let us dance a dance that returns our beautiful planet to a friendly environment for children and animals' (pp.65–66).

Summary – embodiment / transcendence

To summarise, the notion of the body and transcendence are inextricably intertwined in cultures that use music and dance regularly in rituals involving trance. Instruments have musical functions and spiritual significance. Sickness is thought to have a spiritual component and even in societies where Western values are also established, a sickness thought to have a spiritual element will provoke a return to traditional healing.

Summary

The cultures that use shamanic and spirit possession ceremonies for healing use music as a central part of the ritual. Sometimes this is to induce a state of trance and sometimes it is to communicate with the medium through which the spirits communicate. The traditions are essentially communal practices and the healing is carried out in the context of a community which shares the worldview of the healer and the sick person. The ceremonies can be curative or preventative. The shaman uses the music to journey to the other world which is interconnected with the everyday world. In spirit possession cults the spirits are seen as visiting a human being. The training for the role of priest, shaman or medium is rigorous and the vocation is often recognised by a fit of spirit possession which is involuntary. The belief in the existence of another world allows for a certain freedom – a freedom through which the shaman learns to travel freely. But this freedom is carefully contained in the training, rituals and ceremony and the belief system itself. Although there is a tradition of healing songs and rhythms, improvisation is included in the system, the musical ideas being given in dreams and trances. By believing in another world inhabited by spirits, there is a possibility of expressing feelings and emotions unacceptable in the 'everyday' world.

Research, indicating that people liable to possession are often lacking in status, indicates that spirit possession may be a way of containing these people within society and giving them more status. The points that indicate the healing 'vocation' to be a healer may occur at a crisis. So the ceremony can be seen as a communal expression of difficult feelings which are seen as belonging to other beings. As this expression uses the non-verbal forms of music and dance, this acceptance can be public due to the nature of these media. This therefore becomes a therapeutic tool both for the community and for the sick individual. This gives the possibility of self and societal change – a change in status – bringing issues of justice and healing together. The whole system runs on a shared belief system of the interconnectedness of the cosmos but that connection is expressed through the body either by using bodily movements to induce trance or symbolically by using the body to express beliefs about the other world.

This reading of traditional healing through music is necessarily done by an outsider who has been immersed in the culture of Western ways of thinking. By using accounts from the healers themselves as well as accounts from Western anthropologists and ethnomusicologists I have endeavoured to hear the authentic voices within the tradition and to represent them as truthfully as possible within the context of the model.

CHAPTER FOUR

Of a New Consciousness

The founding of Narnia

After a taxi crash, the children and Uncle Andrew found themselves in
Narnia again. In the darkness a voice was singing. The low notes seemed
to come from deep in the earth. It was a wordless song, although it didn't
seem to have much of a tune. It seemed to be the most beautiful sound
that they had ever heard. Then, as if by magic, more voices appeared,
more than could be counted. They had a tingling quality like silver and
although they were high and glittering they were in some way in
harmony with the low note. In the sky, shoals of shimmering stars
suddenly appeared. They seemed to be leaping into the sky, thousands of
sparkling lights – planets, constellations, and galaxies – in response to
the high silvery notes. It was if the stars themselves were singing, called
into being by the first Voice.

That Voice was now getting louder with a feel of triumph. The sky
began to grow lighter and on the distant horizon the first signs of dawn
began to appear. They felt a gentle wind. And still the Voice sang. The
colours of the dawn turned from pink to yellow to orange to bright gold.
The Voice grew stronger and its beauty was overwhelming. In golden
glory the sun appeared above the horizon. Digory was amazed. It was the
most beautiful sun that you could imagine and it seemed to be laughing
with joy as it rose in majesty. Now they could see the nature of the land
that they had entered. Through the valley in which they stood, ran a
wide river, flowing swiftly in the direction of the sun. To the south they
saw mountains; to the north there were gentler hills. But the whole
landscape was bare – bare earth and rock. There was no vegetation to be
seen; but the colours of the earth were exciting. They were glowing,
bright and hot and made you feel excited.

Suddenly they saw the origin of the Voice. A huge, majestic golden
Lion stood facing the sun. The Voice was coming from his wide-open

mouth. He was walking to and fro and now he was singing a new song. It was gently lilting and as it rippled over the scene, grass appeared and spiky arms began to push their way up through the earth. Soon the children realised that these were trees growing. Beneath them flowers were springing up – buttercups, daisies and dandelions. Tangled shrubs were appearing on all sides – flowering currants, rhododendrons and climbing wild roses.

And all the time the Lion was walking; and all the time he was singing adding new notes and new tunes. Polly began to see that his song was connected with the growth in the landscape. He sang a new row of long deep notes and a hedge of tall trees appeared. A fast pattern of notes made primroses spring up all over the fresh green grass...

And still the Lion sang – the most beautiful song she had ever heard. It was changing, growing wilder. She wanted to jump, run, climb, dance and shout. She wanted to rush up to people and hug them. Now the earth began to swell up in humps all over the place. Some of them were small like molehills, while others were much bigger like small houses. They swelled and swelled until they broke open. Out of each hump there came an animal. The Lion stopped singing. He looked straight at each animal as if he was going to consume them with his gaze; and then he breathed – a long slow warm breath; it made the animals and the trees sway. The blue sky now hid the stars, but Polly could still hear them singing their cold sparkling song from beyond the sky.

There was a quick flash of what seemed to be fire. They were not sure whether it came from the sky or the Lion but no one appeared to be burned. It made their blood tingle. At last the Lion spoke: 'Wake up, Narnia. Wake to love. Start thinking. Start speaking. Trees, start walking! Animals, start talking. Waters remember your holiness.' And out of the trees wild creatures appeared. There were the gods and goddesses of the forest and Fauns, Satyrs and Dwarfs. The river god rose from the river accompanied by his daughters, the Naiads... (summarised from Lewis 1955, pp.93–109)

In C. S. Lewis's concept of Narnia lie elements of the shamanic Other World but with a strong admix of the Judaeo/Christian creation story and at the end mythical creatures from ancient Greek civilisation. It contains various elements that were to characterise what is now called somewhat loosely the New Age which has expanded its sources considerably since the middle of the twentieth century. The New Age marks a rediscovery of some of the belief systems that were found in the last chapter, transplanted into a society whose dominant culture is very different. In Western society these systems met with the established Judaeo/Christian systems to produce something radically different. The beliefs and practices have the appearance of being selected at random from the variety of practices outlined in Chapter Three, often depending on the experience of various influential travellers. A popular entry point to Western culture was the west coast of the US, where the beliefs and practices acquired a distinctive character.

The sources for New Age philosophy are, in general, Eastern and indigenous religions combined with a desire to rediscover ancient beliefs and practices. The chapter headings in David Tame's (1984) book *The Secret Power of Music* show the desire to rediscover ancient wisdoms rather than create new ones. His chapter 'Overture: Music and its power' draws on Judaism and Confucianism. Two chapters set out the ancient wisdom of China and India. There is an affirmation of ancient Greek systems, especially Pythagorean. Two chapters – one on 'The twentieth century: The "new music" (which concerns the development of modernism) and 'The twentieth century: Jazz and the blues – Their nature and origin' – show how, in the opinion of the author, Western music has lost its way. A chapter entitled 'Assessment: The physics of the OM' draws again on sources from ancient Judaism, ancient Egypt and Tibet. The final chapter – 'The ancient wisdom revisited: The modern esoteric viewpoint' – deals with the revival of gnosis largely in the area of theosophy and composers interested in this area such as Cyril Scott. It is an interesting book in that it does clearly demonstrate the antagonism to the dominant traditions that underpins much New Age thinking, as well as giving examples of the many sources that are drawn on in pursuit of a New Model for music.

Jonathan Goldman (1992) in *Healing Sounds – The Power of Harmonics* also roots his work in ancient mystery traditions referring to the Egyptian god Thoth and the Alexandrian philosopher Hermes Trismegistus by name and to traditions originating from Egypt, Rome, Greece, Tibet and India. He describes how sound can be seen as 'the primary causative form of the universe' (p.11). He points out how priests and magicians were often musicians and how esoteric knowledge underpinned the principles of Hermetic philosophy, at least two of which involved music. One is the 'principle of vibration', which states that all is vibration, and the other is the 'principle of rhythm', which states that everything flows. He claims that a third principle, that of correspondence, which states 'as above, so below', can be seen to apply to musical phenomena. Here he claims we can listen to the audible frequency of the planet and the human body and 'use harmonically related sounds to influence the vibrations of atoms and stars' (Goldman 1992, p.17).

Firmly based in esoteric tradition is Corinne Heline's *Color and Music in the New Age*. In this she deals with such subjects as the astrological correlations of colour and music, the mystery of black and white, the development of New Age ideas in the areas of colour and music and the relationship of colour and music. Wagner figures prominently as 'a tonal and color sensitive', wearing only silk next to his body and choosing appropriate colours for the piece he is composing. She selects pieces as particularly in tune with the seasons. Spring, for example, is represented by Handel's *Messiah* and Wagner's *Parsifal*. The whole book has a powerful sense of the notion of the initiate who has special knowledge of the Divine mysteries. These grow out of a Gnostic synthesis of Christian and pagan traditions with much reference to the Grail legends.

Hinduism, Taoism, native American spirituality and Celtic traditions have also contributed a great deal to the belief systems that underpin what is really a collection of spiritualities. Each person has a right to choose from a variety of belief systems, and, indeed, is encouraged, in the interests of being 'true to their own energy', to undertake their own search. Some critics have therefore condemned it as a 'pick and mix spirituality'. However, certain elements can be identified as common – such as a belief in reincarnation and in a profound connection between human beings and the natural world and spiritual beings (who may be given a variety of shapes and names).

Anthroposophy as developed by Rudolf Steiner (1970) has also influenced the New Age. His philosophy is in itself eclectic, drawing on Eastern sources as well as Christianity. Notions of a soul, however, tend to replace notions of God. It has a strong sense of the interrelationship of various worlds and the soul as related to these. In this, the arts play an important part. He compares the static form of architecture with the fluid form of music:

> Musical creations, however, must be generated anew again and again. They flow onward in the surge and swell of their harmonies and melodies, a reflection of the soul, which in its incarnations must always experience itself in the onward-flowing stream of time. Just as the human soul is an evolving entity, so its reflection here on earth is a flowing one. (Steiner, quoted in Godwin 1987, p.259)

Here we see the notion of re-incarnation and the journey of the soul through this process. Music is seen as crucial to this journey, both as a metaphor for it and also because of its influence on it.

Steiner's anthroposophy was all-embracing, including medicine, education and philosophy within its remit. David Aldridge (1996) summarises the tenets of anthroposophical medicine as follows:

- Each person is a unique individual and treatment decisions must recognise this individuality.

- Scientific, artistic and spiritual insights, which recognise the whole person, need to be applied together in our therapeutic endeavours.

- Life has meaning and purpose. If these qualities are lost then there is a deterioration of health.

- Illness may provide opportunities for positive change and new balance in a person's life. (p.8)

The tenets of anthroposophy were mixed with ideas coming from the developing tradition of depth psychology, especially the thinking of Jung and research into human creativity and its expression in humanistic psychology (see Chapter One). This tended to follow the lead of neurological research locating logical thought in the left hemisphere of the brain and more creative and imaginative work in the right.

The New Age might be said to have started in its most public form in the UK when the Beatles started their work with the Maharishi Mahesh Yogi and committed themselves to transcendental meditation; they also developed a respect for the sitar player Ravi Shankar, who was to establish a long-standing relationship with the classical violinist Yehudi Menuhin. Such developments were part of wider movement world-wide that included the 'jazz-meets-the-world' movement led by the jazz musician Joachim Berendt in Europe. This brought together jazz players like the trumpeter Don Cherry with Eastern players like the sarod[1] player Ali Akbar Khan. There was a rediscovery of the spiritual dimension of jazz with such works as John Coltrane's (1965) *A Love Supreme* with its supremely spiritual message outlined on its sleeve notes (CLP 1869, EMI Records).

In the UK these developments joined with well-established groups examining indigenous folk traditions which were involved in the exploration of pagan traditions. In these traditions music had been traditionally used in

1   A stringed instrument from the Indian subcontinent.

sacred rituals to promote fertility in many ways through helping crops to grow, promoting birth in animals and humans and helping the process of dying. Within this movement there was also a political strand promoting the insights and rights of the poor and marginalised traditions. The singer Frankie Armstrong worked from 1964 with figures in the folk world such as A.L. Lloyd and Ewan MacColl whose work had a strong political underpinning. Armstrong writes in her 1992 book *As Far as the Eye Can Sing* of her first encounter with skiffle:

> I met artists, radicals and serious musicians and learnt to communicate feelings and ideas through song. I found it easy to identify with the creators of the songs we sang. Initially they were the songs of the black and poor white peoples of the United States. Later they were the songs of the peasantry: land workers of the British Isles and Eire. (pp.15–16)

A concern for women's issues was strong and powerful and women were well represented in this movement. The Women's Peace Camp at Greenham

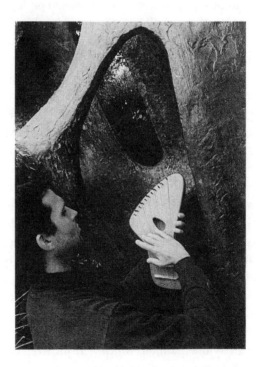

Figure 4.1 Bordun lyre (maker: Choroi) interacting with large Barbara Hepworth sculpture
Reproduced courtesy of the Tonalis Centre for the Study and Development of Music

Common was a formative experience in the lives of many leading figures in the New Age.

Peter Hamel (1978), in identifying the roots of the New Age in a rediscovery of esoteric traditions as we have seen above, establishes links not only with the masterworks of the past but with some developments in the avant-garde classical traditions (see Chapter Two). He sees the beginning of a new form of world music in 'compositions of our own century that have incorporated mystical-magical, spiritual, metaphysical and even non-European elements' (p.11). However, mutual suspicion has characterised the attitude of the classical academy and the New Age activists to one another's activity. There is often an attack on the dominant tradition within New Age thinking. David Tame in his 1984 work *The Secret Power of Music* attempts to define the basis of his attack within the spiritual dimension. This is an area of dispute between the two traditions. New Age spirituality includes a number of diverse elements whose relationship to music can be summarised as follows:

1. There is a strong sense that the universe is basically benign and that all that is needed for a healthy life is to tap into a universal love which is there for all to share. This love can be expressed and received by means of music.

2. This love activates the entire universe including humans whose destiny is inextricably bound up with the universe as a whole. This love is a vibrating force which can be accessed through music. In using music we can be creative in a material, psychological and spiritual sense.

3. Suffering is bound up with a sense of cosmic destiny and is to be learned from. When it has been learned from, it will go. Music can play a part both in the learning and the letting go.

4. Each human being needs to tap into the universal energy of love (sometimes called the 'true' or 'higher' self) which will know how to deal with any suffering. Meditation of various kinds, some involving music, will help this centring process.

5. Human beings can call for help from supernatural beings in the universe, often identified with angels. These are more prevalent than the concept of God. This can be done by means of music.

6. In some groups, there is a powerful sense of the soul, whose sick-
    nesses have effects on the body which can be cured by trance tech-
    niques, some of which involve music.

The rapid growth of the New Age musical tradition can be understood as a
reaction to the dominant musical traditions. To understand how this works
we need to understand what the dominant artistic cultures of classical and
popular musics have marginalised within their traditions (Tame 1984, p.73).

We have seen how spirituality is one aspect of this marginalisaton. Other
significant aspects are:

-   elitism

-   the loss of a certain mutuality and respect for difference

-   commercialism (especially in the area of popular music)

-   materialism

-   a decontextualised view of the arts

-   the loss of a certain gentleness and softness in favour of strong,
    powerful musical styles (some would say of a masculine character).

Chief among these is elitism. The classical tradition (see Chapter Two) has
constructed an innate notion of musical ability set in a hierarchy, at the top of
which is the notion of the genius who composes masterworks. This hierarchical concept is challenged in the New Age by the notion of music for all
and (more importantly) *by all*. All humankind is musical and all are potentially healers. Many courses claim to release everyone's inner potential
through music. This often takes the form of going back to very basic
soundmaking and rebuilding a person's musical experience from inclusive
and affirmative foundations. Vocal practitioners like Frankie Armstrong,
Kristin Linklater, Eloise Ristad, Chloe Goodchild and Jill Purce run
workshops to free people's natural voice, which is seen as having been
imprisoned by the elitism of the classical traditions. Some of these ideas were
developed in performing arts contexts which integrated music with other
performance techniques as in the experimental work of the Roy Hart
Theatre. The inclusion of movement with music, particularly as a way of
relaxing people, characterised the work of many vocal practitioners. This is
in contradistinction to the disembodied nature of much of classical music
performance theory.

There is also a tradition in the New Age of mutuality and respect with
minimal judgement (Gardner 1990). The commercialism of the world of

popular music is similarly undermined (although there is now a lucrative market in New Age music established) by this 'music for all' approach. This concept delights in the process of music-making and downplay the place of the musical product. There is also a return to simple, unamplified vocal sounds and a participatory approach to activities as in the workshops of the singers listed above. The Roy Hart Theatre, for example, extends the vocal range by exploring the full range of human vocal sounds like screams, moans, bird-like chirping and nasal timbres. Such sounds are regularly used in voice workshops designed to unlock people's vocal potential.

The dominant traditions of popular and classical traditions are both patriarchal constructs and, regarded from an essentialist position, reflect a certain aggression and power in their concentration on challenge and excitement (see Chapter Two). This leaves the way open for the New Age traditions to concentrate on nurture and relaxation.

The underpinning philosophies challenge the prevailing materialism by emphasising spiritual values and regarding all activity in a spiritual frame. Indeed, it could be said that in the context of the materialism of Western capitalism and its link with the Protestant work ethic, there was an inevitability about the growth of the phenomenon of the New Age. Nothing within the New Age context is free of spiritual implications.

It is in a spiritual framework that healing takes place in the New Age. There is a great stress on music as healing – healing for oneself, a group and the cosmos. Music is not intended to stand freely as a commercial product. Its fundamental purpose lies in healing the world – spiritually, psychologically and bodily. In this process, the intention of the music-maker is paramount:

> If the intent behind the music is pure, if it is created to heal, or if it is spiritually inspired, it will have a healing or inspiring effect on the listener. On the other hand, if the intent behind the music is purely commercial or, indeed, of a destructive or highly chaotic nature, the effect will be healing. (Gardner 1990, p.8)

Theoreticians of the New Age have attempted to plot the relationship of the classical and popular traditions to their work. Stewart (1987) in *Music and the Elemental Psyche: A Practical Guide to Music and Changing Consciousness* sets out an overarching scheme in his chapter entitled 'The four ages of music and consciousness'. He links these 'ages' with notions derived from numerology. The first he describes as 'Primal', consisting of natural and simple sounds. The second he calls 'Environmental' or ethnic folk music in which natural sounds develop a uniqueness by relating them to their place of origin. The third is designated 'Individual', in which individual creators emerge. He sees the 'Classical' tradition as the last stage, in which in European music 'degenerates into a rigid set of entities frozen upon paper by the notation system' (p.36). He hints at a fifth age with the development of electronic methods of generating and controlling sounds. His analysis highlights the criticism of the dominant cultures, especially in the areas of formalism and commercialism. His solution is to return again to primal music traditions – a return to an intuitive and 'natural' sound world.

The New Age is an eclectic phenomenon. It is dynamic and changing. It has become a route through which new methods are tried and tested, later to find acceptance in a wider world. Because of its debts to the analytical tradition in the shape of Jung, this is often in the area of psychotherapy and music therapy. This is well illustrated by John Ortiz who is a psychologist and a clinical hypnotist. He has synthesised his professional training as a psychologist with principles drawn from the martial arts and Taoist ideas (Ortiz 1997, pp.xvi–xvii). His work shows the combination of psychology with Eastern philosophers, notions of transformation through creativity and the desire to heal to be found in many New Age texts.

Awareness and exploration of new avenues and new experiences characterise a great deal of the work. The New Age is concerned with balancing the dominant culture with certain of the subjugated ways of knowing examined in Chapter One. Frank Perry's (1998) sleeve notes for his cassette *Deep Peace*, 'based upon the tri-unity of the Creator – Father/Mother/Son–Daughter', which was recorded in 1980, illustrate the desire to balance the 'opposites/complementaries of Freedom and Restriction; Chaos and Order; Composed and Improvised etc.' He sees his work as group ritual and goes on to set out a programme that fuses Gnostic ideals with those of other traditions very clearly.

Some New Age thinking has entered the area of popular music. This was particularly true in the rave culture to which many sleeve notes bear testimony. The sleeve notes to the collection *Textures* trace this line quite clearly:

October 1994: Trance Europe Express 3

Sometimes it's just *being* there. In the 60's it was the mud and brown acid at Woodstock for the hippies; when punk speed-powered through the 70's, the Sex Pistols at the 100 Club; for the early 80's Creation-weaned indie kids, chaos with The Jesus and Mary Chain at North London Poly;

and for Thatcher's children the ecstasy re-birthing through acid house at Shoom at the Fitness Centre.

Depending on your generation, these were the events to have been part of. Today, in the age of techno, it's the Love Parade. A demonstration for the cause of 'Peace, Happiness and Pancakes' (a German saying), the Love Parade is much more than a 'techno parade' that brings the shopping centre of Berlin, the Ku'damm, to a standstill on a Saturday afternoon in July. (Wrawicker 1996)

The following section from the Orb Remix Project highlights the spiritual aspirations of this culture as well as the attack on commercialism. Drugs feature, and the writing recalls the shamanic culture outlined in Chapter Three. The traditional journeys also used hallucinogenic herbs in some places but in these cultures strictly under the watchful eyes of the teachers and elders of the tradition:

> It's one of those evenings – the end of the world is just a couple of bus stops away and all that – at Nicky's birthday party in North London... Olivier the terrible is passed out on the settee. The rest of us are peering at the moon which tonight is in eclipse and accompanied by the appearance of the comet Hyakutake... I've been asked to write a few words to go along with the album of Orb remixes you have in your possession... The Orb haven't lost their musical viability, they are far too idiosyncratic and forward looking for that... The chase for the ultimate high...is hitting an all time low, for me anyway.

> I'd like to think that this was merely a function of me being jaded, but it's not quite like that. Ambient, rave, trance, techno, dub, trip-hop, whatever it is that reverberates like a huge ever growing pulsating brain that rules from the centre of the ultraworld, to heist a phrase, is with few exceptions conceptually dead in artistic terms. All the rest is just marketing and sales...

> I listened to The Orb quite a lot in rehab last year. It's *great escape* with a lot of interlinking melodic and rhythmic narratives. Fine for transporting you to a synthetic dubbed-outland. The Orb are a musical looking-glass... Always though you can hear the care involved. You can also hear that despite being pioneers of ambient music they've got some skull-punching drumbeats...

> I see it (death) as a renewal. That's what your genes are there for, you pass them on to the next generation. (The Orb 1996)

Many New Age themes can be seen here – the notion of transcending the present (done by the use of repetitive rhythms), a sense of reincarnation and the idea that the music lost its way when it gave up its original value system in favour of commercialism.

To summarise, the twentieth century has seen the development of easier access to a variety of music and spiritual cultures. The New Age is a collection of spiritualities challenging the prevailing Western materialist Cartesian culture. The music is similarly diverse, drawing on ancient, Eastern and indigenous sources. Within it can be traced powerful notions challenging the elitism, racism, sexism, capitalism and materialism of the dominant musical culture. The notion of healing within it is always set in a spiritual frame within which music has a prominent place.

Community/individualism

In this section I shall examine notions of community-building through music and the place of the individual journey. As we have seen, the roots of the movement lay in movements like 'flower power' and the protest movements of the 1960s. Here collectivism was of the essence. The notion of the large festival to generate the sense of belonging developed from the famous gathering at Woodstock. Present-day festivals such as Glastonbury and WOMAD are prime examples where very large groups of people are unified by listening, sometimes involving dancing and drugs. Around the fringe of these are groups of people forming free improvisation groups, where people 'converse' musically for long periods. Such impromptu groups which started to spring up in the 1970s explore a group unity created by people freely exploring sounds (vocal and instrumental) together. The purpose of the music is not for listening but simply for investigating relationships through improvisation. The sessions often start from 'scratch' with no prior discussion. Some will be more clearly based in drumming traditions, others edge more towards free jazz traditions and so on. The nature of the exploration depends entirely on the background of the participants. They are similar to verbal discussion groups with members getting to know one another's peculiarities and typical musical reactions, but have a very different 'feel' because of the nature of music as a medium. They are examples of community-building through free improvisation.

The spiritual beliefs underpinning the New Age mean that community is often perceived as being wider than a gathering of human beings. Many of the belief systems involve being at one with the earth and the sky and the elements. Many of them in the UK would trace these to Celtic or pagan roots in which sound was an important way of connecting with the natural world. In origin music was seen as a way of influencing the natural world upon which human beings depended – the elemental energy of wind, water and light, rain, wild and domestic animals. The literature will also regularly root New Age practice in such phenomena as the shamans of Mongolia developing their harmonic overtone chanting by listening to the sounds of the waterfall, which is given to human beings in order to help them learn the art (Goldman 1992). New Age recordings merge sounds from the natural world with those produced by human beings. Singers are recorded with whales calling in the background and water sounds are combined with pieces of classical music such as Pachelbel's *Canon*. Connection is of the essence and many groups will involve hugging in some way and chanting together, often in the open air and associated with ritual. The rituals contain notions of ecological healing of some kind.

The Sufi philosopher Hazrat Inayat Khan returns to ancient Christian traditions in the interfaith dialogue that characterises the New Age to show how the sum of group music-making experience is greater than its parts, referring to the use of 'a chord, a sound that is produced by ten to twelve people with closed lips ... It reaches so deeply into the human heart and creates so religious an atmosphere that one does not miss the organ' (quoted in Hamel 1978, p.213).

Music is seen as having the power to create community in a unique and deeper way. Repetitive chants are often used for this purpose. Frankie Armstrong (1992) writes of her own attendance at Balkan singing classes:

> I guess it was the singer in me that revelled in the sounds we made and songs we learnt, while the social worker in me observed with delight the changes that came over individuals in the group. As a group, too, we quickly developed a sense of support and collective identity. Though I had no idea at the time, this was the experience that would eventually change the direction of my life. (pp.84–85)

Dance groups found a similar collective identity through creating a shared space by means of music and dance. Gabrielle Roth (1992) links this with a tribal identity and the rebirth of the feminine:

> Find the thing that's ruling yourself and break through that. In order to do that you've gotta have some kinda tribal space where you can work with mirrors (other people) with support and collective energy... We're experiencing the rebirth of spiritual feminine energy... When I first

started in the sixties, I was in the most far out part of the culture... Now my crazy work has entered into mainstream consciousness. (p.5)

There are many who can point to profoundly healing experiences in the context of such dancing or singing groups. Isolated people are given a sense of belonging and reconnection.

Nevertheless, there is also quite a powerful sense of the journey of the individual soul searching out its own destiny, because of the prevailing reincarnational belief systems. The Graeco-Roman concept of the heroic journey is now transposed to the spiritual plain and concepts of karma and kismet are evident in many of the systems. Within this, music can be used as a powerful tool in working out this destiny, particularly as a way of purifying and of working through problems with relating to people and the natural world in past lives.

Summary – community/individualism

The notion of community is central to most New Age philosophies. This community is often conceived of as being one embracing the whole cosmos. Music is seen as a powerful way to connect with the cosmos and groups use freely improvised sounds to do this as well as engaging in experiences of group-listening at large festivals. Such experiences can heal damaging experiences from the present or past lives by connecting into a larger whole. This is an important part of the soul's journey through its various incarnations.

Containment/freedom

This section will examine how the New Age has been founded on notions of freedom, but has also developed its own patterns of containment.

Freedom is an important concept in the New Age. The tradition grew up at least partly as a reaction against containment, especially in the area of elitism and notation of the classical tradition. As most of the followers of the New Age will have received at least a smattering of, and in some cases a full-blown training in, Western high art traditions there is a real sense of 'sloughing off' the binding structures of this tradition. On a course run by the New Age vocal practitioner, Jill Purce, I met a well-established opera singer doing just that (like the use of notation as discussed in Chapter Two).

The work of New Age vocal practitioners is particularly strong in this area. Eloise Ristad encourages students to challenge the internal critics that insert themselves between the person and their creative spirit, which needs to flow freely for them to find their own natural voices (Ristad 1982). These judges are placed in our heads by our immersion in the classical tradition through the processes of music education. She has developed a number of methods to do this including unusual postures and visualisation. The starting point of Chloe Goodchild's work is the place where 'singing, like living, is...natural, well rooted, spontaneous and free' (Goodchild 1993, p.30). Her work encourages people to explore the full range of human emotion through vocal sound-making, find their own authentic sound and making them aware of a place of silence within themselves from which the inner voice comes. Her students are encouraged to find a place of freedom within themselves.

In the work of New Age voice practitioners like these, there is a deep sense of abandoning rational constraints in the interest of more intuitive approaches:

> It is the nature, the basic principle of sound, that the more it is in tune with nature the more powerful and magical it becomes. Every man and woman has a given vocal pitch, but the voice expert says: 'No, that is contralto', or 'soprano', 'tenor', 'baritone' or 'bass'. He confines what cannot be confined. Are there, then, really so many voices? There are as many voices as souls. They cannot be classified. As soon as a singer is classified, he has to sing at this vocal pitch. If his natural vocal pitch is different, he will not know it... Once a person has been handed over to the composers, and therefore has to sing at a predetermined pitch, he loses the natural voice that he once possessed. But quite apart from singing, one will find, even in speaking, only one... (Hazrat Inayat Khan, quoted in Hamel 1978, pp.213–214)

Implicit in such writing is the belief that in order to be healed at the deepest level we must find our own natural voice, that this is the ultimate musical freedom. Healing is related to finding our own 'naturalness' or, indeed, nature. This thinking underpins the free improvisation groups:

> In spontaneously assembled groups, a communal form of singing and music-making has been developed, using bells, cymbals and gongs... We were told at school and by our parents that we should sing in one particular way, that we must not sing 'wrong' micro-intervals, and in this way we have been deprived of most of the fun of singing. (Hamel 1998, pp.184–185)

Drawing on the work of Steckel (1973) Hamel saw the development of folk-rock traditions as a pursuit of spiritual freedom. He links this with the drug culture: '...through Folk-Rock music... the younger generation have loudly proclaimed their dance to freedom, as well as through countless individual experiences of the magical, mind-bending drugs used by foreign and ancient cultures' (Hamel 1978, p.9).

It is, however, remarkable how quickly a notion of orthodoxy starts to arise even within a tradition remarkable for its freedom. Although there are many differing systems of relating sounds to the chakras (see below, pp. 186–189) we can get writing declaring:

> When our root chakra is in balance, we feel secure, alert, full of active energy, stable, and warm. Because it is at the base of the seven major chakras, the root is the base of the animal energy... The musical pitch related to the root chakra is C; its balancing pitch is the fifth above, G. (Gardner 1990, p.16)

Musical freedom is designed to set the soul free of its suffering. Free of imprisoning suffering, the soul or higher self will be able to achieve miracles, which are only prevented by not following one's true energy or true life's destiny. This is largely a matter of losing excess baggage and travelling light. Jill Purce's clients described a feeling of a heavy shadow being lifted from them by the process of working with their voices with her.

Although there is a great stress on freeing, there is in many of the techniques a sense that the process of freeing has within itself the notion of containing powerful emotions. Leah Maggie Garfield (1987) writes of the traditional women's techniques of keening and wailing (rediscovered by New Age practitioners of toning, in which the body is rebalanced by means of a variety of vocal techniques): 'In practice, keening is a melodic, mournful combination of a moan and a cry done in unison or with overlapping waves of sound. Keening can be done singly or in groups. It's a grief sound without sobs or screaming. While the sound itself brings up sorrow, it prevents hysteria' (p.63). She goes on liken this to how the American women surrounding the Pentagon to protest about the build up of arms and the women at Greenham Common in the UK used this technique based on an upward vocal glissando to excellent effect.

The practitioners of toning recommend the use of groaning to release stress, tension and emotional and physical pain: 'There is a tone which resonates with the pain and relieves the tension... [Toning] is an escape valve for the pain because it is breaking up of the tension which we label "pain", and it brings new life energy to that place. It is an inner sonar message' (Keyes 1973, p.41). Weight lifters' grunts and the cries of karate practitioners are examples of the same phenomenon alongside other gestures in everyday life like sighing, groaning and moaning. The power of this form of release is explored by New Age.

Summary – containment/freedom

There is a strong sense of freeing people from the restraints of the classical traditions. This is done by expanding the range of sounds available. Through such work we will discover our natural voice which will enable our soul to slough off suffering and find its true energy. There is, however, a notion of orthodoxy within the tradition developing which could become as restraining as the classical tradition.

Expression/confidentiality

In this section I shall examine notions of what is being expressed and how this relates to issues of confidentiality. The early thinkers in the New Age had

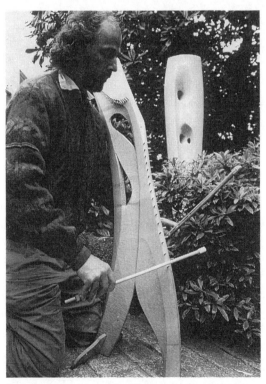

Fig 4.2 Bass double bowed psaltery (maker: B. Weyeneth) The psaltery is inspired by Hepworth's sculpture. It uses two bows to explore breath movements. Each side is tuned to a whole tone scale and when played left and right creates 12 tone music. Therapeutic applications – for dyslexia etc.
Reproduced courtesy of the Tonalis Centre for the Study and Development of Music

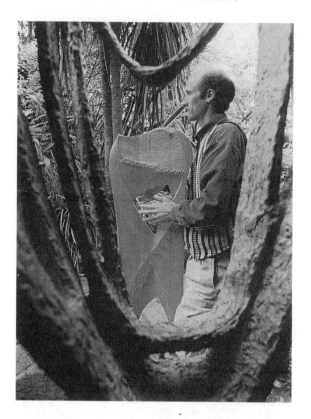

*Fig 4.3 Tone harp (maker: B. Weyeneth). The harp works with pure movement/
continuum forces and is seen through one of Hepworth's harp-like sculptures.
Reproduced courtesy of the Tonalis Centre for the Study and Development of Music*

a strong sense of trying to reach and express new levels of human consciousness, particularly magical/mythical ones. The work of thinkers like Jung,
Teilhard de Chardin (1964) and Jean Gebser (1973) developed these.
Gebser also developed a theory of four modes of consciousness – magical,
mythical, mental and integral. Linking this with music, Peter Hamel sees the
late twentieth century entering the exploration of the integral (Hamel 1978)
in which notions of the individual self give way to expressing the deepest
sounds of the universe.

This search for cosmic sounds has resulted in a search for 'different', often
deeper sounds, especially those that have been associated with ancient belief
systems. The increasing presence of people from those traditions in Europe
helped this musical link. Here the German newspaper *Süddeutsche Zeitung*

(1974) reports on the performance of the lamas (Buddhist monks of Tibet) of Gyoto lamasery (monastery):

> The six monks intone their litany-like phrases – a Ghiaurov or Talvela could well be envious of them – at sepulchral depths (for pedants, BBB), their performance being punctuated during the first section of the two-hour ritual only by small hand-bells and a wooden percussion instrument, later joined by drumbeats and the mighty sound of a Tibetan alpenhorn. What is fascinating about this chanting is not merely its resonant depth, but a special voice technique that accentuates certain overtones so strongly as to give the impression that the monks are singing in harmony...[They reflect] the deeper, mystic links between the proportions of the cosmos, of the human body and of the harmonic series. (quoted in Hamel 1978, p.74)

The connection between meditation and music, often drawing on Buddhist belief systems, have fed a great deal of New Age thinking.

Because there is an attempt to express what is beyond words, beyond human consciousness, the chants often use 'holy' words in ancient languages, names for God or mantric syllables:

> In the case of the mantric symbolic syllables, the minutest vibrations of a sound are of enormous importance... A mantra can be accompanied by a physical sound, but its power is spiritual and cannot be perceived by the outward ear, even if it is perceptible to the heart. Thus the mantra is not actually uttered by the mouth but by the spirit, and consequently it has significance only for the instructed initiate. (Hamel 1978, p.113)

What is interesting here is that in the communicating of the deepest meaning of the cosmos we see the notion of the initiate appearing. This might be regarded as the emergence of a new elite, not based on cognitive knowledge but on spiritual awareness.

In this context there is considerable use of a variety of wordless sounds: 'Toning is the process of making vocal sounds for the purpose of balance... Toning sounds are sounds of expression and do not have a precise meaning' (Beaulieu, quoted in Goldman 1992, p.137).

R. J. Stewart in recommending a return to primal music-making, explores the notion of 'the word of power' pointing to the existence in many spiritual traditions of words that are intended to be 'uttered at length – which means that they were musical' (Stewart 1987, p.103). To illustrate these he cites the 'Aum' of Tibetan buddhism, 'Ama', the name of the 'dark Mother deep' or 'primal ocean', and 'Amen', which he describes as the word of peace. In these he highlights the presence of humming sounds, describing the closing 'n' of Amen as symbolising and stimulating: 'Our understanding of creation moving into an entirely new dimension, by a balancing power that brings all energies to a peaceful union' (p.108).

The process of hearing and listening to meditative music invokes a new quality of listening, very different from classical or rock traditions. The music is seen as being produced by a meditator out of a concern not with product but with process, the end being the state of contemplation achieved *through* the music. In this context, music is seen as having the capacity to replace the mystical states induced by drugs (see Chapter Five):

> An improvisatory or contemplative music…which is not about medita-
> tion or self or God at all…[is] capable of being a vehicle, energy-form
> and magic force for spiritual self absorption, a music which has no
> pre-determined, stylistic function to perform, but which will flow end-
> lessly and will not be listened to as one listens to classical music – indeed,
> which is not there to be perceived at all… (Hamel 1978, p.142)

To reach such states is to assist the soul on its journey by allowing expression of the higher self. Suffering is to be transcended and left behind through music. There is a strong element of release in New Age thinking, releasing old hurts, present anxieties, and fears for the future. Paul Newham's work in voice/movement therapy was based on the work of Alfred Wolfsohn, who, as a German Jew in World War I, was fascinated by the vocal sounds of the wounded and dying soldiers. After the war he suffered from a mental illness that medicine could not cure, and he could not forget these sounds. He developed his own cure, which was to emulate them with his own voice, which he calculated would have a cathartic effect. This was successful and, having escaped the Nazis, he set up his own school of singing training in London. Here he put into practice his belief that singing was a way of over-coming trauma and was similar to psychotherapy. In his therapy Newham (1997) uses vocal techniques drawn from many cultures to diagnose and treat the effects of such illnesses as stress, anxiety and depression. He explains,

> Because the human voice is a physiological, psychological and social
> phenomenon, negative factors in any of these areas can cause depleted
> vocal expression. Therefore, in order to release the voice from constric-
> tion it is absolutely necessary to utilise a method that pays attention to a
> person's physical make-up, their psychological nature and the social
> environment in which they live. In Voice Movement therapy the client
> begins by making his or her most effortless natural sound… It is…an

artistic medium of freeing the voice and body from restriction and liberating a person from difficulties which hinder a freedom and fluidity of expression. (Newham 1998)

There are similar themes in Jill Purce's (1998) use of chant: 'Through the therapeutic use of the voice we are able to bring these areas of hurt and pain safely up into the light of clarity and illumination, often ridding ourselves of traumas which have beset us since early childhood.' How often words are used to interpret such experiences varies from group to group. Some New Age groups adopt a model of sharing both the music and the experiences with the group in some way. This represents a merging of Western psychotherapeutic practices with the communities that characterise the shamanic systems described in Chapter Three. New Age musical practitioners often work both individually and in groups, where confidentiality and trust are stressed. Some are groups which meet regularly, while others like sweatlodges (drawing on indigenous American traditions, see p.59) meet intensively for a weekend on a pagan festival to perform certain rituals involving music and other elements to purify the energy.

There is also a stress on the intention of the person expressing the sound and a notion that true feelings cannot be hidden; even if the person produces a pleasant sound, if they are angry the anger will be part of the sound. This is particularly important when training people to use sound to heal. This was part of the work of Dr John Diamond who is most famous for the development of behavioural kinesiology through which he tested muscles. He also worked on music, but saw the intention of the person making the sound as more important than the sound itself. Goldman (1992) summarises Diamond's theory: 'FREQUENCY + INTENTION = HEALING' (p.20).

Summary – expression/confidentiality

Notions of expression often concentrate on expressing the deeper aspects of the cosmos rather than the self. Music is often linked with meditative practices using wordless sounds or holy mantras in ancient languages. Healing is achieved by managing to reach this integral form of expression. Music is seen as an important part of this process, which often results in a different sort of music-making and listening from other traditions. Group work is common but there is little need for notions of confidentiality as the intention is to reach a shared or cosmic level of consciousness. In keeping with this theory, the intention of the music-maker is seen by some as more important than the actual sounds used.

Unity/diversity

We shall see here how the notion of unity has underpinned much of thinking about the soul, but that the tradition of respect and mutuality has led to a deep respect for diversity at a communal level. The New Age is built very firmly on notions of peace, harmony and interconnection. There is, therefore, a great stress on unity within the personality and the wider cosmos.

The renewal of the soul is central to the belief system. There is a notion of a reintegrated 'cured' soul; however, some see the process of healing as a shedding of undesirable aspects of the self. This pursuit of concord can lead to a sweetness in the music and a desire to exclude discord. Some systems contain an element of catharsis or 'emptying' to achieve this and arrive at a sense of peace. One of these associated with drumming and dancing, developed by Gabrielle Roth and called 'drumming the five rhythms', is discussed below (see pp.182–183).

However, as we are all pursuing our own truth, which we must discover and uncover during our lives (and sound is an instrument for doing this), there is a great stress on respecting other people's truth. Respect for difference characterises a great deal of New Age thinking. Although the individual soul strives for unity, society is enriched by the diversity of souls, confident in their own energy.

This notion has enabled the New Age to keep within itself a wide variety of musical styles. It has never forgotten its eclectic origins and is always seeking new sound experiences. Respecting the music of poor and marginalised cultures is an important part of large festivals in the wider vision of world peace.

Summary – unity/diversity

There is a great stress on unity in the tradition and this unity extends beyond the individual psyche. The cosmos flourishes in the right relationship. However, within this, there is also stress on respect for diversity, which results in a great stylistic diversity within the New Age. In cosmic terms, integration is seen as the peaceful co-existence of diversity.

Challenge/nurture

In this section we shall see how New Age music has filled a gap left by the classical tradition in the area of nurturing through music. This is greatly stressed, while more challenging musical traditions are often seen as aggressive and destructive. The notion of entrainment (see Chapter One) – of starting where people are and moving them gradually to a greater sense of power rather than jolting them out of their position by a sudden shock – underpins much thinking. The underlying philosophy is that people will be empowered through nurture rather than through challenge. The notion of reincarnation has the idea of the soul moving through a series of episodes within it, but these will be dealt with ('healed') through the nurture of others, which can be achieved musically. The notion of being held by a group musically is quite well developed (see 'A humming bath' in Appendix I). There is a stress on being able to hold and be held, often related to Taoist notions of yin/yang.

Repetition is deemed to be supportive and nurturing. The popularity of repetitive chants often drawn from the Native American tradition bears testimony to this. They are contemporary sung mantras, used to calm and quieten: 'Repetitive musical phrases, if created with healing intent, also have the power to help the listener become receptive to whatever healing procedure is being administered' (Gardner 1997, p.59).

This nurture is seen to lead to the realisation of your own power. The vocal practitioner Susan Lever believes singing leads to encouragement of general empowerment. She laments the passing of communal singing as a natural part of daily life, claiming that in an age of personal stereos, televisions and dwindling church congregations most people sing only at harvest festival, Midnight Mass or when drunk:

> It's a great shame because making sound can really change your mood. If you feel low and you make happy sounds, it will, without a doubt, lift you. Your breathing will automatically change and so will your physiological state. You will have a lot more energy, a lot more confidence and a lot less stress (Lever, quoted in Alexander 1994, p.5)

Many of the vocal practitioners running voice workshops can point to experiences where they first felt the power of singing. Jill Purce in her publicity for her 'intensive week' on 'The Healing Voice' writes:

> My own first transmission of the power of the voice came in early childhood in Ireland. We were visiting a remote island off the west coast. The only other people in the boat were the old women of the island returning home. A violent storm blew up and it seemed obvious that all of us were going to drown. Suddenly the women began to sing with an ancient power and deep passion. Almost at once our fear dissolved, waves of strength surged into us and finally we were overcome with feelings of bliss and enchantment. (Purce 1998)

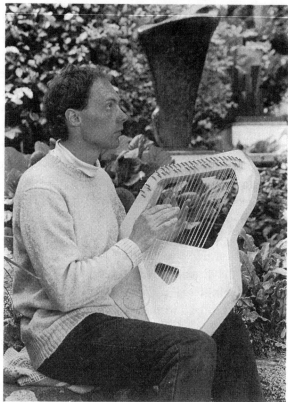

Figure 4.4 Lyre player
Reproduced courtesy of the Tonalis Centre for the Study and Development of Music

Jill Rakusen (1992) claims to have distilled musical power in a particular song. Her song is about an old man walking who is 'pacing steps of peace...speaking words of peace...breathing breaths of peace...living his dying in peace' (publicity leaflet). It was written for a dying friend and she recommends its use by people struggling 'to cope with pain of any kind, with illness, with death and dying, with uncertainty, with violence, oppression, with war', offering to send her card with the song on wherever it is needed. It is an unaccompanied tune in the Aeolian mode. The notion of a power song bears resemblances to shamanic practices described in Chapter Three.

Much of the material coming from the US, particularly that aimed at women, is concerned with power and the right use of it. Starhawk, 'a feminist peace activist', for example, has produced a tape entitled *The Way to the Well*, subtitled *A Trance Journey for Empowerment*. It consists of a guided visualisation accompanied by a repeated rhythm on a drum. The visualisation takes the form of a journey to a well where participants will find their own power. The tape includes a chant for women's voices about finding your power, which is repeated several times. The purpose of the drum is supportive and is intended to create the trance state advertised in the subtitle. The repetitive nature of the drum rhythm and the chant is designed to support people in a transformation process:

> Now I think of these drum stories as free-form improvised poems, a type of theatre in which the listener becomes the protagonist and faces an opportunity for transformation. The story focuses on power; the three wells let us encounter power-from-within, power-over, and our collective power to heal and nurture.

There is quite a protesting streak within such writing which encourages people to claim their power instead of denying it. The thinking is often seen in relation to traditional Christian attitudes to power which are perceived as asking already powerless people to give away what power they have in the interests of submission to a divine will or a hierarchical church. It is in this system that the early link between the New Age and the protest movement is still apparent. There is a real encouraging of the democratisation of power, including musical power.

Practitioners like John Ortiz use music to enable people to take control of their lives:

> The songs chosen played a significant part in helping Donna get in touch with the core of her depressive mood…After a few weeks, Donna looked forward to the bittersweet feelings and memories the introductory songs evoked, and smiled with a sense of geniality in anticipation as the more lively 'in between' songs came on. The progression, she felt, served to remind her that things change – life wanes and waxes – that taking responsibility and initiating movement in one's own situation can 'feel pretty good'. The concluding bouncy, energetic songs progressed from providing a sense of much needed energy to becoming 'theme songs' to her new-found animated self. In a sense, the tape became a sort of compact 'auditory metaphor' for her own life. (Ortiz 1997, p.5)

This is an example of the process of entrainment at the level of practitioner and patient described in Chapter One.

Notions of nurturing and caressing through sound have found their way into the *Trance* culture. The sleeve notes to *Textures* include the following:

> Textures is about feeling…is about **music** that makes you *feel* real. What feels right to you? **Textures** is about…Motion. Sound. Vision… **Textures** is a music made by **machines** for people who can't stand the

way things are. **Focused** on conscious **evolution**, pushing through into the future... **Textures** is a state of mind. Reflecting the **duality** of life, there are two sides to the coin: mixes lift you up and caress you down in the firm grasp of **Darren Emerson** and the cradling but never cosseting arms of **Alex Paterson**. (Wrawicker 1996)

Summary – challenge/nurture

Notions of nurturing dominate the musical scene of the New Age. This is often done with sung repetitive patterns or repeated rhythms on the drum or finding your own singing voice. This is seen as a route into empowerment and of taking control of your own life.

Excitement/relaxation

This polarity can be related to the yin/yang idea – the strong and the vulnerable. Many catalogues of New Age cassettes distinguish between the two sorts of music. One is music for relaxation, especially in the context of massage and aromatherapy, where examples abound. Here there is the development of electronic music using sweeping, expansive soundscapes consisting of sustained chords changing very slowly, sometimes allied with natural sounds. In general, the pieces are characterised by an absence of discord. What discords there are are resolved in keeping with the Western harmonic systems. Music designed for energising, in general, differs from its relaxing counterpart in the areas of volume and speed. The daring adventurousness of the pitch combinations of the contemporary classical tradition is not explored.

The sleeve notes often concentrate on the intention of the music. *Sea So Serene* consists of the sounds of the sea with the instruction: 'Take a break from your day...relax, as so many do, to the warm, caressing sounds of mother earth. Close your eyes and let the sound embrace you with pleasure and serenity' (Lifetime Cassettes 1993). It has also an indication that it does not contain subliminal elements. These are introduced on some recordings to make the effect deeper, and such tapes usually carry a warning about their presence.

In 1997, Beechwood Music issued three cassettes entitled *Spirit of Relaxation*. The music combines natural with electronic sounds. The individual tapes are titled *Ocean Surf*, *Rainforest* and *Dolphins and Whales*. An overall instruction for use runs:

Okay, you've just got your first *Spirit Of...*album. You can listen either with the complete intention to relax i.e. lying down, with no disturbances in a cool, calm room with the lights dimmed, making yourself as comfortable as possible, allowing the music and sounds to totally wash over you. Or you can safely play it as an accompaniment to whatever pursuit you happen to be doing. Unlike spoken word relaxation tapes, *Spirit Of...*is a musical listening experience and completely safe to use anywhere.

You will find an instant effect on your mood and stress levels. The depth of this effect is entirely up to you. Complete concentration with no distractions, coupled with relaxation breathing techniques, you will arrive at another dimension of the mind. Total tranquillity and a feeling of deep, deep relaxation will follow. Listen closely and concentrate. Treat each tape as different levels or unwinding mental stages to reach a perfect state of sublime relaxation.

By listening whilst performing another task, *Spirit of Relaxation* will have a far more subtle effect. Your general mood will become calmer, more peaceful and much more relaxed.

The surrounding atmosphere will immediately change, also becoming serene and harmonious. Other people coming into this atmosphere will also be positively affected; feeling somehow soothed and instantly de-stressed. (Beechwood Music 1997)

Other companies are using indigenous recordings or artists, attempting to cement the link between the traditional culture and the New Age. Panoramic Sound, for example, issued in 1988 a recording called *Visions*, which 'has the flavor of a more contemporary sound, mixed with the seasoning of times gone by'. This puts together the flute sounds of J. C. High Eagle with guitar and dulcimer and natural sounds. The sleeve notes both describe the piece and also indicate the intended effects on the listener: '*Midnight Waters* – Soft flute, a harp-like strum of a guitar and the midnight trickling sounds of a gentle brook revived with life are captured as it brings a soothing message of the importance of flowing with the currents found both within and outside of us' (Panoramic Sound 1988).

Such sleeve notes show a recovery of a contextualised view of music. Music is seen as linked with the listener and the environment, sometimes linked with the seasons or particular times of the day. Hamel (1978) refers to the work of a German percussionist and a psychologist who worked together to produce a meditation music that interpreted the cycle of the time of the day as an aid to relaxation and meditation. Books in this area often contain lists of recordings with their probable effects. Lingerman's 1983 Work, *The Healing Energies of Music*, for example, offers suggestions for pieces to combat insomnia, boredom and cowardice and to enhance love and devotion. The second chapter entitled 'Music for better health and well being' sets out its theory at the outset, suggesting that certain pieces affect the physical body and are appropriate for manual work; others affect the emotions and the mind, bringing clarity and creativity: 'Finally, there are those pieces of music that penetrate through all outer layers. This kind of music speaks directly to the heart and soul, reminding you of your whole, divine connection and highest selfhood in God' (Lingerman 1983, p.13).

This chapter also consists of a categorised list of pieces. They are taken from a range of sources including classical (mostly pre-1920), jazz, folk and New Age. Other chapters offer 'Music for daily life', 'Music for home and family', 'The music of nature', 'Angelic music' and 'Music to God and Christ'. Chapter Nine, entitled 'A gallery of great composers' describes the work of the male composers of the classical canon, giving their star signs and also including Gregorian chant. 'The deeper mysteries of music' deals with colours and music and the book ends with a long list of pieces with their effects carefully described.

The influential Sufi philosopher Hazrat Inayat Khan calls for a rediscovery of the natural voice and a rediscovery of our own powers to influence our moods, setting out spiritual exercise involving music (described in Hamel 1978, p.213).

Gabrielle Roth (1992) developed a musical system that reflected the flow of human rhythm in life.

> As I observed people I became aware of the rhythms in other people's dance and began to articulate them (**flowing, staccato, chaos, lyrical and stillness**) and the psychological maps that these represented. I got a real hint of freedom because I realised that you could discover your own unique dance, your own maps, through your consciousness via your body. Our story lives in our bodies – all the shapes are in there and dance is a gateway to express and understand ourselves. (p.1)

Roth develops the wave form which is accompanied by drumming patterns. It starts with flowing movements in 3/4 time; then it moves to staccato (sharp, disjointed movements) in 4/4 time. Chaos is represented by 6/8 and movements are well rooted by the feet with more chaotic movements of the upper body. Lyrical movements follow using 4/4 time, floating away from the earth. Stillness is accompanied by gongs and involves the dancer being still in a comfortable position. The wave format is seen to be the pattern of the flow of human feeling. By entering into it in this way through movement we experience a catharsis.

As seen in the section on expression, the aim of meditative music can be seen as profoundly different from the rhythm of excitement and relaxation. Peter Hamel (1978) sees how such ideas sit uneasily with the public concert and many attempts to introduce that element within the Western concert format have been doomed to failure:

> The conventional attitudes and expectations are too alien to it, concentrating as they do 'on the dramaturgy of tension and relaxation, "high point and low point" thinking, fortissimo upheavals and pianissimo murmurs'. The 'action' of a Rock group, the 'necessary' excesses of the percussionist and the familiar rigmarole of a Jazz concert are inimical, in most cases, to real meditative self-absorption. (p.153)

There is a deep sense in all New Age thinking that music has a profound effect not only on human beings but also on the cosmos as a whole:

> Music can even transform matter into spirit, into its original state, by touching every atom of a whole, living being, through the law of harmonic vibration...But music penetrates our innermost depths and thus creates a new life-force, a breath of air that lends joy to all existence and leads one's whole being to perfection. Therein lies the fulfilment of human life. (Khan, quoted in Hamel 1978, p.215)

Because the effects of music are seen on a cosmic rather than a purely human scale, books in this area can be extraordinarily prescriptive and condemnatory, declaring certain styles as globally evil. David Tame (1984) in *The Secret Power of Music* sees Morton Subotnik's electronic piece *Silver Apples of the Moon* as taking people's power away:

> ...dangerous in a perhaps surprisingly tangible and immediate way. It as though there exists a chasm within each of these electronic compositions: a dark yawning crevasse which, if we allow it to, will gladly swallow up whatever portion of our mind we offer it by the directing of our attention towards it. (pp.102–103)

Other writers link the healing power of music with style:

> One factory, in particular, a manufacturing and repair plant for sophisticated electronic equipment, where concentration and clear-headedness are essential, was playing a great deal of rock on its continual music broadcast system. It was recommended that this be eliminated. The man-

agement changed to different music and found to their delight an immediate increase in productivity and an equally pleasing decrease in errors,
even though the employees were quite vocal about their dissatisfaction
at having had their favourite music removed. (Diamond 1980,
pp.103–104).

Summary – excitement/relaxation

There is a real sense of the profound effect of music in all New Age thinking
which has a very contextualised view of music-making including links with
seasons and times of the day. People are encouraged to be aware both of these
effects and also of one that transcends simple excitement and relaxation and
affects them and the cosmos at a profound spiritual and material level. This
has sometimes led to a view of certain styles and sounds as intrinsically evil.
These are often associated with loudness, discord and commercialism.

Embodiment/transcendence

This section will examine how the notions of the relationship of the soul to
the body are worked out in this tradition: 'Originative music, which is equivalent to primal music in both human consciousness and society, is *physical* and
metaphysical, biological and psychological, material and spiritual. It is rooted
in the unknown, yet utters forth its presence into the material world as sonic
vibration' (Stewart 1987, p.44).

The New Age is often regarded as a search for transcendent value systems
in the face of rampant materialism. However, it aims also to see the body and
the transcendent as connected. Hamel (1978) draws on the work of Jean
Gebser and Lama Govinda in seeing how this search was evident in various
developments in popular music and how each phase then yielded to commercialism. He refers to the first recording of the group Pink Floyd – 'which still
conveys a feeling of open joy' (p.36) – and then to the beginning of
underground and psychedelic music. All of these as they became commercial,
in his opinion, lost the sense of 'creating a powerful attunement experience'
(p.37).

The notions of embodiment and transcendence are carefully worked out
and well integrated in many New Age systems. The notion of the aura is an
important diagnostic tool in much of the thinking. Rudolf Steiner, in all his
writings, distinguished between physical, etheric, mental and astral bodies. A
case study on the effect of Wagner's *Valkyrie* on a young woman includes the
following descriptions (which uses Steiner's terminology):

Before the performance began she seemed rather listless and indifferent. The health aura showed signs of delicate health. The astral body was full of the usual colors, with signs here and there of irritation...her mental body was replete with thought-forms of music [she had been studying the score before the performance]... Before the first act was half over a great difference in her health aura was noticed; it now glowed and scintillated with new vigor...I noticed some streams of light protruding from her mental body like long, waving tentacles: on the end of each was a spinning thought-form similar to a vortex-like whirlpool in water, caused by suction. As some familiar motif floated up from the general vibrations of the music...these tentacles in her mental body sucked the vibrations into themselves in large proportions... The thought-forms already there, from the previous study of music, were strengthened until they filled the body with beautiful light. It seemed to relate her to the deep pulsations of the Law of Rhythm in all nature, and the experience made the separating walls (the vibratory difference) between the lower and higher mental bodies to disappear and the ego was able to approach nearer to the personality and to impress it with loftiest ideas...

What was the effect on the astral body? ...It was not very long ere it was great boiling mass of beautiful color – a mighty many-hued bird beating its wings against a cramped cage to escape...It found its way of least resistance and rushed through that – into tears... the young girl wept violently for a while, until some of the pressure of it was exhausted, then she grew calm and for the rest of the evening was benefited – in fact she was a 'new being' when she left the hall. (Heline 1964, pp.136–7)

A common system underpinning much New Age thought is the notion of chakras. The word comes from the Sanskrit word for 'wheel' and traditionally gifted individuals, including yogis and clairvoyants, have seen whirling vortices of light in the aura around a person's body. The aura is usually defined as an electromagnetic field which is being validated by such techniques as Kirlian photography, a method devised in 1939 by the Soviet electrician Semyoin Kirlian for capturing the aura on film. It involved passing a high-frequency energy field through an object and a piece of unexposed photographic paper. The result was an image of the 'bioluminescence' of the object on the paper. It is claimed that disease can be detected in this light field before it manifests in the body. The field is seen to be constructed of seven layers, and these auric layers correspond with seven energy centres within the body.

The energy can be blocked at any of these points and it is the task of the healer to unblock them so that the energy can flow freely. Healers are always exhorted to visualise their own chakras opening to allow the flow of energy to pass through them freely before embarking on healing work. The system I am familiar with describes the chakras thus:

- the base chakra at the bottom of the spine is associated with sexual energy
- the second chakra, associated with the spleen, contains our creativity
- the third chakra, located in the solar plexus, contains our identity
- the fourth chakra in the centre of the body at the heart level is associated with feeling
- the fifth chakra, located in the throat, is associated with speaking out and expressing our true energy
- the sixth chakra in the middle of the brow ('the third eye') reflects wisdom
- the seventh chakra at the top of the head is where we connect with the Divine.

Some systems claim that there are two further chakras. One is situated about a foot above our heads – the so-called 'transpersonal point' or 'cone of power'. The other is situated 12 or more inches below our feet and represents our connection with the earth.

Connections are often made between the chakras and the endocrine glands. These are associated with the production of hormones and links back to the 'humours' of medieval medicine can be made. Certainly, notions of balance are very much around in this New Age system as they were in the humours system which saw humans as being inextricably linked with the natural world (Helman 1994). As such the rediscovery of the chakra system may be seen as much as a rediscovery of lost elements of European culture as an importation from the East. There is often an attempt to link the ideas with those of ancient European figures such as Pythagoras:

The mathematician Barbara Hero, working at MIT [Massachusetts Institute of Technology], has found that the colours Pythagoras (Greek philosopher, geometrician, and musician, 600B.C.) is said to have ascribed to the musical tones, when generated by computers, actually produce their complementary colours (opposites). Hero's interpretation, one with which I would agree, is that chakras absorb the seven spectrum colours in sequence and emit their complements. (Gardner 1997, p.13)

Besides colours, connections are made of certain perfumes and musical tones with the opening of the chakras, which are often seen to be like flowers with opening petals. Composers have linked the notions of the perfumes and sounds together (Boyce-Tillman 1998b, 1998c).[2] One system of relating the vowels to the perfumes runs:

Oo (as in moon) to the base chakra
Oh (as in show) to the belly
Aw (as in paw) to the solar plexus
Ah (as in far) to the heart
Eh (as in weather) to the throat
Ih (as in wit) to the brow
Eee (as in seen) to the crown.

There are, however, a variety of ways of relating the vowels, pitches and colours as outlined in Goldman (1992). Barbara Hero (see p.186) has based her system of balancing the chakras through sound on the Lambdona diagram, a mathematical table said to have been discovered by Pythagoras. What is clear is that we need the full range of sounds to cleanse all the chakras. The full range of these vowels is found in ceremonial words like 'Hallelujah' as well as in the young child's invocation, 'Why?'

Using this system, practitioners will ask participants to sing low notes to cleanse the lower chakras and increasingly higher notes to cleanse the upper ones. Remnants of this thinking are still found in Western culture with such phrases as 'Tune your music to your heart' or designations like 'head voice' and 'chest voice' regularly used by singing teachers. In the New Age systems we find a potential unity between embodiment and transcendence carefully worked out through the system of chakras. Participants in workshops are often encouraged to drone single notes associated with a particular chakra requiring healing.

The theory of the chakras is found also in the trance 'scene'. It is fully worked out in the sleeve notes of *Return to the Source* (Dekker 1999):

As we dance as one with the forces of creation
The sleeping serpents will be awakened

2   These publications were written for the Society of Perfumers and link some of their commercial fragrances with the notions of chakras, which are in turn linked with the notion of the labyrinth.

With these snakes of creation our souls will entwine
To dance this ritual buried deep
Within the collective mind
Opening our hearts we surrender to the dance
One tribe united
We journey into trance…
Let the journey start…

… As we raise our arms with an ecstatic cheer we feel our connection to each other as one tribe united in spirit – the power of the collective. The euphoric dance floor release is as ancient as human existence stretching back through time to the original campfires. It was our community ritual, our rite of passage into ecstatic oneness. The chakra journey is our attempt to focus this powerful energy of the techno dance floor into a contemporary ritual for today.

Inspired by dance therapist and 'Sushumna' choreographer Antara, it is the culmination of many years of research and practice.

A multi-sensory dance floor event using lights, colour, sound and smells – we will be taken on a journey through the seven centres of our being.

Some of the leading producers within the psychedelic trance scene have made music especially for this journey creating special tracks for each chakra which are featured on this compilation. To complete this dance floor experience, computer visual artists have produced specific images. Essential oils and herbs are burnt that further stimulate each chakra.

Like the priestesses of ancient temples the Sushmna Ritual Dance Co work within the dance floor to create sacred space, facilitating crowd participation, breath awareness and energy exchange.

The chakra journey is a ground-breaking project that stretches the parameters of the techno trance scene to new levels of awareness.

The rest of the booklet consists of a variety of well-illustrated writings about the notion of the chakras.

Altered states of consciousness associated with the phenomena of ecstasy culture and acid house are the subject of Matthew Collin's (1997) book entitled *Altered State*. His detailed description of a culture that brought music, dance and drugs into an exciting and risky mixture draws attention to the relationship of this culture to the dominant one:

The eighties were a long way away now, almost innocent in hindsight. For the children of ecstasy, gulping down their first pill in pleasure domes of the late nineties, the euphoric frontiership of acid house must have seemed like ancient history, its roots in black gay culture all but forgotten. Many weren't even ten years old during 1988's Summer of Love. But for all that had changed, old uncertainties and contradictions remained – between a commodified culture and the illicit drugs that fuelled it, between rhetoric and reality, between knowledge and ignorance. And underpinning it all, still, was the restless search for bliss. (p.316)

Here Collin underlines that the fundamental search in ASCs (altered states of consciousness) was for transcendence. This we found in Chapter Three, but in the societies examined there the use of the hallucinogens was under the control of experienced elders. The commodification of all aspects of Western capiltalist society has produced a situation where money is the only value system. This has opened the way for the exploitation of what is a fundamental need in human beings – the experience of transcendence. The combination of drugs, music and dance to produce this is not a new phenomenon. What is new, however, is its alliance with a capitalist economy and its associated value systems, which allow for the exploitation of human need.

These traditions are not, strictly speaking, part of the phenomenon of the New Age, but are included here because they have been influenced by its thinking. ASCs have been part of New Age thinking, especially in the rediscovery of shamanic traditions. Gareth Frowen-Williams (1997) describes how the initial encounter of Western anthropologists with shamanism led to the assumption that shamans were psychotic. He charts how developments from the 1960s onward saw the meeting of notions from the human potential movement and transpersonal psychology with the developing New Age ideology to assure a revered place for shamans in New Age communities as 'one of the most integrated members of his or her community' (Frowen-Williams 1997, p.8). He identifies how music operates to create these altered states, defining the shaman's view of the origin of music: 'To the western mind music is essentially something created by man [sic], although it may be an unconscious process. For the shaman, music is something separate, a form of spiritual power that has an autonomous being apart from human minds' (p.51). Following on from this he describes the shaman's drum as a 'functional tool rather than a musical instrument as such':

> The drum is of prime importance in shamanic ceremony – it is the 'horse' or 'reindeer' upon which the shaman rides to the realms of the spirit. A most potent tool for bringing about ASC, the drum acts as a focus, creating an atmosphere of concentration, thereby allowing the shift of

attention from the everyday outer world to the inner world of the mind's eye. The lightness of trance characteristic of the SSC [shamanic state of consciousness] calls for the maintenance of a strong steady beat, without which the shaman might lose concentration and therefore fail in his or her mission. (p.52)

Research has already been cited in Chapter Three into the origin of the shamanic state of consciousness. In the New Age too it is often attributed to a combination of the shaman's psychic state and the effect of the drumming which is linked with 'delta' brain waves, neurological activity associated with

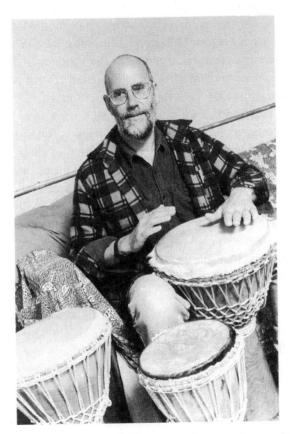

Figure 4.5 Chris Southall with the drums that he uses for trance dance and drumming the five rhythms (see pp.59–60)

dreaming. Frowen-Williams (1997) cites scientific research which says that drumming at a speed between 180 and 220 beats per minute can elicit states often deemed shamanic, including such features as:

- Sensations of flying and energy waves in the body
- A sense of energy
- Out-of-body experiences
- Imagery like journeying and meeting animals. (p.53)

Many of the shamanic ideas are drawn directly from the ideas explored in Chapter Three. So the drum is seen as a symbol derived from the World Tree, connecting the world of the spirit with the physical world. The New Age shaman will still sometimes make his own drum under spirit guidance, having reverence for the tree that provides the wood, acknowledging the animal whose skin makes the head and making offerings of food and song to the instrument. Along with the drum the rattle is also used. It too focuses attention and acts as a link with the natural world:

> The rattle is the shaman's other tool of choice. The technology is simple, yet the aural payoff is emotionally complex. Shake a rattle and you hear the rustle of the brush outside the fire circle, or the scrape of branches in the wind, or the dry warning cough of the rattlesnake. Its distinctive voice, full of high frequencies, is said to serve as a focusing device. (Hart and Lieberman 1991, p.130)

The shamanic songs are power songs and are

> usually simple and monotonous... Tempo increases as the shaman gets literally carried away and the relevant state is approached. Singing in this manner may affect the human organism in a manner similar to that of yogic breathing exercises. I have found singing a shamanic journey aloud 'solidifies' the experience, making it more vivid – it is as though one sings it into being. (Frowen-Williams 1997, p.57)

There is a powerful belief, founded in systems like that of the chakras and in the work of neo-shamans, that music can have a direct effect on bodily illness. Many claims are made on the efficacy of music to break up kidney stones, stimulate the immune system, cure (as well as prevent) cancers and prevent or relieve pain:

> In a 1984 paper delivered to the International Society of Music Medicine (Germany), he [Olav Skille] reported that a series of simple tones (a bass tone, then a fifth above, and then back to the bass tone), each played for five minutes, effectively treated the pain of such dis-ease as rheumatism, Bechterev's disease, and menstrual cramps...

> A medical machine invented in Germany, the lithotripter (literally meaning 'stone crusher') [is] designed to destroy kidney stones without surgery…The patient is placed in a large tub of water with the kidney area just above a 'belt' through which explosions of sound are aimed. Within these explosions are the frequencies, or vibrations, which duplicate the frequency of the kidney stone mass. Gallstones, too, may be pulverised by the lithotripter. (Gardner 1997, p.29)

This is founded on a strong belief of the relationship between sounds and the very essence of the material world: 'Sound reaches down to the cellular level. It is most likely that sound patterns are really the dance of molecules and atoms' (Dodd 1989, p.25).

Jonathan Goldman (1992) links sound with the crystal therapy so popular in New Age medicine. His theory of the link between sound and light develops this relationship further. He quotes from Marcel Vogel:

> The quartz crystal is an oscillator. You can tune it with pressure. You can cut it to a specific configuration so that when you tune it, it produces a sound that is subsonic. That sound induces luminescence in the body of an individual. It is cold light produced by an electronic vibration change. (p.144)

Such belief frames allow for the development of medical systems using sounds which have a bodily effect. Many of these are being developed. Some represent a fusion of scientific research with New Age thinking and therapies. This is clear in the work of the American acupuncturist Dr Robert Friedman, who has worked with Kelly Howell from the organisation Brain Sync to produce a series of tapes called *Sound Techniques for Healing.* These are designed to help with such diseases as arthritis, abnormal blood pressure, insomnia, headaches and depression. On these tapes he combines healing imagery with visualisation techniques to calm the energy in the nervous system and revitalise the circulation with guidance on how to apply finger pressure to acupressure points and sound waves designed to soothe away pain: 'Pure and precisely tuned frequencies combined with deeply relaxing music guide you into the euphoric theta state, releasing a rush of *endorphins* – your body's natural pain blocker and relaxant' (Friedman 1993).

Friedman recommends daily listening to the tape for six to eight weeks, and then as needed afterward. There is a warning not to use it while driving or operating machinery, that it is not a substitute for medical care and to stop using it if uncomfortable feelings are aroused. Here there is real faith in the power of sound to heal in the same way as conventional medication. It declares its scientific basis in terms of brain function:

> When pure precise audio signals of different frequencies are delivered to the brain through stereo headphones, the two hemispheres of the brain function together to 'hear' not the actual external sounds, but a phantom third signal – a *binaural beat.*

> EEG research results shows that parts of the brain begin to resonate sympathetically to this 'phantom' binaural beat, like a crystal goblet vibrates in response to a pure musical tone, in what is known as a *frequency following response...*

> The program uses *window frequencies.* Window frequencies are extremely precise frequencies that fit through narrow biological windows and have a direct effect on the cells, causing the release of healing-specific neurochemicals. (Friedman 1993)

Another system which uses the idea that sound waves directly affect the cell tissues of the body is Cymatics, developed by Dr Peter Guy Manners, a British osteopath. This involves the application of sound for bodily healing through the use of harmonically related tones. For Manners, disease is an 'out of tuneness' in some part of the body. The sounds resonate with particular parts of the body that are in imbalance and restore them to their natural frequency. He states:

> A healthy organ will have its molecules working together in a harmonious relationship with each other and will all be of the same pattern. If different sound patterns enter the organ, the harmonious relationship could be upset. If these frequencies are weak in their vibration, they will be overcome by the stronger vibrations of the native ones. If, on the other hand, the foreign ones prove to be stronger, they may establish their disharmonious pattern in the organ, bone, tissue, etc. and this is what we call disease.

> If therefore a treatment contains a harmonic frequency pattern that will reinforce the organs, the vibrations of the intruder will be neutralised and the correct pattern for that organ re-established. This should constitute a curative reaction. (Manners, quoted in Goldman 1992, pp.90–91)

To do this, he invented the Cymatic instrument, a machine which is capable of producing a huge range of composite harmonics designed for every organ of the body and many specific diseases including emotional problems and physical diseases such as anaemia, diabetes, sciatica, kidney disease and multiple sclerosis. The art is to find the right combination of sounds for the person and the disease. It is always a group of frequencies that are fed into the body. Some of these relate to the organ and others to the person him or herself. His system is based on research that he has carried out since 1961 on the effects of sound on body chemistry. Some of his sounds are worked out by scientific methods, but for others he uses radionics, which is based on the premise that everything radiates an energy. Although there is little scientific evidence for the efficacy of the therapy, there are many individuals who can point to healing by this method.

The French physician Alfred Tomatis (1991), who was the son of a French opera singer, developed a system based on his belief that some sounds cause fatigue in people while other sounds can energise them. His background was in otolaryngology and he had been working on the human ear. To the functions already discussed in Chapter One – that is, to keep the body in balance and also to process movements inside (cochlea) and outside the body (vestibular) – he adds that of charging the body with energy. His research revealed that sounds can charge the central nervous system and the cerebral cortex. The most famous story associated with him is that of a Benedictine monastery, which, following the reforms of the Second Vatican Council, discontinued its practice of chanting the Office. The monks became tired and depressed. Tomatis suggested that they reinstate their practice of Gregorian chanting and the health of the monks was restored. The reason for this, he states, is that Gregorian chants contain all the frequencies of the vocal spectrum – that is, from about 70 cycles per second to about 9000 cycles per second. He identified the effects of various frequencies in the range. Two thousand hertz, for example, will stimulate the resonance of the bones. He writes: 'The sound produced is not in the mouth, not in the body, but in fact, in the bones. It is all the bones in the body which are singing and it's like a vibrator exciting walls of the church which also sing' (Tomatis, quoted in Goldman 1992, p.76).

He regards the upper resonances as particularly beneficial and trains his clients to use the higher harmonics of their voice. He invented an 'electronic ear' which helps listeners hear high frequency sounds, an ability often lost in ageing. He recommends listening to carefully chosen sounds for four hours a day. You can also discover how to create your own sounds which will then be fed back through the electronic ear with timbre optimised to recharge the brain. Deficits in particular areas of the sound spectrum are identified and associated with particular disorders and traumas. He has successfully treated thousands of people including Maria Callas, Benjamino Gigli and Sting. He himself manages on little sleep, claiming that this is due to his practice of recharging his brain by using sounds. Goldman (1992) links the frequencies he uses to those used by Tibetan monks in overtone chanting. Tomatis went on to develop the theory to produce treatment programmes for the conditions of dyslexia, learning and hearing disorders, autism, pregnant women, musicians experiencing problems in performance and people suffering from depression, stress and anxiety. The theory includes that of one dominant and one passive ear which in right-handed people is the right ear, linked as it is with the left brain. His theory of dyslexia and stuttering is that such a clear dominance has not developed, leaving the brain unable to process information clearly. Another theory sees some children as 'listening-damaged'. Treatment for this replicates in audible form the situation in the womb four and a half months before birth when the auditory nerve is fully developed. This is used with insecure, anxious, aggressive, autistic and dyslexic children.

The link between embodiment and transcendence is worked out in many New Age traditions that link dance and movement with music. In shamanic work, ecstatic dance, like the drum, is a functional tool in the journeying technique. Gareth Frowen-Williams (1997) describes his own experience:

> Earlier this year I underwent a weekend of Terpsicore Trance therapy (TTT) with Leo Rutherford, one of Britain's leading shamanic practitioners. Based upon the Afro-Brazilian traditions of Candomble and Umbanda, TTT is a technique developed by Dr David Akstein and Dr Jacques Donnars. My induction into the trance-dance involved hyperventilating whilst Leo spun me round and round. It was an extraordinary experience and one I am unlikely to forget. The drums were pounding and I was spinning and jumping. It was like riding on a tidal wave of energy with nothing but a tiny rudder to guide me. I became a bird soaring in the heavens. I was filled with power and potential and then I was lying on the floor exhausted in a heap of perspiration. This was undoubtedly one of the most intense ASC's I have ever experienced. (p.58)

So the greater use of the body in the ASC intensifies it; the shamanic state is produced by a combination of music, psychological state, willingness and bodily activity. While the West discovers shamanism, it is declining in traditional societies. Neo-shamanism is in general regarded as different from traditional shamanism: 'Perhaps Shamanism in the west is more of a luxury than the necessary aid to survival of many traditional societies' (Hill, quoted in Frowen-Williams 1997, p.60). This is challenged by the psychologist Roger Walsh (1990) who postulates that human beings may have a need to enter altered states of consciousness. In this frame the New Age is making available to Western people an important area of human experience and teaching them how to handle it and interpret it.

Gabrielle Roth's (1992) development of the 'wave' and the five rhythms described above (see pp.182–183) is one of the most worked out of the systems using dancing and drumming in combination. She describes how, after an accident, she could no longer pursue the dance tradition she had experienced:

> It was devastating, but what kept me alive was my work with kids theatre and movement with therapy groups...What I had to figure out was how to seduce people into their own dance as I had no hope of teaching them the steps. How do you seduce a human being into their own brilliance? (p.2)

When she could dance again she found her approach had changed profoundly. The concentration on structural approaches to dance that she had learned gave way to trance-dance (in a way that echoes Chapter Three):

> I'd go off on these trance dance dreams. I wasn't controlling the dance – I was being danced...The dancer disappeared inside the dance and I'd find that divine part, divine spirit, the spark of infinite beat...Every time I was letting go of more and more, I was getting high and suddenly that released me from all drugs, from everything... I'd found the part of myself I had a desperate hunger for... This was my prayer. I was sweating my prayer. (p.2)

So, for her, the experience of transcendence is an embodied experience. The spirit is freed through the action of the body. For this reason, she strives to rectify the divorce of body and spirit through developing her dance form: 'The fastest way to still the mind is to move the body; the fastest way to open the heart is to move the body; and the fastest way to get into the soul power is to move the body' (p.3). She praises the adolescent dance culture in this respect:

> I have great hope for the next generation, the dance culture generation. They have the weight of the result of planetary unconsciousness on their shoulders. They can't hold all this in their bodies, so they dance because they have to. The dance gives them something to fall back on when it all falls apart... The traditional Church, combined with the 'powers that be', were obviously threatened by people reaching ecstatic states of consciousness ON THEIR OWN so they tried to wipe it out. (pp.3–4)

She sees dance as a safe womb-like state. The workshops that she runs are a way of protecting the form of her dance and provide a safe place for others' exploration. We see many of the themes of the New Age in this writing – the attitude to the Church, the notion of a safe place and the desire to unite body and spirit as in traditional cultures.

It has already been seen how popular chanting traditions are often associated with meditation in New Age groups. They are also associated with breathing techniques; indeed singing is a place where we take control of breathing, which is normally an involuntary activity. The uniting of music and breathing in simple exercises has been seen to have profound effects on very disturbed individuals:

> Meditative music, long sustained sounds, gentle movements or even a single note can be appreciated and accepted for the first time, even by the most rigidly intellectual or drug-saturated 'nit-wit', if only he gives in to the task of observing his own breathing: when it comes in, when it goes out, whether it is regular or restricted. Body-awareness is certainly a capability, or rather a gift, which is diametrically opposed to our competition-orientated upbringing... Ways need to be found...that will allow man [sic] to find his own vibration... (Hamel 1978, pp.174–175).

The chants are drawn from a variety of traditions. Hindu traditions have always seen the use of mantric syllables as a way of opening the chakras. Hamel quotes a mantric sequence from the Chandogya Upanishad that shows clearly how the transcendent and the material world are linked and relate back to the primeval sound of the universe – the OM:

> The essence of all beings is earth,
> The essence of earth is water,
> The essence of water is plants,
> The essence of plants is man,
> The essence of man is speech,
> The essence of speech is the Holy knowledge (Veda),
> The essence of Veda is Sama-Veda (word, tone, sound),
> The essence of Sama-Veda is OM. (quoted in Hamel 1978, p.111)

There is a revival of an interest in Gregorian traditions (see Tomatis, above) and the popularity of the chants of Hildegard of Bingen (1098–1179) reflects their capacity to induce transcendent experiences. The practice of overtone chanting has been adapted from traditions found among Tibetan monks. The practice is one of singing one note while changing the shape of the vocal cavities so that the different harmonics are accentuated. This gives the impression that two notes are being sung simultaneously. Goldman (1992) calls it a 'one voice chord'. Dr Huston Smith reported on the Gyume and Gyote monks in the film *Requiem for a Faith*:

> They discovered ways, we still don't know how, of shaping their vocal cavities to resonate overtones to the point where these became audible as distinct tones in their own right. So each lama thus trained could sing chords by themselves. They are singing D, F# and A simultaneously. The religious significance of this phenomenon derives from the fact that overtones awaken numinous fields, sensed without being explicitly heard. They stand in exactly the same relationship to our hearing as the sacred stands to our ordinary mundane lives. (Smith, quoted in Goldman 1992, p.66)

There are groups of overtone chanters meeting regularly with spiritual and healing intentions. Jill Purce runs regular workshops helping people to develop the technique for their own healing, which include group overtone chanting as well as a range of vocal techniques to connect with oneself, with others and with the cosmos.

> There is a profound sense of disenchantment in Western society. I think this is because, quite literally, there is no chant in our lives anymore. All the situations in which members of traditional cultures came together to chant have been eroded away, so we fell disempowered and helpless in a desacralized world. My aim is to re-enchant the world, to make it more magical through people chanting together again. The workshop gives us a real sense of what a literally enchanted community could be like. (Purce 1998)

Other chants are taken from indigenous traditions, particularly those of native Americans. The use of these repeated chants is also designed to encourage transcendence.

Many of the traditions are tightly linked with mystical traditions and present themselves as the rediscovery of traditions of ancient wisdom. One of these is the Kabbala, the Jewish mystical tradition. This is based on a mystical diagram called the Tree of Life. The various points on this have been associated with different vowels. From it, Israel Regardie developed a system called tonal chanting. In this he toned the 'God names' in a way that reinforced the harmonics: 'There are certain sacred names associated with specific spheres. These are names which, chanted like a mantra, will cause the reciter to resonate to the frequency of the sphere. This is another aspect of sacred sonic entrainment similar to the practices of tantra utilised by the Tibetan monks...' (quoted in Goldman 1992, p.42).

Summary – embodiment/transcendence

The New Age has well-developed systems for balancing the embodiment/transcendence polarity drawn from a number of different traditions. Steiner's notions of physical, astral and etheric body are used by some practitioners but more common is the notion of the chakras. There are many systems relating these to music and sound is seen as important in healing any imbalance in one of them, which is seen as the origin of physical disease. These techniques include the use of pitches, colours, vowel sounds, mantric syllables and chants from a variety of traditions. Breathing techniques and movement are often used with chanting to enter meditative states. A belief that sound has a powerful effect on the body has led to the development of techniques like Cymatics using vibrations of various frequencies to treat bodily illness and the wide-ranging systems of Alfred Tomatis treating a variety of disorders through enhancing the energy of the brain.

Summary

The New Age is a many faceted collection of traditions that has drawn on a variety of sources – both ancient and modern – to balance contemporary trends such as elitism, commercialism, materialism, racism and sexism. It has produced a variety of musical practices, many of them syntheses of ancient traditions and contemporary ideas. Communal music-making can represent healing at a personal, ecological and cosmic level. The interconnectedness of the cosmos can be accessed and expressed in music. There is a stress on the discovery of 'natural sounds' including those from the natural world which are included on recordings with human sounds. These represent freedom from the restraints of the Western classical tradition and the amplified sounds of popular music. In making this music, a 'true energy' is discovered which will connect the soul to the universe and so produce healing effects. There is a belief in the journey of the individual soul associated with re-incarnational belief systems. However, the task of this soul or higher self is to express the energy of the cosmos, which results in a close link between meditative practices and music. Here the stress is on the process of music-making or listening, the meaning of which is often construed as cosmic rather than as solely personal or communal. There is a powerful sense of a need to create unity and the true self is seen as united within its true energy. However, there is a real notion of an acceptance and respect for diversity within a cosmic whole.

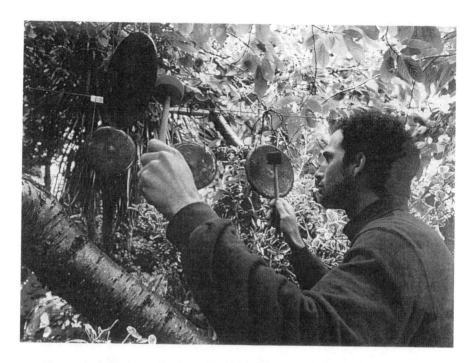

Figure 4.6 Soundscape work using gongs and Tibetan bowls
Reproduced courtesy of the Tonalis Centre for the Study and Development of Music

Nurturing music is favoured above challenging music which is sometimes regarded as intrinsically evil. This leads to a predominance of softer and concordant sounds, a re-valuing of melodic traditions and a preference for calming timbres. Chanting and repetitive patterns are often seen as a way of nurturing people and enabling them to find a sense of empowerment. The sense of the transcendent dominates the traditions although this can be linked with a variety of mystical traditions or a syncretic belief system. The notion of chakras is widely used to link the transcendent with the body. These can be opened and 'treated' musically by means of various forms of chanting including overtone chanting, the use of vowel sounds and mantric syllables. Because of the overarching belief of the effect of music on matter, systems for treating the body using sound have been developed. Breathing and movement are also combined with music to produce transcendent states which are regarded as intrinsically healing.

The New Age has developed healing systems within the context of a strong sense of the spiritual. It can be understood as balancing the dominant classical and popular traditions of the West, which it does by drawing on ancient wisdoms and the practices described in Chapter Three. These take on a different character in the context of a culture which has no shared value systems. It can be seen as an entry point and testing ground for new ideas which are later adopted by classical and rock traditions and music therapists. It is often combined with other holistic therapies. The various worldviews that make it up attempt to contain notions of individuality and diversity within an overall cosmic scheme.

CHAPTER FIVE

Of Doctors and Therapists

'Old Harry's Game'

In this popular drama on the UK's Radio 4, Satan is training a young devil called Scumspawn in hell. Scumspawn calls him up, saying that there is a problem in the Reception Pit. 'Master, we need your wisdom and experience!' When Satan responds, Scumspawn explains that following a gas explosion at the Grand Ole Opry, they have taken unexpected delivery of a country and western band. 'Obviously we set about giving them their introductory scourging but now we are in trouble, because every time we subject them to more suffering and pain...they just write a song about it.' In the background the country and western band are singing

> We're standing in a lake of fire
> And the flames are a-getting higher

'You see how horrendous it is,' says Scumspawn. 'At the moment they're stuck for a rhyme for "inferno", but it's only a brief respite.' Satan responds with offering the help of his new assistant, Nero. Scumspawn protests: 'But he is a mere mortal.' Nero retorts that actually he is a god. At this Satan is cross: ' No, you're not actually a god, Nero.' Nero protests: 'I am a god. The Senate declared me a god.' Satan invalidates this claim by retorting that his status was only given by a certificate from a bunch of fat Italians wearing sheets. Nonetheless he dispatches Nero to deal with Scumspawn's problem. 'Any idea how you're going to deal with it?' ' Simple' says Nero. 'I shall just remove their vocal chords.' Satan praises Nero's natural aptitude for his devilish role. 'You can't teach that. Logic combined with sadism.' Scumspawn protests that the other demons will not be very keen on obeying a mortal. The female singer of the country and western band embarks on a singalong song about her 'D-I-V-O-R-C-E' becoming final today. Other souls in hell join in with 'Me and little J-O-E'.

She continues:

Will be going away
I love you both and this will be
Sheer H-E-doubleL for me.
I wish that we could stop this D-I-Eurgh!

Nero has succeeded in his task and the singing stops (based on Hamilton 1998).

I use this story from a comedy radio play because deep in music therapy is the notion that somehow suffering can find an expression in music and that it can be used to overcome obstacles. Here, people are in hell and some would see the unconscious at least as some form of personal Underworld (in some cases, a place of torment where personal demons need a measure of exorcism!). The central tenet of music therapy is that 'the music is not an end in itself but is used as a means to an end' (Bunt 1994, p.8).

This chapter will concern itself with associations between music and healing that have found a place in mainstream Western medicine. Most significant of these is music therapy. The development of music therapy in the UK is charted by Leslie Bunt at the beginning of his seminal book *Music Therapy – An Art beyond Words* (1994). Before the twentieth century, music had been used for of its sedative and stimulating effects on patients. In 1891 the Guild of St Cecilia was founded by Canon Harford to explore the use of music in medicine. Although it was supported by prominent figures including Florence Nightingale it attracted considerable criticism from the mainstream medical press. This was followed by its use as a morale-booster and a way of occupying patients. In the US the main thrust of the development occurred after World War II, where the medical authorities wanted to meet the challenge of the returning veterans. The evidence on which the work was based in the 1940s and 1950s was largely anecdotal.

In the UK it was pioneered in the 1950s and 1960s by Juliette Alvin, a concert cellist and teacher. It was used in two main areas:

- for adults with learning disabilities (previously designated 'mentally handicapped')

- for adults with mental health problems, falling under the auspices of adult psychiatry.

To these were added as the work developed:

- children with learning disabilities, physical disabilities and mental health problems
- adults with neurological problems
- adult offenders
- hospice residents
- care of cancer patients
- people with HIV and AIDS
- survivors of sexual abuse
- pre-school assessment centres and day nurseries
- special schools
- day centres, hospital and residential homes for the elderly
- people with chronic difficulties in communication.

Because of this wide range of contexts the practice became underpinned by ideas from a variety of sources. Some (and this is particularly true of the US) of these ideas owe a great deal to medical models, drawing on developments in physiology and neurosurgery. Another strand drew on developments in psychotherapy (following Freud, Jung and their successors). This is reflected in this quotation from Hanne Mette Kortegaard (1993): 'The function of the music in music psychotherapy is to provide a space for the exploration of feelings attached to transference, countertransference and the new symbols created through the therapeutic relationship' (p.60).

This highlights an important difference between music therapy and classic psychoanalysis. There has always been in the concept of music therapy the notion of a relationship in which the therapist necessarily plays an active part. Indeed many interpret the meaning of the music in the therapeutic encounter in terms of this relationship (Pavlicevic 1997).

In contrast to this, other therapists rooted their work in behaviour therapy. Because this proved easier to assess and monitor, this was an important strand in the 1950s, 1960s and 1970s; in the US, music therapy found its place in the behavioural sciences. The development of humanistic psychology from the work of Carl Rogers (see Chapter One) provided a middle way between the two poles of analytical and behaviourist frames. The stress was on the therapeutic relationship and such qualities as empathy, acceptance and genuineness with the end goal of 'helping individuals to realise their potentials' (Feder and Feder 1981, p.43). The ideas influenced the work of Paul Nordoff and Clive Robbins (Nordoff and Robbins 1977; Robbins 1993). In the 1960s and 1970s the developing cognitively based therapists and work on the mother–infant relationship influenced the work, especially with children.

There is a call today for more eclecticism and a greater degree of openness. The profession is now better established in mainstream medical practice with accepted job structures for music therapists. It no longer needs to establish its credibility by means of discrediting some work as 'too deterministic or, contrarily, too vague' (Aldridge 1996, p.10). Music therapy is now drawing on a variety of sources: 'It is, therefore, essential to accept, and more, respect the diversity of viewpoints and approaches among music therapists. It is mandatory to get beyond individual prejudices' (Robbins 1993, p.7).

Cheryl Dileo Maranto (1993) lists a whole range of techniques for use in music and medicine to be added to traditional therapeutic techniques (some drawing on the New Age techniques outlined in Chapter Four):

- Music listening
- Music vibroacoustic therapy
- Toning
- Entrainment
- Music-elicited imagery
- Music and directed imagery
- Guided imagery and music
- Music and verbal relaxation methods
- Music and biofeedback. (Maranto 1993, pp.164–167)

There is also an increasing literature associated with general rather than psychiatric medicine. This has much to say on the calming effect of music and also of music as an alternative to technological or medication-based approaches. The involvement of community musicians in the health services is also developing.

Aldridge (1996) develops the notion of an 'ecology' of ideas and calls for orthodox and complementary medicines to work together for a medical model that 'considers the whole person' (p.8). The sources for these ideas he identifies as 'colleagues, both near and distant, patients, students and hospital practitioners' (p.8). It is significant that his own practice is in the context of a

German hospital based on the anthroposophical principles of Rudolf Steiner (see Chapter Four). He describes his own approach as developed from the Nordoff–Robbins (1977) approach:

> It is an approach…that actively involves the patient in making music creatively. The therapist encourages the patient to improvise music using percussion and tuned percussion instruments, by singing with the patient, and by encouraging the patient to play with the therapist at the piano. No attempt is made to interpret the music psychotherapeutically. The process of creatively improvising music, and the development of a musical relationship between therapist and patient are seen as the vehicles of therapy. Visual arts and eurhythmy are also practised within this hospital. Health is seen as an activity that occurs within an environment of creativity. (Aldridge 1996, p.9)

The stress on an active approach, the limited use of words and the special relationship are found in much of the literature. He links health with creativity: 'What emerged was the idea that in music therapy, being creative may not have anything to do with the illness, but it may have something very important to do with regaining health. Categories of illness were going to tell us little about becoming healthy' (Aldridge 1996, p.11).

The earliest models were drawn from psychotherapy. In individual work the normal pattern was of a confidential one-to-one relationship between client and therapist. Just as analytical techniques owed a great deal to Freud's technique of free association, so music therapy was based on improvisation on the part of both therapist and client which was the musical equivalent of free association: 'Music improvisation offers a free-flowing awareness, in contrast to the focused awareness in verbal dialogue' (Kortegaard 1993, p.61). The ability to improvise at the piano is still an important prerequisite of much music therapy training. In group work, too, improvisation is the central technique.

Because the profession is relatively young, there are still many debates about the nature of the profession and, indeed, the nature of music therapy itself. Leslie Bunt (1994) selects three of these as containing crucial constructs:

- Music therapy is a systematic process of intervention wherein the therapist helps the client to achieve health, using musical experiences and the relationship that develops through them as dynamic forces of change. (Bruscia 1987, p.47)

- Music therapy provides a framework in which a mutual relationship is set up between client and therapist. The growing relationship enables changes to occur, both in the conditions of the client and in the form that the therapy takes... By using music creatively in a clinical setting, the therapist seeks to establish an interaction, a shared musical experience leading to the pursuit of therapeutic goals. (Association of Professional Music Therapists 1990)

- Music therapy is the use of sounds and music within an evolving relationship between client and therapist to support and encourage physical, mental, social and emotional well being (Bunt 1994, p.8).

There is a concern that music therapy should develop its own research methodology. Summarising music therapy research, Josee Raijmaekers (1993) claims that the research has focused on the three areas of emotion, cognition and communication.

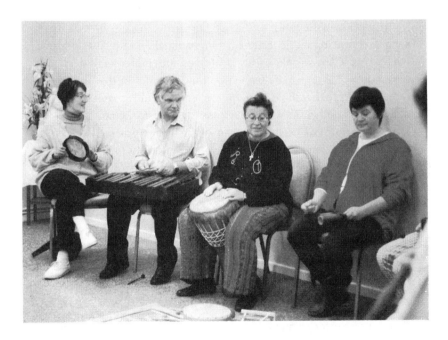

Figure 5.1 Sharing sounds

Therapists vary in their opinions on how far the music needs to be interpreted in words. This is sometimes linked with the rediscovery of memories central to some schools of psychoanalysis: 'Music therapy offers a particularly potent modality for bringing children's musical memories into expression and communication' (Robbins 1993, p.14).

Now more group practices are employed using a wider variety of musical activities. Denise Erdonmez (1993) attempts to classify these by using Gardner's (1982) analysis of tasks as top-down or bottom-up processes:

> Tasks which involve a wholistic approach to music (basic perceptual, responsive tasks) can be termed top-down tasks, in that they work from a global perspective. Improvisation is one method we use in music therapy...and so do other music therapy methods where there are no directives or instructions, and where the 'gestalt' of the experience is of paramount importance.
>
> Consider a group improvisation session where there are no directions, no instructions, and where clients are free to explore not only the music sound, but the musical and non-musical interrelationship with others in the group. There are no analytical processes here, but there is an enriched 'gestalt' experience.
>
> In specific music tasks, such as asking clients to sing the melody of songs, sequencing music material and rehabilitation of piano skills in a client post-CVA (stroke), the strategies are more analytical and demanding. These may be termed bottom-up tasks, in that they work from specifics to the whole. We require clients to build up, as it were, from one skill to another. As we set our aims for a music therapy session (or series of sessions) we need to be aware of the hierarchical nature of skills. If we take our client's pre-morbid level of musicality into account, we might more accurately gauge the higher potential of some clients. (Erdonmez 1993, p.123)

This highlights how early music therapy started with top-down tasks, holistic in concept. As therapy moves to include more bottom-up tasks, it moves more into an area that was once the province of education.

It is also important to remember that, in general, the musical experience of the founders of the movement was in the Western classical tradition. Clive Robbins (1993), placing music therapy in the history of music, writes:

> Throughout history mankind [sic] has created music for self-expression, for socio-political and religious rituals, and for artistic and cultural experience... Now, in music therapy, there is a new purpose – the contemporary act of music being created specifically to influence an individual's condition or state... The conclusion is inevitable: here in this individualised realisation of music is the next stage in the evolution of the deepening relationship between mankind [sic] and music. I venture to assert that

much of the essential value of the role of music in human life in the future will be the creative realisation of music in therapy. (p.8)

He is clearly here referring to Western music and ignoring the shamanic and spirit possession traditions described in Chapter Three. It is clear that the thinking in music therapy is related to the dominant Western classical tradition and Western medical models which tend to concentrate on the mind and body and exclude a spiritual dimension.

To summarise, music therapy has developed gradually in the twentieth century. The early work was with people with learning disabilities and psychiatric problems. Initially it drew on the models established in psychotherapy. Patient and therapist interacted in a one-to-one confidential relationship by means of musical improvisation. The ability to improvise at the piano is central to music therapy practice. Behaviourist techniques found favour because the effects were easily measurable and satisfied an increasing demand for research to justify the area. To these two schools of psychology were added notions drawn from the development of the humanistic psychology of Carl Rogers. This led to the wider use of group work. The profession is now better established with a pay and career structure, and techniques are now drawn from a wide variety of sources including the practices of the New Age. However, these concentrate on the areas of body and mind and the practices are usually stripped of their spiritual dimension. There is more interest in applications for music in general medicine and the use of community music agencies in health care.

Community/individualism

In this section I shall examine the notion of community in terms of relationship through music-making and how this relates to individual well-being. 'The general objective of music therapy is to give all patients an opportunity for communication and socialisation' (Berruti et al. 1993, p.66). Such statements are common in the literature. Because of the already-constructed models of psychotherapy, the early setting for music therapy was often a one-to-one situation with a music therapist relating to the client by means of music, largely through the medium of piano improvisation: 'In the early days of training, there was no reference to groups, other than more formal groups such as choirs. Our only experience of being in a group was the classes in movement and improvisation' (Towse and Flower 1993, p.74).

There was a powerful sense of relationship between the therapist and client but it was a closed and confidential one like the relationship between the patient and the psychoanalyst. There is within music therapy, however, a far greater sense of relationship than in the harder, psychoanalytical talking traditions. The use of music with two people improvising together encourages a greater degree of intimacy than is possible through the essentially sequential medium of words.

Deep in the Jungian concept of the personality is the notion of individuation. The process leading to individuation is carried out internally and in response to internal threats and opportunities. The journey is to the subconscious and unconscious with a view to finding a real self, freed from the neuroses created by early traumas. However, there was also in the Jungian system the notion of the universal unconscious and the utilisation of images and symbols which were viewed by Jung as being of a transcultural nature (Jung 1964b). Within the Jungian philosophy there was a great sense of becoming a unique person within the context of culture.

Part of this process is the establishment of boundaries, knowing the limits and the edges of the person and being able to distinguish these from those of other people. The very structure of the profession – exposed to the dangers of sitting alone in close dialogue with a client who is very 'sick' – led the therapeutic world to develop this concept as much for the safety of the therapists as for that of their patients. The notion of the individual journey is still quite strong. This can lead to the breaking up of existing relationships, where individual selfhood cannot be achieved, and the establishment of self-sufficiency. Had the models developed with a greater stress on community involvement, it is debatable whether the emphasis on the individual journey would have been so great.

However, isolation is often a cause and symptom of mental illness, and the task of a music therapist is to create a sense of belonging. Group work is now better established and lays great stress on musical interaction:

> Music is very much a social act: people can listen, imitate, learn from each other, even trying out and discarding different styles of interacting. Alternative ways of behaving can be explored in the safety of the musical setting... Each member can begin to find an individual place and role in the group and to explore ways of feeling increasingly comfortable in relating to others... Many observers, even of one session, comment on the fact that music can quite quickly bring people together and provide a sense of group cohesion, a sense of immediate belonging. People appear to be attracted to music and will stay with it for quite some time before becoming overwhelmed or satiated. We may not need to draw attention to this verbally, as in the cohesive silences that often bind people together

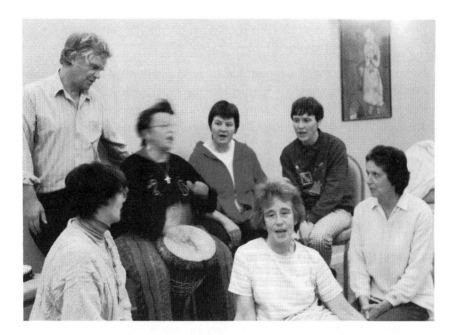

Figure 5.2 Creating community, with the author playing the drums

at the end of a shared musical experience. Whether we listen to music or make music together, the very structure of organised sounds themselves provides a unique opportunity for such integration. (Bunt 1994, pp.27–28)

From such writing we can see quite clearly the subtlety of the relationships encouraged by group improvisation.

As part of his series of television programmes on *Music and the Mind*, Paul Robertson (1996) plays an impressive videotape of Paul Nordoff working with an autistic boy. Initially the boy was only able to produce screams and shouts. By working with these (starting where the boy was) Nordoff is able by the end to enter into an impressive musical dialogue with a sharing of musical ideas.

Used in group sessions, the creation of community is often regarded as central to the therapy. Amelia Oldfield (1993) writes of working with families:

Each family member is 'equal' in this activity and the usual conflicts regarding control can temporarily be laid aside... It usually helps parents to focus on one or two areas of difficulty, such as controlling aggressive behaviour, giving their children more praise, allowing themselves to relax and improvise with their children or dividing attention between several siblings. (pp.49–50)

Work with a patient with symptoms of anorexia was developed to encourage 'a balanced human contact' that includes the experiencing of equality and the giving of feedback on the contact. Music is viewed as a more subtle way of relating than words, the use of which should be limited (Oldfield 1993, pp.49–50).

David Aldridge (1996) links therapy with social concerns:

The European tradition influenced Western post-war culture both in the arts and psychotherapy. Such a culture has emphasised the individual as self and recognised a need for personal expression. What we are attempting to address in our work is the existential quality of the arts where the self finds expression. This stands in contrast to the scientific movement which seeks to understand the individual according to the group. However, as we know from twentieth century history, the cultural tradition that enlivens self-expression can be used for good or evil. The expression of the self unfettered by social concerns can lead to tyranny. So too, the music therapist who says listen to my work as a work of art alone, without concern for its clinical relevance, imposes an individual tyranny apart from indulging in solipsism. (p.17)

In one-to-one therapy, the notion of a musical relationship between therapist and client is central to much of the writing about music therapy. Here the individuation of therapist and the patient are seen as important:

The development of the patient and the self-realisation of the therapist are symmetrical phenomena. Only insofar as the psychotherapist by her meeting with her patient is capable of moving towards her own individuation, will the patient be put in the position of establishing a world in communion with her psychotherapeutic partner. (Benedetti, quoted in Kortegaard 1993, p.62)

The establishment of 'communication' between therapist and client is essential to the efficacy of the therapy. This is done by means of the process of 'interactional synchrony' (Condon 1980) which characterises normal human communication. As rhythm is the way in which this synchrony is organised, music has a very special role to play. Aldridge (1996) also refers to the centrality of phrasing:

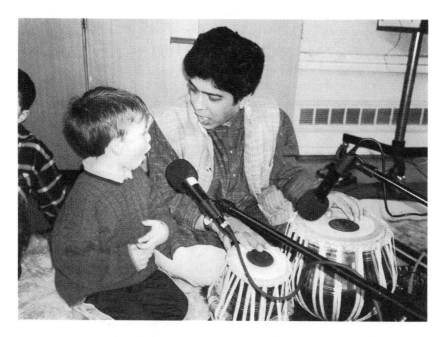

Figure 5.3 Indian music being used to encourage health
Reproduced courtesy of the Gurukul Institute of Indian Classical Music

A central feature of both musical and biological form is phrasing. When we speak in dialogues then we must know when a phrase is ending, and how to begin another. This occurs in speech by accented differences in a rhythmic context... Synchronisation is achieved by a shared interaction in a rhythmic context known to both participants. (p.55)

This has been particularly important in work with autism, which can be described as a state of self-absorption. People's innate musical ability has been used by many therapists to encourage essentially isolated individuals relate to the wider community (Temmingh 1998).

The relationship of GPs (general practitioners) to the wider community is beginning to include music. A pioneer in this area is Dr Malcolm Rigler. His experiences as a doctor in the centre of Birmingham enabled him to see that health for his patients could only be achieved in the context of a healthy community. When he started in a new practice in Withymoor, West Midlands, in the early 1980s he initiated ten years of community arts projects, including transforming the waiting room at his surgery into an arts activity area (Rigler 1998).

Two GPs in Gosforth, Newcastle, Dr Anand and Anthea Anand, have established Gurukul, The Arts for Health Project. This teaches Indian classical music through performances, workshops and lessons which take place in community venues and schools. It draws on the relationship within Indian traditions between the cycles and rhythms of nature and healing, commending its spontaneous and unwritten nature. The weekly workshops have two elements:

- The teaching of a holistic approach to health. This includes stress, the mind–body connection, the meaning of illness, methods of self-help and the place of arts in this.

- A practical interactive drop-in workshop for you personally to learn to express your feelings and relax through the much forgotten instrument – your voice.[1]

Healing Arts on the Isle of Wight provides arts programmes in St Mary's Hospital. The director, Guy Eades, is unhappy with the notion of 'disability', with its individualistic focus, and has established links with the Isle of Wight's Quay Arts Centre to allow people to move more easily between the health-care world and the arts world. He co-ordinates a programme of performance arts at St Mary's and 11 other venues within the island's community health services. These include weekly music reminiscence sessions and music performances. 'Art is all about communication – people being able to say things they haven't otherwise found a way of expressing.'[2]

In New Zealand, the Arts Access Aoteroa Trust is using arts to help sick people re-integrate into the community. It has initiated a programme of creative spaces for people with psychiatric and intellectual disabilities. The first two were set up in 1986, one in a psychiatric hospital and one for patients moving from a psychiatric hospital into the community. In the Starship Children Hospital in Auckland:

Children are encouraged to use creativity to personalise their own space in hospital. Donated pillowcases are painted with permanent fabric paint, and artwork is displayed on notice boards above the child's bed. This provides the child with a sense of belonging and positive self-esteem...

1   From Gurukul publicity leaflet 1999.
2   From Healing Arts publicity leaflet 1998.

Music sessions are also a regular feature of the programme and occur spontaneously. Children and their families are invited to share ideas about how these sessions develop. Recorded music from a variety of cultures is provided for familiarity and to introduce children to new sounds. (Sarah McDonald, hospital play specialist, quoted in Eames 1999, pp.22–23)

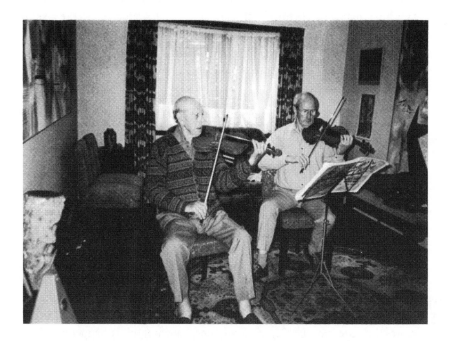

Figure 5.4 Eric Lawson (former deputy leader of New Zealand Symphony Orchestra, 1948–1971), now 94 and blind, plays with John Dodds, a recently retired member of the NZSO.
Reproduced by kind permission of Arts Access Aoteroa

Summary – community/individualisation

Although one-to-one situations characterised early music therapy practice, the use of the group is now well-established. Even in one-to-one practice, relationship through music is regarded as central. However, the very fact that the work, in the context of Western society, is often located in separate institutions such as hospitals means that issues of relationship with the wider society are problematic. There are an increasing number of arts schemes starting to address this split.

Containment/freedom

These two meet in a real partnership in the work of music therapy. The background of the early music therapists was in the classical tradition; this is also the situation for most of their client group because of the way music education is constructed. Because of this, early music therapy was conceived of as being a freeing from a tradition. The stress was laid heavily on improvisation and, moreover, not on improvisation within a particular set tradition, but within whatever style the client seemed to lean towards. It was the task of the good music therapist to be able to follow the patient and, to some extent, to lead the patient in any path. This account illustrates well the need of the therapist to respond and adapt the improvisation to the minutest of changes in the client's performance:

> I am in the middle of an improvisation with Noel, an artist who has come for six music therapy sessions to help him to 'loosen up'. Noel is surrounded by the temple blocks, bass and conga drums, two cymbals and bongos, as well as marimba and xylophone. His playing is busy, rapid and 'tight', and my own spontaneous playing at the piano meets and reflects his 'tight busy-ness'. I listen to his ongoing rhythmic play, his small melodies, made up mostly of adjacent notes on the marimba, going up and down, up and down. I listen for change. For three sessions we have been playing this tight busy-ness, and my musical and interactive expectations are all but hypnotised...
>
> Something changes, he extends the (monotonous) rhythm, and at the same time he does an interval leap instead of the preceding adjacent notes. My attention is caught. Something 'meaningful' is happening. I not only think it, I feel it. I have a flush of excitement, because even though I have been waiting, what Noel does is unexpected, and our joint spontaneous playing can begin to move on. My change in level of arousal is triggered by something within the music – it has to do with the change of rhythm, the melodic leap, and the succeeding gradual build-up in intensity. (Pavlicevic 1997, p.18)

Such a passage has no sense within it of a pre-set system, a pre-set tradition to which the two participants conform. The emphasis is on the ability of the client to be free and (perhaps more important) the ability of the therapist to respond to that freedom with subtlety, using any appropriate style. This section of a session with John, a three-and-a-half-year-old boy with talking difficulties, shows the therapist struggling to find an appropriate style:

John comes in, moves quickly to the drum and cymbal, takes up the drumsticks that I offer him and starts to play. The contact with the instruments is immediate. He plays in short, sharp loud bursts of sound. I explore on the piano a variety of musical ideas and try and match some of the excitement and energy that he is generating. I am trying to find some point of contact and to meet these short bursts of expressive energy… Music based on alternating intervals of fourths and fifths in the bass with clear, short melodies that I play or sing seems to attract his attention and to support and sustain his drumming. (Bunt 1994, p.18)

There is a clear sense here that it is the responsibility of the therapist to find the musical structures that are most able to contain the ideas of the client. Indeed the training of the therapist is in this intuitive grasp of musical structure: they must learn to trust their own feelings and their grasp of musical structure. All music therapists need musical training or experience of some kind, for it is on this that they will draw. This could be likened to the traditional healer learning the melodies of the various spirits as discussed in Chapter Three.

Leslie Bunt (1994) stresses the importance of the clients' desire to make their own choices:

Of all the elements timbre seems to have a direct associative potential… What this element does teach us is that in therapy people of all ages are disturbed by imposed choice. People have a right to explore a range of musical sounds and experiences for themselves… As music therapists we are in a privileged position to observe other people's choices…offering people a range of choices, so that preferences can be observed, does take time, often a great deal of time, and patience. (p.50)

However, drawing on work with an anorexic patient, the therapists Henk Smeijsters and Jose van den Hurk (1993) construct a list of guidelines to encourage or check the expression of anger:

- Continue the release until the anger has 'worn off', which means that vehemence is passing over – audible in dynamics, rhythm and tempo – and that a balance between musical tension and relief develops after not too long a period (at any rate within one session).

- In case the vehemence does not pass over, and one can expect the released anger to escalate and degenerate into uncontrolled regressive behaviour, this release should be stopped by guiding the musical play into another direction. Should this fail, then have the client stop playing the instrument concerned and offer another one.

- After the process of release, stimulate the client in 'knowing where to draw the line'. This is releasing oneself without having an uncontrolled breakdown, by keeping one's playing within bounds. For this purpose, offer work situations that include elements of structured release. Work situations in which elements of form, characterised by musical tension and relief, alternate with each other.

- Stop using release if it does not increase the understanding in relation to experiences and feelings (if the release does not produce new material). (pp.355–356)

Here we see a mixture of musical and some non-musical techniques for containing potentially destructive emotions. The notion of musical form is seen here as connected with containment and this is also allied with the associations of some instruments. Guidance is also given as to how to read the presence of anger in the music.

There is in the literature on music therapy almost an accepted sense that the art forms are able to contain potentially destructive emotions. This is why a number of doctors who have used verbal therapy are turning to the arts. In the analytical systems there is a sense in which the powerful emotions aroused cannot always be contained in words. Unless there is some way of expressing the powerful (often infantile) emotions safely, the client is at more risk than before. Later developments have taken the role of the arts very seriously for this reason.

Freud's notion of sublimation is also present in some therapeutic writing about the process of musical creativity in this area: 'Music is a third step in the therapeutic relationship which carries part of the unbearable burden of emotions, making some of them more acceptable by sublimation to a musical creation' (Priestley, quoted in De Backer 1993, p.36). The containment is sometimes seen in non-musical terms. The music-making may be free but the surrounds of therapy sessions are always tightly held. Bunt (1994) describes the setting up of a group session in an acute admissions ward in a psychiatric unit in a general hospital:

Some musical structures will be set up, in the hope of providing a sense of security. But within such structures there is freedom to improvise and explore... Boundaries are established at the start of the group. The group is scheduled to run for an hour and a quarter and people are free to come and go as they wish. (p.23)

Jos De Backer (1993) entitles his chapter on his work with an ego-weak boy called David 'Containment in music therapy'. The containment is a result of the process of projecting his chaotic feelings onto the therapist which enables him to bear them (projective identification). It takes away the defence he has constructed in silence and the therapist is able to respond through music: 'He will, as it were, stretch a skin over the patient's experience – an acoustic skin – which binds and shapes the expression of chaos' (p.36). The fact that the therapist is improvising with the patient means that someone is helping bear his difficult and painful experiences. De Backer describes the therapist as acting as a 'psychic container' for the patient and says that in group therapy both therapist and group act as a container together. This notion is found in much of the literature. In developing this, Gianluigi di Franco (1993) links the lack of containment of painful feelings, which characterises the psychotic patients with whom he works, with a model of the physiological structure of cells. The healthy cell has a structure in which the membrane contains the nucleus and its sub-nuclei, whereas in the pathological cell the sub-nuclei are no longer contained by the nuclear membrane.

A group of Italian music therapists use listening as a way of freeing painful memories in psychotic patients: 'During one session the listening caused a fit of discomfort and the patient asked to interrupt the listening. The melancholy melody of the excerpt had aroused in Paola memories related to her tragic childhood and strong emotions' (Berruti *et al.* 1993, p.71).

Claire Flower (1993) describes how music was used with a group of adolescents in special care who needed to take control of their lives. She adopted a non-directive approach which enabled the clients to make choices musically and in other ways. Many of the clients in therapy have a sense of being trapped and one of the 'curative factors' of the therapeutic session highlighted by Irvin Yalom (1985) is the installation of hope. This is done musically by the abandonment of a sense of right and wrong responses and encouragement to 'play' in a secure environment.

Work with patients with Alzheimer's disease shows how people can be freed from the limitations of their diminishing world:

As their lives seem to ebb away, and their faculties fade, music appears to be a ray of light in their dimming world. It beckons them slowly out of their anguish, out of their 'absences'. It touches them, and gently nudges them into song, speech, movement, moments of alertness, peace and pleasure. When caught in their frantic, rapid shuffling along the corridors, it slows them down to a comfortable pace. When their joints and limbs seem to freeze and block, music brings about a thaw. It gives them glimpses of the past, as memories emerge, prompted by songs, sound and rhythms. (Gaertner 1998)

Summary – containment/freedom

In music therapy freer structures have been developed than those of the Western classical or popular traditions. Free improvisation, tailor-made to the needs of a particular client, has been the core skill developed by music therapists. Music is seen as being able to contain potentially destructive emotions as well as release difficult memories. This can be done in individual and group situations where the music of others is seen as a container for the emotions of a client. However, structures, both musical and extra-musical, have been developed that provide limits.

Expression/confidentiality

This section will examine how the notion of expression in a confidential situation is worked out in music therapy. Self-expression is central to music therapy. One might say that the whole of therapeutic 'industry' of the twentieth century is based on the old adage that 'a trouble shared is a trouble halved'. One of Yalom's (1985) 'curative factors' in group psychotherapy is catharsis. Bunt (1994) confirms how central this is to music therapy:

> Cathartic moments are a clear feature of making music and are very likely to occur in moments of free improvisation... Group members can learn how to channel and express such feelings in constructive ways, supported by the therapist and the group in a safe and consistent place. Music-making is very much a physical and releasing activity. (p.28)

Paul Robertson (1996) in *Music and the Mind* describes Tony Blois, who is a musical savant. This means that he has very limited intellectual resources in most areas but an immense musical gift. For Tony, who is blind and autistic due to brain damage at birth, music is his chosen means of expression and for some time his only one. His immense talent became apparent when he was given a keyboard at the age of two. His mother describes how at first he embarked on an intense programme of musical exploration. After six weeks with help from his mother he mastered *Twinkle, Twinkle, Little Star*. He now has 7000 songs in his repertoire and his musical talent has enabled him to expand his other abilities so that he now has more conversation:

> His language may be rather literal, but through his music he can directly express very powerful feelings… When I asked Tony how he felt about his mother, he played 'Twinkle, twinkle little star' as a Bach two-part invention (a short piece working out a single idea). It was both impressive and beautiful and showed how profound musical communication can and should be. How could many of us express our emotions so eloquently? (Robertson 1996, pp.13–14)

Music can be used to support children's coping efforts when hospitalised by allowing them to express their fear, anger, sadness and loneliness. In McDonnell's (1983) study they shared their experiences of home and school through improvised songs and so decreased their sense of isolation. Grimm and Pefley's (1990) study used an audiotape of children talking and singing about their hospital experiences to encourage other children to communicate their feelings of helplessness. This increased their resilience and their ability to cope.

Music therapists often have to work with emotions that Western society has difficulty in expressing publicly. Without the rituals that characterise the societies described in Chapter Three, grief is a problematic emotion for the West. Two Dutch music therapists give guidance on how to work musically with 'various emotions that occur with mourning', giving advice on the selection of instruments and how to relate the length of the music-making to the intensity of the emotions, concluding:

- Stimulate the client to bid farewell symbolically, in a musical way in the music therapy and in a non-musical way outside the music therapy, for example by performing a ritual.

- Have the expression of emotions dependent on the fact whether the client has had too little opportunity to express emotions in the past. (Smeijsters and van den Hurk 1993, p.255)

Here we see a rhythm about the expression, a process of deintensification that is audible in the music. We see certain associations with instruments and motifs that can be provided by the therapist to encourage the release of emotions.

Aldridge (1996) distinguishes between catharsis and expression. He describes how the move from one to the other can be used to facilitate change:

> At the centre of therapeutic work is the creative act in performance or composition. The creative expression is not the same as cathartic expression. Whereas personal emotive expression may be the first step in the process of healing, the continuing therapeutic process is to give articulation to a broad range of human feelings. While passionately playing music can lead to an emotional catharsis it lacks the intensity of form which articulates the whole range of personal aspiration. (p.18)

In relating expression in sounds to words, there is an acknowledgement that music can express what is not expressible in words, especially pre-verbal experiences:

> Since ego-weakness genetically finds its origin in the pre-verbal stage, it is obvious that music is very closely connected to this world of experience. What cannot be put into words (these chaotic feelings and experiences) can primarily be addressed and expressed through a non-verbal media. (De Backer 1993, pp.36–39)

Hanne Mette Kortegaard (1993) describes how 'schizophrenia can be understood as an inability to find meaningful symbols for emotions' (p.56) and how, in therapy, 'the musical expression becomes a symbolisation of the pressing feelings expressed during improvisation, whether this be an expression of the transference, countertransference or newly created symbols of the therapeutic relationship' (p.61).

Ann Sloboda (1993) documents how her music therapy with a man with an eating disorder acted as 'a bridging process between musical expression and the conscious expression of feelings': 'In a ten minute improvisation entitled simply: "How I feel", Brian played the metallophone throughout, in a way that resembled the "sad" voice mentioned above... For a client who struggled to make sense of his emotional world, music therapy provided an alternative way of exploring it' (pp.103–111).

Others highlight how problems played out in words can be worked through in a different medium: 'The structured, non-verbal nature of many musical activities and improvisations can be very reassuring for families who have become entangled in verbal conflicts, and the delicate issues of control can then be readdressed' (Oldfield 1993, p.54).

In relation to words and confidentiality, some liken therapy to the older practice of the religious confessional. It is possibly for this reason that the notion of confidentiality has grown up as being central to psychotherapeutic practice. Like the priest, the therapist hears, understands but cannot pass the information on. In the area of words, when what is being discussed is often of the most private and intimate kind, this is clearly a necessity, but may not be necessary in musical work. We have already seen how a debate around how much music therapy must be interpreted in words crops up regularly in the literature. 'It is important that a musician knows what he or she is expressing' was one therapist's comment to me. The implication behind the words was that unless the specific events, traumas and experiences were identified in words, the music-making would not be therapeutic. In this model, the music-making is simply a trigger for more verbal forms of psychotherapy and there are some therapists who operate in this way.

However, the problem of interpreting musical events is well documented. Here is one of many examples: 'Loud playing could indicate a release of physical tension or a desire to communicate aggressive and frustrated feelings. It could also indicate confidence, focused attention and internal strength' (Bunt 1994, p.52).

In their listening programme for psychotic patients a group of Italian therapists (Berruti *et al.* 1993) appear to establish what are normal connotations for music: '[Alberto] proposed that the group listen to some pieces of music to which he attached special significance: pieces of jazz music. He expressed associations that conflicted with the possible connotations of the excerpt. These were felt to be delusional' (p.70).

But Ruth Bright (1993) highlights cultural problems in the 'reading' of musical meaning. She played items of European and Asian origin to three groups of people of Caucasian origin – students, working people and ageing people. Her findings were that:

- When listening to music in the idiom with which they were familiar, most members of all three groups perceived it in the same way as the composer.

- When listening to music in an unfamiliar idiom, there was discrimination, but far less marked than with music in a familiar idiom.

- A large proportion of the participants, particularly in the student group, failed to recognise any mood in the music; they saw it as stupid and meaningless.

- In one particular case…most of the participants perceived it as sad and lonely, despite its being a joyful piece in the ears of the people of the culture from which it originated.

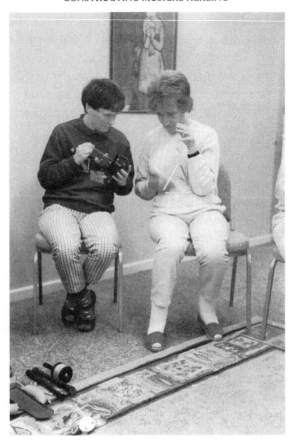

Figure 5.5 Listening

- For whatever reason, the members of the student group were far less willing to assign moods to the Asian items than were the members of the 'adult' groups. (p.206)

In the area of personal meanings, Bright (1993) has several examples of how personal associations can interrupt 'normal' reactions:

For example, the song 'Danny Boy', because of its words and its harmony pitch, speed of performance and general structure, is generally perceived as a sad song. In one seminar, a participant began to laugh when the song was played. He explained that in his office it was used as a request for someone else to answer the phone whilst you went to the bathroom, based on the line in the song, 'The pipes, the pipes are calling.' (p.199)

I was working with a woman finding calming music. The woman had found slow, baroque pieces particularly helpful and it would have seemed a logical step to Bach's *Air on a G string*. However, on hearing this, she became extremely agitated. It transpired that the piece had been associated with a traumatic memory. These examples recall aspects of the debate about musical meaning set out in Chapter Two. In these cases, the music had clearly developed personal meanings.

This enables it to play an important role in reminiscence therapy with older people. Both pleasant and painful memories can be recalled by carefully chosen pieces of music. Creative arts activities in Wellington, New Zealand, are personalised to meet clients' needs. One 83-year-old resident uses playing the piano as part of reminiscence therapy to evoke visual memories (Eames 1999).

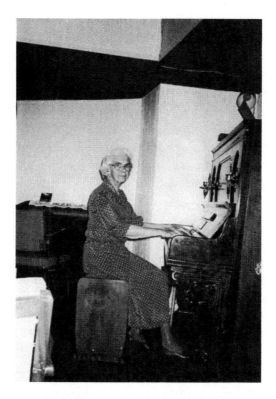

Figure 5.6 Mrs Mills (aged 83) of Longview Rest Home, Wellington, New Zealand, finds playing the piano evokes visual memories for her

Dr Elizabeth Kubler Ross (1983) gives a moving account of the effect of a live performer dancing to a piece of Tchaikovsky in an old people's home:

> They were all sitting half dead in their wheel chairs, mostly paralysed and just existing, they didn't live. They watched some television, but if you asked them what they had watched they probably would not have been able to tell you. We brought in a young woman who was a dancer and we told her to play beautiful, old fashioned music. She brought in Tchaikovsky records and so on and started to dance among these old people, all in their wheel chairs, which had been set in a circle. In no time the old people started to move. One old man stared at his hand and said, 'Oh my God, I haven't moved this hand in ten years.' And the 104-year-old, in a thick German accent, said, 'That reminds me of when I danced for the Tsar of Russia.' (p.2828)

The relationship of music to recall makes its use to resolve problems associated with grieving a real possibility. This is particularly true of older patients where confusion can be caused by unresolved grieving. Music can help to recall these events and the associated emotions. The music needs to be carefully and sensitively chosen, as the meaning of it will differ from person to person. What is clear here is the multiple meanings that a single piece of music may have (see Chapter Two) both when listened to and when improvised.

Whether music is used alone or in association with words it is important that the expression is accepted, encouraged and even praised by someone. Here the therapy may have recourse to words. But it can happen through the music itself:

> The group members were beginning to show signs of accepting and encouraging one another. Over a period of time, in more extended work, some of the patterns and habits from earlier in life that may have contributed towards particular problems can be explored in the trusting setting of the group. In music it is possible to try out different ways of playing. Taking risks may be easier for some people in a musical rather than a verbal medium. For example, a timid person may risk getting very angry on the drums, without setting in motion reactions that might occur using words. (Bunt 1994, p.27)

Such a position is closer to that of shamanic practice described in Chapter Three, where the community holds the rhythm while the shaman works in the middle of the circle. Indeed, in the context of dramatherapy, Roger Grainger (1995) describes a similar process. He calls it group holism where 'the group is felt to be more than the sum of the interactions of its members' and how one person can become the focus of group awareness within the 're-lational area' which he claims represents the 'spiritual identity of the group' (p.31).

Summary – expression / confidentiality

Notions of expression are central to music therapy. Music opens up the possibility of expressing ideas and emotions inexpressible in words. Catharsis can move towards artistic expression and this represents a change in the personality. Although words are sometimes used to interpret musical offerings, it is difficult to ascribe meaning to the music with certainty. Words may also be used in the all-important acceptance of the musical expressions by the therapist but this can be done powerfully through the music-making of the group itself. Despite this, there is still a great stress on confidentiality, based on psychotherapeutic models.

Unity/diversity

This section will deal with transformative effects of music and what part unity and diversity within the self plays in this process. Here again there is a central debate: do they merely express what is there or are they able to transform it? Following the argument in the previous section, the process of expression *which is accepted or received by someone else* can itself transform what seemed unacceptable into something potentially useful. Amelia Oldfield (1993) describes how difficult but how important it is to get families to accept the rather chaotic piano playing of a young child.

The notion of integration and reintegration is deep within the heart of Western therapy, and deep in the Jungian concepts is the notion of integrating the shadow. What part can music play in this process? How far can the therapist, working with the client, use or suggest or guide him or her into musical ways in which this might happen? De Backer (1993) sees music as useful in the treatment of what Melanie Klein called 'splitting'. The term means that good and bad parts of the personality are separated. He describes how, through music, his client (David) joins these elements together in his personality:

> David expresses his synthesis: death and life...death is a chaotic and alarming game, life is a peaceful and melancholic one. Thus, the presence and absence is not expressed in words, but symbolised in a musical

game… In this way one is no longer a victim of these circumstances and no longer subject to the contingency of the parents' absence. (p.37)

The concept of integration was central to Jung's theory of the personality and yet others such as Michael Fordham (1986) have emphasised a rhythm of integration and de-integration. We have already seen in Pavlicevic's statement above (see p.216) that sometimes it is necessary to change a fixed pattern in order to initiate the process of change. The application of behaviourist principles to music therapy might suggest that certain behavioural patterns can be changed musically; in other words that a change in musical patterns may effect change in the behavioural pattern. In the Pavlicevic account the change was initiated by the client. The literature is filled with examples of changes effected by music therapy.

The concept of integration includes that of the peaceful co-existence of diversity. Smeijsters and van den Hurk (1993) relate this to musical motifs and instruments:

- Stimulate the client in the improvisation of forms consisting of different elements.

- Encourage the client to the variation of motifs.

- Include isolated expressions for the client, for example, releases, in a form.

- Have the client act out persons to whom perhaps parts of the client projected…

- Encourage the client to improvise several unknown or impenetrable parts of herself.

- Select instruments that enable demonstration of opposite behavioural patterns and expressions of emotion. (pp.257–258)

Summary – unity/diversity

Notions of integration were central to Jung's thinking. That this can be achieved by means of music has been a central tenet of music therapy. It is necessary sometimes to de-integrate in order to re-integrate. This can be achieved through improvisation. The notion of integration contains within it the peaceful co-existence of diversity. The use of small motifs of different character can be used to achieve this.

Challenge/nurture

The therapeutic relationship can be seen as a nurturing relationship. In this section we shall see how far notions of challenge have been part of the tradition. The notion of empowerment is deep in the Jungian version of the heroic quest. The personality rid of its neurosis or with its shadow integrated will be stronger than the embattled, beleaguered 'sick' personality. The goal of the therapy might be seen as empowerment. The sense of therapist as nurturer is deep in the literature. The improvising music therapist might be seen as holding and supporting the client on his or her own particular journey. Indeed, the passage from Mercedes Pavlicevic above (describing the changing of an obsessive behaviour) is a musical expression of the good parent feeling and being sensitive to the changes in his or her child.

In the treatment of David, a boy with a weak ego, Jos De Backer (1993) identifies a return to humming and singing like a mother comforting a child as a regression to an earlier phase when David needed love and security. Claire Flower (1993) describes how a client used the theme from the British soap opera *EastEnders* as 'a musical hand to hold' (p.42) and a safe starting point for exploring more difficult areas.

In a series of guidelines for working with feelings of uselessness and worthlessness the notion of musical nurturing is prominent:

- Express the feelings musically. If the music therapist does this both for and together with the client, he/she uses empathetic techniques or empathetic counter-transference.

- If necessary, present the client with a musical gift by using musical means that affect the client emotionally...

- Adopt symbolically the role of the very first guardian...

- Try to compensate the feelings by structuring the musical improvisation in such a way that the client realises that a personal contribution is necessary. (Smeijsters and van den Hurk 1993, p.256)

There is an ongoing debate about music therapy and skills. The introduction of the notion of skill acquisition into therapy might be seen as introducing an element of challenge. It is one of the main distinguishing features between music therapy and education: whereas education is concerned with the imparting of skills, therapy is concerned with the use of skills for therapeutic ends. However, some clients can benefit from acquiring musical skills and information and to a certain extent will automatically acquire greater musical skill by engaging in music-making activities.

The encouragement of non-musical skills through music-making is well documented:

> During this group session a sense of caring for other members of the group was beginning to emerge. The suggested theme for the final improvisation took account of some of the feelings expressed by certain members of the group... Group work provides many opportunities for supporting each other; in this example we noted the beginnings of such sensitivity in the musical dialogues developed between people in the group. (Bunt 1994, p.27)

Later Bunt adds: 'Music is more than a temporary diversion: it presents people with a challenging opportunity to look at aspects of themselves in a different light. As in any therapy, such a process can be painful' (1994, p.35).

Therapists draw attention to the difficulty of balancing challenge and nurture within a session:

> I feel it is important for them to perceive music therapy sessions as a time to work and face up to challenges but overall as enjoyable and fun... I try to introduce gradually challenges which I feel the family are ready to deal with in order to make it possible for them to succeed and to gain a sense of achievement at each stage. (Oldfield 1993, p.48)

In these guidelines for the increasing of self-confidence we see ways of supporting and challenging as well balanced:

- Support the client musically in such a way that the client's play becomes an important ingredient of the music.

- Allow the client in time to take initiatives and adopt a leading role.

- Confront the client with deviant musical material after she has repeatedly been confirmed in her choices. (Smeijsters and van den Hurk 1993, p.257)

Kortegaard (1993) likens it to the process of feeding: 'This way of working with schizophrenics requires empathy on the part of the therapist. She must continually relate to her manipulating role, in order that the patient may meet a gratifying mixture of gratification and frustration or nourishment and poisoning' (p.60).

Summary – challenge/nurture

The role of nurturing is greatly stressed in the literature. This can be effectively done through music-making both by the therapist and by the group itself. The role of challenge is less apparent. Music therapy has traditionally used clients' existing musical skills rather than embarking on a process of skill acquisition with clients, which might be seen more as the province of music education. However, the acquisition of social and personal skills can be encouraged through music. There needs to be a balance of challenge and nurturing within sessions.

Excitement/relaxation

This section will deal with the effect of music on the mood of patients. Listening in audience played little part in the construction of music therapy in the early days, but it is becoming more common. I have known therapists who have recommended that clients use calming music at certain times in their therapy, and others that have discussed with depressed clients music that will energise them. One patient discovered that a cure for her depression was to see the film *Chorus Line* with its enlivening musical score. There is an acceptance that music affects pulse rate, blood pressure and heart rhythm (to an extent measurable by an ECG).

Johannes Kneutgen in the collected volume *Neue Wege der Musiktherapie* (*New Ways of Music Therapy*) used tape-recorded lullabies in place of sleeping tablets to soothe debilitated children at night and reduced bed-wetting by two thirds. George Hengesch in Bonn allowed schizophrenic psychotics to play classroom percussion instruments. This calmed them enough to enable him to resume his speech therapy programme with them (Hamel 1978).

Ruth Bright (1993) identifies cultural considerations that must be taken into account in this area. In defining culture she indicates that the following areas need to be examined:

- Ethnic origin
- Religious culture
- Educational, family and social culture
- Chronological age
- Cultural aspects of personal preference
- Psychiatric illness. (pp.194–195)

Wheeler (1988) found five characteristics that would affect personal musical preference and therefore the effect of music. These were gender, age, musical training, personality and mood. Other researchers have linked personal preferences with personality characteristics. Extroverts, for example, were found by Stephen Dollinger (1993) to prefer arousing music like jazz.

Cheryl Dileo Maranto (1993) identifies a number of ways in which listening is used in the treatment of physical illness. She identifies several considerations in selecting music for what she terms 'passive/receptive methods':

- Familiarity with the music
- Preference for the music
- History and associations with the music
- Characteristics/elements of the music. (p.157)

The methods she distinguishes include:

- music listening free-field or with headphones to reduce pain and anxiety
- music-elicited imagery, a technique involving 'listening to music in a very relaxed state in order to elicit spontaneous imagery to thera-peutic goals…[with] no interaction between client and therapist during the music listening'
- music and directed imagery, in which 'music and specific sugges-tions for imagery are given to the patient who is in a very relaxed state…relevant to the therapeutics goal, for example enhancement of immune functions'
- guided imagery and music, in which 'a person in a relaxed state listens to carefully selected music', during which 'spontaneous images are reported to the therapist who provides suggestions for focusing and deepening the experience'
- music and verbal relaxation methods, in which music is used to enhance 'traditional verbal relaxation methods, such as progressive muscle relaxation, autogenic training and/or suggestion'. (pp.164–167)

Some of these techniques are related to techniques found in the New Age tra-ditions as described in Chapter Four.

A group of Italian music therapists at the University of Genoa (Berruti et al. 1993) tried using listening programmes with psychotic patients. They identify how peace and well-being could be induced and the release of strong emotions be encouraged. Josee Raijmaekers (1993) in her work with psycho-geriatric patients investigates the effect of associative listening on her patients. She chose five musical extracts 'representing a set of values': 'old age, action, religion, childhood, warmth' (p.131).

It is clear that one cannot be prescriptive about the effects of music on patients. Hamid Hekmat and James Hettel (1993) emphasise this finding in their work on the *Attenuating Effects of Preferred versus Non-preferred Music Interventions*:

> [The] choice of preferred music may assist the client in pain coping above and beyond listening to music that is pre-chosen for them and possibly non-preferred. The control of music selection may have profound effects on the ability of participants to cope with pain because of an increased sense of control and self-efficacy. (p.170)

Cathy Chatten (1997) describes how finding the right music played an important part in the treatment of Elsie, who was exhibiting challenging behaviour in her demented state. By trying to understand this behaviour, which was violent and antisocial, it was discovered that Elsie had been a piano teacher, preferring classical music, had loved animals and had been a very private person, living alone. A tailor-made regime reduced the number of different people who cared for her, allowed her time in her room and the ward quiet room, away from the television. They found out that the quiet second movements of piano sonatas and string quartets were her favourites and that she became agitated in louder sections. These soothing passages often sent her to sleep in the quiet room. These were not optional extras for Elsie but 'a vital part of her care' (pp.22–23).

Other investigations of the use of music with patients with dementia have stressed the negative effects of an environment completely filled by music. Jeannette Morrison (1997) in a survey of residential units that included older people with dementia often found music playing on a cassette player, at the same time as the radio or television. These sounds were often loud and competing with others such as those of the vacuum cleaner and raised voices. 'Nor,' she adds, 'was it clear that anyone was listening to it' (p.18). She identified that the residents had no control over their noisy environment for three reasons;

- they cannot operate the cassette player/radio/TV themselves
- they cannot move away independently
- they cannot communicate their preferences verbally. (p.18)

She goes on to link this lack of control over one's life with feelings of hope-lessness and suggests that it is an area where the patients might be given some control. But: 'Many staff did not seem to understand the implications of a question which asked whether staff and client needs – to listen to music – might ever be in conflict. However, some had obviously thought carefully about the way they used music in the home' (p.18).

She concludes her research with the following guidelines:

- The loudness of the music should be carefully monitored.

- It might be more appropriate not to have background music at times when residents need to focus on something in particular.

- Staff need to find by some means the music to which residents best respond (e.g. by asking, and finding some way of giving choice, by talking with the family, by making careful observations of responses when music is playing or not playing). (p.19)

Various forms of imaging to music have been developed. Professor Leuner of Gottingen used music to intensify the mental images of the patient. He called the technique 'katathymic image-experience' and found it to be effective in both 'ill' and 'healthy' patients. In the latter group he saw 'deepened self discovery and the clarification of personal identity' (quoted in Hamel 1978, pp.167–180). Symptom severity was reduced, including stuttering. Other doctors have had groups of people imaging to music and interpreted the images, a method developed by Helen Bonny (see Chapter One).

Music has been combined with therapeutic hypnosis. This has drawn on the notion that music can lead to altered states of awareness such as col-our-synaesthesia, the awakening of colour images while listening to music. In this work (Hamel 1978) it was established that patients tended to have negative experiences before the music appeared but after the introduction of the music, happier images appeared. It was also found that several years later the same pieces of music could be used to induce the feelings of happiness; the music seemed to have been retained in the memory following the hypnotherapy. Therapists are aware that reactions to pieces vary considerably from group to group. Leslie Bunt (1994) cites a number of studies in this area showing, for example, that fast music affects children's play activity and linking calming and exciting music with changes in the electrical resistance of the skin.

But the qualities of excitement and relaxation are not only associated with listening. Instruments are also seen as endowed with particular qualities or as evoking particular reactions: 'The bass drum and the cymbal can be very frightening for young children, or feed into uncontrolled chaos for older children' (Oldfield 1993, p.49). In the treatment of a patient with the symptoms of anorexia the therapists found: 'The instruments got a different emotional charge. While beating the gong, the client became extremely angry. The vibraphone made her peaceful and calm, but also lonely. The cymbals became the sign of resistance against her being well-adjusted. (Smeijsters and van den Hurk 1993, p.241). The music therapist Auriole Warwick said in an interview with me: 'If they are excited, put the tambourines at the back of cupboard.'

Music therapist Liz Wilcock studied the reactions of 120 clients at the Bristol Cancer Help Centre to Tibetan bowls. These are metal bowls coming from Bhutan, Nepal, India and Tibet that can be played in two main ways. One of these is a sonorous gong-like sound and the other a humming-type sound made by circling the wooden stick round the outside edge of the bowl:

> In the surrender of the ego to this overwhelming and penetrating sound extraordinary images and feelings can occur, however those who fight against the sound and remain separate from it experience emotions ranging from mild irritation to 'murderous rage'. As we cannot shut our ears, non-acquiescence to the sound can feel like rape. Care has to be taken to check that no-one is upset by the sound before using it in groups. The sound floods all resonating cavities in the skull with vibrations and successfully dominates any sensory feedback information. (Wilcock 1997)[3]

The effects evoked in these patients and also on some in hospices and day care centres were quite remarkable. They include powerful images like 'a monk on a hillside', 'a stone cave with a high dome with water beneath' and 'like sitting on the edge of a mountain'. What is interesting in the light of this polarity is that sounds were 'exciting and relaxing at the same time'. This was confirmed by another music therapist, Cathy Richards who states:

> The strong vibrations emitted have a simultaneously calming and stimulating effect on the body and emotions. This type of sound both relaxes the body, lowers blood pressure but also provides a form of cerebral stimulation. Overall this produces both a sense of well-being and increased energy. (quoted in Wilcock 1997)

3   *Tibetan Bowls and Their Uses in Music Therapy* (unpublished study).

Wilcock cites another example of autistic patients who were encouraged to achieve a sense of unity and connectedness by working with the bowls, and a patient with cerebral palsy who stopped shaking for the first time in years when the bowl was played. She identifies effects in the areas of mind, body and spirit and summarises them as follows:

- the bowls are felt by the skeletal system so are useful with stroke and deaf patients

- they resonate well with minimal physical movement so can be used by patients with cerebral palsy, palliative care and post-operative patients

- the singing sound encourages the patients to reflect at a deep inner level so being suitable for patients with emotional crises or a sense of disintegration

- the concentration required to play it encourages imagination and opens the group up for deeper work. (Wilcock 1997)[4]

In the area of improvising, there is a real importance placed on establishing the right beat for the client. Robbins (1993) describes the problems of Walter, a trainee music therapist who was a pianist with experience of jazz and popular music:

> His [Walter's] years of playing as a provider of background entertainment, and the continuous repetition or earlier popular music in his work with elderly patients had combined to set him playing in constant tempos... Habituated styles of playing were displaced as directive freedom and clinical resourcefulness developed hand in hand... The more Walter developed clinical freedom in playing for Karyn [his patient], the more his personal music history surfaced. The emergence of this new clinical resource and its relevance to Karyn at this time reflected their interrelated paths of development: she moves to him to grow and as she grows, she moves into the space he creates for her. (pp.20–23)

Leslie Bunt (1994) develops the notion of 'rhythmic entrainment' (discussed in Chapter One): 'In walking to our own comfortable tempo with musical support, for example, we are learning to synchronise a movement with a sound. At such moments the response produced occurs in synchrony with the

---

4   *Tibetan Bowls and Their Uses in Music Therapy* (unpublished study).

appearance of the stimulus: this is often described as "rhythmic entrainment"' (p.62)

The effect of the influence of behaviourism on the practice of music therapy has resulted in quite a large body of research literature on the more generalised effects of music therapy, especially the value of music in enhancing self-esteem, socialisation and energisation through rhythmic activity (Gfeller 1987).

Some of the most systematic work on the use of music to control the excitement of the body in clinical settings has been carried out by the German doctor Ralph Spintge. He is in charge of a pain clinic at which he has constructed a database of the effects of music on 90,000 patients (Robertson 1996). He makes music available to his patients through high-quality sound systems all the time; his research has found that anxieties about being in hospital are calmed by it and recovery is improved. It is in surgical procedures that its use is most systematically used. He and his team have composed pieces which are designed to put patients in the optimum condition, both mentally and physically. So effective is the fifteen minutes of soothing music that lulls the patient that only 50 per cent of the recommended doses of analgesics and sedative medication usually used are required for painful surgery. Some procedures are even carried out without anaesthetic. This is followed by more invigorating music which is designed to encourage the patient's systems to respond actively to the surgical procedures. When these are completed the music takes the patient back to a relaxed state for recovery:

> Ralph Spintge believes it is the rhythmic components of music that are most effective in his work. Pieces composed to create specific physiological change in his patients are designed to lock into the innate neuro-physiological and biological rhythms that underlie the vital functions of the body.
>
> Ralph Spintge agrees that part of the value of music is that it distracts the mind and allows the patient to escape into the imagination. However, the potency of music actively to change the physiological state goes beyond mere distraction. (Robertson 1996, p.27)

This is an example of extremely systematic research into the effects of music on the body. It goes far beyond merely designating music as exciting or relaxing.

Summary — excitement / relaxation

Music therapy has used the ability of music to encourage excitement and relaxation in a variety of ways. This has become more apparent as listening experiences are becoming more common in therapy. Here cultural factors play a part and it is difficult to be entirely sure of the effect the music will have on individual patients. The use of music and imagery has been exploited in a variety of ways, sometimes involving the interpretation of images, sometimes combined with techniques like hypnosis. The use of music in surgery has resulted in decreases in the use of medication, but it needs to be carefully related to the surgical processes being undertaken.

Embodiment/transcendence

This section will examine how the constructs of Western medicine affect music therapy's approach to the effect of music on body and spirit. Western medicine is based on a separation of body, mind and spirit (a separation which is sometimes construed as being of debatable existence). These are divided up into different areas, with different people and different institutions or sections of institutions responsible for them.

In terms of treating the body, music therapists work with physically disabled patients of every age, using music to diagnose disability and treat it. I was once with the music therapist Auriole Warwick at an assessment centre for children with multiple disabilities. Her task was to find out if a particular three-year-old child who had no speech could hear. She went from side to side with a variety of instruments, playing them in each ear. The child's face was expressionless, but when she played a small glockenspiel on one side a seraphic beam lit up its face. It was the only sign of emotion or any relationship with the world in the entire session.

Because the early music therapists worked in the area of people with learning disabilities there is a clear strand of music being used to encourage motor movements of many kinds. Certainly motor observation is part of music therapy practice. In his reflections on a music therapy session with John, a withdrawn three-and-a-half-year-old boy,

> [the physiotherapist] observes a whole range of both gross and fine motor skills. She sees John handling both one or two beaters while drumming and three while dancing. She is quick to comment that his whole body seems to come alive with the sounds, resonating throughout in response to the physically stimulating music he hears and makes. His movements appear to be the mainstream of his music. At times his move-

ments are fast and active, even somewhat chaotic, but he is also able to be more focused and still. She notes, with some concern, that he finds it difficult to pick up the sticks from the floor. He tends also to have some problems in hand and eye co-ordination, especially when playing very fast music... (Bunt 1994, p.21)

The use of movement is recommended by therapists. Amelia Oldfield (1993) describes how she gets parents and babies to do *Row, Row, Row your Boat* or gets parents to lift toddlers in the air and how it is important to do this in each session.

In the area of psychotherapy the mind is often regarded as separate from the body. To dismiss an illness as psychological was once to dismiss its bodily component altogether; today the reality of psychosomatic illnesses is increasingly recognised. There is little work done with music in the treatment of the two really embodied psychological diseases – anorexia and bulimia nervosa – although this is developing (as seen above – see p.222).

David Aldridge (1996), in his research in the Herdecke hospital where he works, chose to concentrate on the physiological implications of improvising music with a therapist. He co-operated with the professor of physiology in the work:

> The initial part of this programme monitored the heart rate of the patient and the heart rate of the therapist, and the recorded playing of the therapist on the piano and the playing of the patient on the drum. These parameters were recorded in real time onto a videotape. Each interaction was structured as a series of episodes: rest, playing a composed work, and creative improvised playing. In some ways this was an attempt to monitor *the physiology of creative dialogues* (p.13)

In her article on music therapy in the *New Grove Dictionary of Music and Musicians*, Natasha Spender (1980) documents the effects of music on comatose patients, who regained consciousness after a long programme of listening to music. Similarly, there are examples of the harmful effects of certain musical experiences, particularly in the world of popular musics and its capacity to induce fits (Critchley and Henson 1977). This interest in the effect of music at the influence of the basic level of the body's functioning is increasing.

Another area of research is the effect of music on babies, especially premature ones: 'In studies on premature babies, music has been shown to promote weight gain, reduce movement, reduce irritability and crying behaviours, increase feeding behaviours, stimulate development, increase blood oxygen levels, reduce stress-related behaviours, and subsequently decrease the length of hospitalisation. (Wigram 1993, p.143).

Maranto (1993) explores the use of music therapy in the treatment and prevention of physical illness and disease. Here she draws heavily on Engel's (1977) biopsychosocial model of illness, emphasising the interrelationship of mind and body and the influence of the earth on both. She summarises the main goals in this area as:

1. Elimination of stress and anxiety

2. Elimination of pain

3. Elimination of depression, helplessness etc.

4. Enhancement of immune function (p.156)

She sees the advantages of music as affecting biomedical and psychosocial levels simultaneously and, compared with most other medical interventions as being non-invasive and painless, with few contra-indications and side effects. She makes the important proviso that it is impossible to establish a consistent one-to-one relationship between a musical procedure and its effect. This is because responses to music are unique to each individual. Her work includes summaries of research of the efficacy of music in the following areas:

- Surgery

- Neonatal intensive care units

- Paediatric medical care

- Physical rehabilitation

- Respiratory care

- Burn care

- Pain management

- Stress reduction

- General hospital or intensive care unit

- Labour and delivery

- Oncology/terminal illness. (pp.161–164)

To take one example from Maranto's list, in the area of physical rehabilitation music has been show to:

- Structure rhythmic movement
- Improve motor functioning
- Reinforce desired movements
- Decrease muscle tension
- Improve motivation for therapy
- Enhance acupuncture efficacy. (p.162)

She sees the area of research into music and the immune response being a significant area for future research.

Tia Lodewijks (1998) combines work on physical and psychological symptoms in her use of musical mini-plays with blind children and those with cerebral palsy. Her work is structured to help children in the following areas:

- Physical: agility, balance, body awareness, copying, fine- and gross-motor co-ordination, flexibility, increased lung volume, fitness, muscle strength and range and speed of movement, interaction, looseness of joints, posture awareness, sequencing and relaxation.

- Musical: sense of rhythm, awareness of note values and changes of tempo, interpretation, taking cues, listening and using silences.

- Psychological: stimulation of the imagination, between the individual and the group, increased confidence, concentration, and self-image, all accompanied by joy and fun.

Yoshiko Fukuda (1998) has been running the asthma music programme in Japan for 17 years. Asthmatics are taught how to master abdominal breathing easily and correctly using a variety of methods: 'Knowledge of the asthma music breathing methods can make both children and guardians feel mentally prepared and secure against a possible asthmatic attack' (conference report).

Another well-explored area is that of music and the brain. Denise Erdonmez (1993) entitles her chapter 'Music – A mega vitamin for the brain'. She looks at the effects of music on patients with Alzheimer's disease, Parkinson's disease and a stroke victim, comparing these effects with the use of music as therapy involving visualisation to music.

The mind/body/soul split on which Western medicine is based has not left much room in music therapy for the concept of transcendence, with its implicit concentration on the disputed terrain of the spiritual. There is more indication in the work of Jung of the possibility of a soul but in contemporary psychiatry the pursuit of selfhood is seen by some to have replaced the pursuit of spiritual or divine wisdom. A book with the revealing title *Psychology as Religion: The Cult of Self-Worship* (Vitz 1979) sets out this argument very clearly.

Peter Hamel (1978) distinguishes between two approaches to music therapy by means of mysticism:

> First of all, two principal schools of music therapy need to be distinguished – that which seeks to work through listening, and that which would bring help to the patient through his own involvement in communicative music-making. Behind these two aspects stand two different ways of looking at the problem. The representatives of the original one place their faith exclusively in the spiritual powers of music, while the others maintain that the 'anthroposophical mysticism' of countless music therapists is to blame for the fact that music therapy is seen as vague and suspect by rationally-trained psychotherapists. The latter regard the 'magical use' of music as a heresy, and further maintain that music is incapable of curing a patient through any purely musical realisation-experience, whether of spiritual or of mental illness' (p.166)

There are a few examples of the use of techniques drawn from religious traditions in therapy. The German clarinettist and psychotherapist Ernst Flackus used Zen meditation music in his treatment programmes for drug addicts in the 1970s. Here he combined music listening with methods of autogenous training:

> During the exercise I played the Zen meditation music softly over a loudspeaker system, but nevertheless made it clear beforehand that the patient should not listen to the music but simply concentrate on the weight and warmth of his body… This introductory exercise was successfully carried out, and encouraged me to introduce specially chosen electronic music from the tenth session onwards. Particularly suitable were tapes on which experiences of nature, such as the pattering of rain with the sun coming out, were represented electronically. (Flackus, quoted in Hamel 1978, p.169)

In the same paper Flackus describes trying to use the music of the Beatles, both because of the strong beat and the association with drugs, alcohol and ecstatic dancing. Classical music proved unsuccessful because it recalled bad experiences of music lessons and the training patients had received in listening in the classical tradition. Clients perceived classical Zen music and electronic music 'virtually as abstract sounds' and Flackus distinguishes this from the listening style of western concert:

> [The subjects do] not listen to them, but merely half-perceive them in the background and in this way…allow them, so to speak, to flow into them… The music hovers in the air as a vibration, as 'tone-colour'. For the young person this resistance is so soothing, and also removes distortions and excesses, be he never so at home in other familiar 'noise scenes' at home, Beat-dive, café or discotheque. Of course, the participants first had to learn the other way in which it is possible, and necessary, to appreciate sounds, if these were to mean any gain in strength to them. It also dawned on them that one perceives and listens to a concert differently, and more deeply, in a state of relaxation than through any activised or agitated form of participation. (Flackus, quoted in Hamel 1978, p.170)

It is interesting to compare this work with the cultural issues in listening described above. It would seem that the sounds need to be different from those of the culture of the clients in order to achieve this abstract quality. Sounds of their own culture, be they popular or classical, cannot achieve the level of abstraction for this combination of meditation and therapy.

There are also indications in current literature on music therapy that major breakthroughs in self-discovery or healing are described in the language of transcendence. These are brought together in a passage in which Clive Robbins (1993) links the notion of transcendence with joy and self-realisation. In the fifth session with a four-year-old autistic girl with severe learning disabilities called Nicole, he writes: 'Stepping rhythmically from foot to foot, she throws her body as far as she can from one side to the other. Her face shows utter joy and release matched in spirit by the joyfulness in Carol's [the music therapist] stimulating and playing' (p.15). He comments:

> It is important not to undervalue *joy*. Joy is more than fun, more than just having a good time. There is something transcendent about the purity of joy, something that relates to an original realisation of one's full humanness. For a child as developmentally disabled as Nicole, joy in discovering self-expression or in achieving musical creation with a therapist can be momentous… Joy is nourishment. (pp.15–16)

He also extols the virtues of the capacity to 'wonder' which he calls 'the root source of both scientific enquiry and creative endeavour' (p.16). He links this with 'a romantic attitude' on the part of the therapist which he sees as essential to the nurturing of 'hope, caring, compassion and insight'. The last of Yalom's (1985) 'curative factors' were existential factors which include major issues such as recognising our own mortality. It is interesting that Bunt, who uses Yalom extensively in relation to music therapy, does not expand on the possibilities of music therapy in this area.

Anthi Agrotou (1993) links religion with her music therapy work in using a theoretical frame drawn from this area to examine the link between 'religious rituals, certain ritualisms, certain kinds of ritualisation and ritualised play' (p.75). She ends her chapter with a passage untypical of therapeutic literature:

> This, then, is the connecting link – or rather the biggest contrast between ritualism and religious rituals of mourning such as those of Christ's or Adonis' death and resurrection. Those rites give the space, under the strength and shelter of the united community, to mourn for all the losses and abandonments, even for the ultimate one of death; and when the community is satiated to its fill with grief – to use a Homeric phrase – it rejoices over its resolution that death had actually been conquered. (p.191)

However, the visionary experiences that characterise the experiences of some musicians of many cultures do present a problem for contemporary psychiatry. Often associated with imbalance of some kind, there is often an attempt to ban them all to the realm of madness and insanity and therefore to unwholeness or ill health. In some areas now there is an attempt to discriminate between the helpful and unhelpful or healthy and unhealthy vision. But it is because of the traditional problems of psychiatry with this area that some creative people experience an unease with psychiatry (including music therapy insofar as it operates within these limits) which would deprive them of the wellsprings of their creativity. It is difficult to know what contemporary psychiatry would have made of the visions of Hildegard of Bingen (1098–1179) or Handel's visions of the angels while writing *Messiah*. Contemporary psychiatry treats the 'crisis' that characterises the call of the shaman (see Chapter Three) very differently from traditional societies which have a spiritual frame within which it can be regarded as 'normal'.

Summary – embodiment / transcendence

The traditional mind, body and spirit that has characterised Western allopathic medicine has not encouraged the presence of notions of transcendence within the therapeutic tradition. There is an increasing literature of the effects of music on the body. Some have explored the linking of music with meditation in relation to the treatment of drug addiction and others the use of music for the development of motor skills. However, there is an increasing use of a language suggestive of transcendence to express breakthroughs in therapy and the use of religious terminology to describe the therapeutic situation.

Summary

Music therapy grew out of work with psychiatric patients and people with learning disabilities. It has been influenced by psychoanalytic traditions, especially Jung, behaviourist traditions and the humanistic psychology of Carl Rogers. Now well-established as a profession in the UK, music therapy has a growing interest in an 'ecology of ideas'. There was a strong sense of an individual journey to be undertaken and early work was usually in one-to-one situations. However, it has always laid great stress on relationships. In the early days these were established between a therapist and a single patient through free improvisation and improvisatory skills on the piano were the bedrock of training courses. Now, group music-making is increasingly used to encourage social skills. Hospitals and GPs are establishing links with the surrounding community by means of music which is seen both as a means of promoting health and of re-integrating 'cured' people into the wider community. Freedom from the dominant classical and popular traditions characterised the development of the free improvisation on which the work of Juliette Alvin, Paul Nordoff and Clive Robbins was founded.

However, the notion of boundaries has always been important in psychotherapy. These are sometimes musical but more often extra-musical, especially in terms of clear beginnings and endings to sessions. Expression is central to notions of therapy, and music is felt to be able to express emotions and ideas inexpressible in words. Although cathartic expression is part of therapy, the move to more aesthetic expression can be seen as in itself therapeutic. Notions of confidentiality prevail because of the underpinning health models, and yet it is clear that therapists find it difficult to ascribe precise verbal meanings to music. Therapists are divided in how far they see it necessary to use words to interpret the experience. The notion of the integration of the personality are deep in the underpinning philosophies, especially those of Jung. However, there is a sense that change is induced by a process of de-integration that can be encouraged through music-making. The process of integration can be seen as the state of the peaceful co-existence of diversity which can be encouraged musically by the use of diverse motifs and instruments.

In this process acceptance is important and this is an essential part of group work. Nurturing is a prominent theme and music therapy can be seen as musical nurturing. Musical challenge is not so evident and the teaching of musical skills is not part of the tradition although music is seen as a way of encouraging social and personal skills in a group music-making context. Music is widely used to relax patients. This is often done through listening, which might be combined with imagery techniques of some kind. Cultural and personal issues need to be addressed when using music in this way. More subtle programmes are being developed to enable patients to co-operate with doctors during surgery. The effects of music on the body are increasingly the subjects of research programmes. Notions of transcendence are less common because of the mind/body/spirit split that characterises Western medicine. However, they can be found in descriptions of breakthroughs in treatment and in describing the overall context in which therapy takes place.

Music therapy is possibly the only improvisatory tradition in the world that encourages total musical freedom and has no underlying musical structures to underpin it. Nevertheless, the fact that most therapists were experienced classical practitioners before becoming therapists has meant that their own work is necessarily underpinned by that tradition. It represents a process-based tradition with little concept of a musical product at all. It is an area of applied music in which the music is valued in its relationship to personal well-being rather than for its own sake.

CHAPTER SIX

Of Connection and Change

Music and power – a story from the Amazon

From the Mundurucú (see Amazonian people) comes a story that links
the loss of women's power with their loss of their musical instruments.
The sacred trumpets of the Mundurucú, called the karökö, now cannot
even be seen by women; but the story goes that the women once owned
them. Indeed, the women first discovered them. Three women named
Yanyonböri, Tuembirú and Parawarö regularly went to collect firewood
in the forest. While they were there, they often heard music but didn't
know where it came from. One day they went off in search of water
because they were thirsty. They came upon a beautiful, shallow lake,
deep in the forest, which shone clear in the sunlight. They called it
Karökö boapti, or 'the place from which they took the karökö'. The next
time the women heard the music in the forest, they realised that it came
from the direction of the lake. When they investigated the lake further
they found only jiju fish in the water; but they weren't able to catch any
of them.

In the village, one of the women thought up a plan to catch the fish
with hand nets. They knew of a nut which would make the fish sleepy.
They rubbed the mouths of the nets with it and returned to the lake with
their nets. Their plan worked. Each woman caught only one fish; but at
the moment of capture, each fish turned into a hollow, cylindrical
trumpet. All the other fish swam away. That is why there are now only
three trumpets in each man's house. Everyday the women went secretly
to play the trumpets which they had hidden deep in the forest.

They were so devoted to their forest music-making that they
neglected their husbands and their housework. The men sent one of their
number to spy on them but although they heard the music they did not
see the trumpets. When the women returned they asked them about their
music and told them they could no longer play in the forest but must

bring the trumpets to the houses. While the women possessed the trumpets they had power over the men who had to do the housework. The trumpets needed feeding with meat and sweet manioc drink. On the day chosen for bringing the trumpets to the village, while he women sent the men out to hunt they made the sweet manioc drink. When the men returned from the hunt, all the women of the village went to the forest to fetch the trumpets. The leader of the women, Yanyonböri, said that all the men should shut themselves securely in their houses and sent a messenger back to tell the men. Rebelliously, the men insisted on remaining in the men's house. Finally, Yanyonböri went back herself and reached a compromise with her brother, Marimarebö. He agreed that they would go into their houses for one night only, saying: 'We want the trumpets and tomorrow we'll take them.' And so the next day the men took the trumpets from the women. The women were forced to go back to their houses, but they wept at the loss of their music. (summarised from Young 1993, pp.242–243)[1]

I have used this story about power relations between the genders (which is intertwined in its original form with sections on domestic and public roles and sexual politics) to illustrate the link between music and power. It also illustrates well the connection of music to the natural world, the mysterious origins of music (in this case in the use of the lake image), public and private music-making and the exclusiveness of some group musical traditions – themes which run through this book, which this final chapter will summarise. In the opening chapter it was suggested that some illness is due to imbalance at least partly caused by areas of mismatch between the personality of the individual and the prevailing values of the society. The outcome of such thinking is that at both a personal and cultural level healing lies in the achievement of balance in the light of the values of the surrounding society. This process of exploring a wide range of human experience will lead us to tolerate and respect as great a diversity as possible, personally and culturally. This includes value systems as well as musical styles and individual pieces.

This chapter will, therefore, also suggest how the findings may be used in various healing contexts. The cultural context for this chapter is in a society in which there is widening access to different cultures by a variety of means –

---

1   Based on a story from *University of California Publications in Archaeology and Ethnicity 49*, 89–91.

transport, the Internet, the recording industry, the mass media and community music-making activities. This chapter addresses particularly the areas of health (of the individual) and education (which sets up the dominant values of society) (Illich 1976, 1977). Underpinning it is the notion that music can transform potentially destructive situations into areas of growth – it is a way of recycling. The chapter argues for a higher profile for music in debates about such areas as law and order, violence, creativity and personal growth.

Individuation

The balancing of the community/individualism polarity at an individual level is to do with exploring solitude and relationship – to acknowledge that individuality is in the context of a wider society and, indeed, cosmos. How do we avoid, on the one hand, a community that stifles individuality and rebellion and, on the other, a competitive individuality that has no roots or responsibility?

The balance between these two has been expressed in different ways in different traditions. The Western classical tradition had a notion of community that included the cosmos and, in particular, God or gods up to the Renaissance. During this period notions of healing through the creation of community were widely found. Post-Enlightenment, the heroic journey model gained prominence with the individual composer set over and perhaps against the community. This has led to an increasing division between the audience and the high art composer in Western Europe. Notions of the aesthetic replaced God and notions of healing were replaced by those of personal enlightenment and amelioration. Theorists have downplayed the relationship of the music made to the culture that generated it, although interest in this area has developed in post-modern debates which have applied cultural theory to classical music.

This has not been as true of popular and folk traditions. Shamans and traditional healers have always practised in a community context, although the training of the shaman has contained notions of an individual journey into different worlds. The New Age has recovered notions of community that includes not only a spiritual dimension but an ecological one. Healing takes place in this context. With concepts of reincarnation there is, in these systems, a notion of the journey of the individual soul. This is often coloured by notions of karma and kismet, which give a frame of reference for suffering in this life within past lives. Music has an important part to play in the healing.

Music therapy, growing up in the context of the Western classical tradition, has always stressed the importance of relationship. This has often been, however, in the context of a relationship of two people out of the context of the wider society. Group work has become more common and music is regarded as a unique form of connection. Health authorities are now increasingly using community arts projects to link health-care institutions with the wider society.

Personal identity

The prevailing values of Western society might be summarised as a 'normalised individualism'. On the one hand, people are conceived as individuals in competition with one another; on the other hand, each individual is treated in the same way by simple cause and effect principles operating in health care and education as if they were all the same. In the light of this, music can offer a person the possibility of belonging to a group of people listening, performing or improvising/composing within a common tradition. Those who favour more individualised approaches may feel drawn to the Western classical tradition while those looking for more communal systems may seek out the New Age traditions. Nevertheless, in performing groups such as choirs and orchestras the classical tradition can offer a real sense of community.

Sonia Gergis, a North London music teacher, ran a 'Music in Harmony' festival. For this, the youngsters (and they were mostly young and included so-called recalcitrant teenagers) could only enter in a group – there were no soloists. The result was a tremendous quality of co-operation. It was good to see piano duet teams and accompanying pianists developing their skills in sensitivity. They were learning to tune their music to other people, learning how to get their rhythms together, to blend their tone colours, to tune their notes to one another, to support others in difficulty rather than compete with them.

The New Age also offers opportunities for individual journeys in learning shamanic traditions and in personalised journeys through a wide range of groups such as drummers, dancers, overtone chanters, singing groups of various kinds and so on. It offers a place for new syntheses of ideas and the formation of new traditions.

Music therapy offers opportunities for an individual journey alongside a supporting therapist. This will help the person who has difficulty in relating to others and could provide an entry into the wider world of music-making. Such links could be developed between therapists and other music-making communities.

More health trusts are exploring links with the wider community. Projects like Exeter Health Care Arts, East Sussex Arts in Healthcare scheme, Hastings and Rother Art in Hospital Project, the Waterford Healing Arts Trust, Stockport Arts and Health, Artlink West Yorkshire and Isle of Wight Healing Arts involve programmes of concerts in hospitals and work in community health contexts. The programmes include people in and out of hospital with the aim of helping a generally healthy lifestyle.

Cultural identity

We cannot reconstruct the tightly knit communities that characterise the cultures in which shamanism and spirit possession cults flourished in a society which is very mobile and where family and kinship patterns are increasingly diverse. For some, friendship and interest groups will play a more significant part in their lives than these traditional groupings. We can construct groups of people who function as once family and kinship groups functioned and through these, we can construct our own identity. Music can play a significant part in this.

Music is important in the maintenance of cultural roots. There are interesting stories of the relationship between traditional musical healing in Africa and its relationship to allopathic medicine. In a conversation with a Xhosa singer in South Africa I asked him how he decided when to go to the Western hospital and when to go to the traditional healer. His reply was that when he (and his immediate family) decided that the sickness was due to alienation from his Xhosa culture, he would go to the traditional healer. We saw a similar phenomenon in East Africa in Chapter Three. So, in this view, some sickness is diagnosed as cultural alienation and the cure is to return to ways of healing that include music.

Just listening to music can give people an experience of identity that is healing. Alice Walker describes her experience of listening to Noel Pointer's version of *Many Rains Ago*:

> But – what were your feelings when you wrote it? Of whom, of what, were you thinking? But it's obvious, in the music itself, isn't it? What I felt was the incredible tenderness and longing between African-Americans as they remembered they have loved each other for centuries, through all kinds of barbarity and distance and time.

To me it is a music of healing. At first, every time I heard it I would cry. With grief and loss and longing. Then gradually I began to feel what was still left between us, as black people. Black women and men. So now when I play it I'm healed by the confidence that a lot of love is left. (Walker 1996, p.138)

Such concepts were alive early in this century in singing traditions in Western culture. Music can bring alive memories that re-root uprooted people, thus helping to reinforce the notion of identity. There is a moving letter from World War I showing how singing was used to strengthen the cultural roots of a young soldier who was aged 25 just before he died of his wounds on 7 September 1918:

Dear Mother and Sister,

I received your kind letter safely today and also the newspaper. I was glad to hear that you are well as I am here at the moment but was sorry to hear that Rich is in hospital. It is better for him to be anywhere these days than on the front. Well, Mam, I haven't got much news to tell you only that we are at it day and night. Well, the food is rather scarce and very little time to eat what you are given. Well, Mam, I understand that you are rather down hearted. Here we try to keep our spirits up through all the firing. We have short services here in the trenches and in all the mud. I turn to sing the verses that I learnt at dear Mynydd Gwyn. I hope that I will be back there soon... Well I haven't got anymore to say, but please try to cheer up, as I will soon be home with you... [I] send you my best wishes as a faithful son and brother,

Goodnight,

Griffith[2]

Exclusivity and inclusivity

Musical groups vary in the degree of exclusivity they operate. The classical tradition has constructed itself as quite elitist with groups of people traditionally excluded from its higher rankings on grounds of gender, race and class. Elitism is about power; it is about control and dependence-creation. The pursuit of excellence is closely linked with it and we see it in every area of contemporary society. It is a form of aggression and often leads to a lack of

---

2   I am indebted to John Roberts for this translation from the Welsh of an unpublished letter from Griffith Roberts, written 3 September 1918, which John Roberts possesses.

partnership between individuals. Competition is inbuilt and discourages many from starting on the process of entering the classical tradition. The perfection of the classical CD (which cannot even be reproduced by those who recorded it in real life) sets impossible standards that can be disempowering. For every Young Musician of the Year, there are not only thousands of discouraged competitors from the preliminary rounds, but also thousands of disenfranchised musicians, half asleep in their armchairs, confirmed in their belief that they never got under starter's orders when the music race got under way.

The classical tradition has constructed itself with a limited range of sounds that are regarded as acceptable and beautiful. Systems promoting uniformity have developed along quite authoritarian lines. The good unison singing sound (the sound of plainchant and choristers) has been encouraged. Even when we have a choir including different voices, we encourage singers within each line to develop a good unified sound, where individual differences are limited in the interest of a group sound. The orchestra, similarly, is a coherent group of players with soloists in some sections (like the woodwind, for example). Here large groups of stringed instruments are encouraged to make the most unified sound possible. Over both of these phenomena presides the figure of the conductor, the symbol of externalised, imposed authority who has the power to dictate what sort of sound is acceptable and to hire and fire people whose 'sound' does not 'fit'. These groups are like a very secure family in which the members voluntarily give up some of their individuality for the greater good of the whole, or the equivalent of government by a benevolent despot with a unified vision of the state he proceeds to create. In general, the smaller the group, the greater allowance there can be for individuality, as in chamber music. There are an increasing number of groups around the fringe of the classical tradition enabling access but in most areas there is a need to have acquired notational and instrumental/vocal skills.

The New Age and music therapy have validated a wider variety of sounds and offer, in general, more inclusive musical communities. The groups are in general non-hierarchical and organised on more democratic lines.

Inclusivity develops structures that encourage and contain diversity for individuals, minorities and the underprivileged. There is a famous saying from the philosopher Thoreau: 'If you look at your brother and he appears to be dancing rather strangely, he may be dancing to a different drum.' The more different the pattern, the more difficult it is for others to make sense of it and the more creativity is required in the inclusion of difference in a musical structure. In our multi-cultural contemporary society, we need to create structures in which these different drums can fit together. If reconciliation through music-making is to be achieved, fundamental to it is respect for the position in which the other person is standing. Within our communities, we need to work at structures and events in which we can co-operate musically.

Ecology

New Age group music-making may well include an ecological relationship and conceive of itself as relating to and influencing the natural world through music-making. Arts Access Aoteroa, in New Zealand, uses harakeke (flax) as an icon for ecological relationship in artworks in the ART and Health Partnership. The story of the origin of the flax is of how the plants lost the power to sing as they learned to live above the earth and become human. Only the flax retained it and reminded humans of their roots. The story is used to symbolise health, family and wholeness and singing is seen as a symbol of this connectedness (Eames 1999).

A pluralist society

Community musicians are now working at more democratic ways of bringing cultures together on a more mutual basis (see the work of Roger Watson in Chapter One), attempting it in a variety of ways. In engaging in musical activity together we engage deeply with one another. If we can resolve problems musically, we may solve them in other ways as well. Conflict resolution in this area is not about establishing a unity based on a single style, but rather about the creation of musical and sociological structures that encourage the peaceful co-existence of diversity (Boyce-Tillman 1996).

In my own piece *The Call of the Ancestors* (Boyce-Tillman 1998a) I used Western classical traditions, leaving spaces for improvisation by groups from other cultures – at the first performance, Kenyan drums, Thai piphat and rock group. The use of a mixture of notation and improvisation enabled the traditions to be true to their underlying principles.

Dr Svanibor Pettan, a Croatian ethnomusicologist, set up an imaginative project to help integrate Bosnian refugees into Norwegian society. He worked with Norwegian university music students and also visited Bosnian clubs to get to know Bosnian folk musicians. He encouraged the Norwegian and Bosnian musicians to work together, learning each other's repertoire and creating new pieces from the fusion of the cultures. The music groups then played in the Bosnian clubs and at the university. All those involved in the project felt it had aided the integration process considerably, as well as helping each group to value its own indigenous traditions more highly. Esteem at an individual and cultural level is closely bound up with acceptance.

In South Africa musicians have had similar aims in music-making. West Nkosi released in 1992 a CD entitled *The Rhythm of Healing*. The sleeve notes reveal the aims of community-building through music. His aim is one of community-building and empowerment:

> The music is a powerful and thoroughly updated mbaqanga version of Sax Jive, Kwela (penny whistle jive) and Marabi (gritty local jazz). The music brings back memories of places like Sophiatown, Alexandra, George Goch, Lady Selbourne in Pretoria, Mikhubane – Durban, District Six in Capetown, New Brighton – Port Elizabeth, and Duncanville – East London. It started way back in the 50's with mbube music, marabi, kwela, tsaba tsaba, and phata phata. In the early 60's Mbaqanga music swept the country by storm, marked by the first use of electric guitars and solid drumsticks instead of brushes. People started dancing differently to a rhythm that forced them onto the dance floor and momentarily wiped away their depression about oppression – that's why this album is entitled 'RHYTHM OF HEALING'.

So great is the healing intention of the disc that one of the pieces is even called 'Staff Nurse'. Here we see a group attempting to fuse the very varied traditions of South Africa and seeing it as part of the wider notions of healing society. *Nkosi Sikel' iAfrica* (the hymn which has become associated with the anti-apartheid struggle in South Africa) has been seen as having a similar function in Chapter Two (Cook 1998).

Musicians in Northern Ireland have been integrating groups of children in music-making activities throughout the conflict there. Their work has often been unreported, sometimes deliberately so. A reporter, invited to the carol singing in Belfast City Hall, asked where the Protestants and Catholics were sitting. On being told that they were all mixed together, he decided that it was not news and left. Such projects could be developed by politicians to help create national unity in a way that respects diversity.

Globalisation

Intercultural projects showing a respect for diversity offer models for a globalisation that is different from the global peddling of a normalised individualism. There is much work to be done in ways of bringing cultures together on a basis of equality and not through the colonisation that has characterised the Western classical traditions in particular. Sadly, the hierarchical classical tradition not only operated a hierarchy within itself but also beyond its boundaries. The subjugation of difference within the tradition spilled over into regarding other traditions – popular, ethnic, folk – as of lower standing. The high art Western musical traditions were spread across the world with an imperial zeal akin to the missionaries of Christianity; it has been seen as 'better' than that of other cultures, and attempts have been made to unite the world musically, as well as politically, by destroying other traditions. A powerful scene in a production of the Pan-African dance company *Adzido* portrayed a black man and woman taken away from the drums they were playing by a stereotypical white explorer (perhaps based on the musician/doctor Dr Albert Schweitzer). They are twisted into the positions necessary for playing the organ and the violin in which they were encouraged, even forced, by the white man. Meanwhile two other black men pick up the drums they have left, and start playing them. The man and the woman stop playing their violin and organ and listen. They look from their Western instruments to their African drums. To and fro their glance wanders. Their dilemma is clear.

And yet the intentions of the classical musicians were honourable. They were bringing 'good' music to the Africans, in the same way as they were bringing the 'truth' of Christianity. Insofar as they made diversity available it was a process of expanding people's horizons. Insofar as they exported value systems which devalued the traditions that they met, they set up the conditions for a musical imperialism akin to political imperialism. It is as difficult to sort out post-colonialism in music as it is in politics. Classical orchestras tour the world and examining bodies operating worldwide, like the Associated Board, promote Western classical traditions in a way that sometimes devalues indigenous musical traditions.

Value systems

Popular music is similarly endangering diversity by the globalisation of capitalistic value systems. Advanced capitalism deals only in products, each with a price tag. Not only does this devalue more process-based systems, it also establishes money as the only value system. It downplays communal systems of ownership as evidenced by the structure of Western copyright law. How appropriate is the model of individual ownership, embodied in these systems, for traditional musics passed on by the process of oral transmission?

Composers and performers are being forced into the position of individual ownership because of the prevalence of the heroic journey myth in the West. The legal structures that govern Western music-making (and threaten now to control the world) have this individualism enshrined within them. How can we both protect the art works of the Third World from exploitation, and also conserve their value systems? How can we value communal systems of knowing, and encourage respect for difference in world traditions? If we do not do this, we may find the musical world filled by a popular tradition (which acquires a few national characteristics as it establishes itself in different parts of the world) and a classical tradition arrogantly spreading the values of a Western elite.

Education and pluralism

Such thinking raises real issues for music education. It will become increasingly inappropriate for schools to pass on a single cultural heritage. The classroom will become a place of sharing diversity and making sense of the similarities and differences between traditions (Boyce-Tillman 1998d). Culture will be instilled by the wider society and the task of education will be to reflect on this and enable young people to make sense of it and develop a respect for musical diversity. Courses embracing a variety of traditions will need to be developed (Boyce-Tillman 1996b).

Questions for exploration

How can music:

- Reinforce a sense of identity and belonging to a community?
- Help construct an identity by musical networking?
- Help re-integrate the sick into the wider community?
- Create inclusive communities?
- Have an ecological role?
- Play a part in peace-making/keeping at a political level?
- Encourage pluralism in the growth of a global community?
- Create educational structures that value diversity within communities?

Incarnation

We need sufficient containment to feel safe, and sufficient freedom to realise our aspirations. With too much containment we feel stifled and trapped and with too great a freedom we feel out of control and unsupported. The balancing of these needs has been the substance of this containment/freedom polarity, both at a cultural and at a personal level. Any musical utterance results from the containing of the inexpressible and the potentially destructive (however this is perceived) within an audible form – incarnation. Most musical traditions have developed systems of containment. The degree of control over them, and how this is exercised, differs widely. The Western high art tradition has developed its notation systems and a pattern of instilling culture that concentrates a great deal on musical form. It has, since the Enlightenment, restricted the amount of improvisation on the part of the performer. Here, improvisation is limited to the composer. He or she can improvise in their head, on paper or at the keyboard but must emerge from this with a finalised product contained in notated form. Within the Western avant-garde there have been moves to greater freedom in the twentieth century especially with the development of chance/choice structures and the intermingling of jazz and classical music.

Shamanic and spirit possession cults also have a rigorous training, which includes both spiritual and musical aspects, for its musical healers. However, they often take place in the context of societies where music is more likely to be regarded as a universal human trait than in the West.

Both the New Age and music therapy have developed as a counterbalance to what was perceived as the excessive containment of the classical tradition. New Age practitioners try to rediscover the 'natural' voices of people, so challenging the limited choices validated by the classical world.

Music therapy has developed free improvisational skills to enable therapists to follow the diverse results of the musical freedom offered to their patients. There is an absence of an audience, which means that the stress can be wholly on the process. It enables the feelings of the participants to play a greater part in the musical form of the session (especially in the case of therapy).

Like the shaman's training (which includes the knowledge of other worlds and different states of consciousness) the training of music therapists includes an equal amount of psychology and music and the constraints operating on the tradition are as much extra-musical (in the form of boundaries or rituals) as musical. Music therapy might well be seen as the one totally free improvisatory tradition in the world, where the players are completely free. It is, however, important to remember the surrounding constraints on the situation and the fact that it is likely that the therapist has had a Western classical musical training. If so, certain constraints will operate from their own training.

The role of tradition in improvisation

Improvisation would seem at first to represent musical freedom. Work needs to be done on how the formal elements of traditions contain the feeling/emotional elements, comparing traditions such as the Western classical, jazz, and various New Age groups. The relationship between improvisation, notation and product needs examining. People need to be enabled to move freely between notated and non-notated traditions. Whereas classical musicians may embrace the freer structures of jazz, many popular musicians wish to learn classical notation.

But improvisatory traditions have internal constraints. Francis Silkstone's work on Thai traditions shows how students have at first to learn the melodic gestures which are used to generate the longer structures of the pieces. 'The musician in an oral tradition has mastered a technique of composition based on the manipulation of formulas, which allows him to perform and compose at the same time' (Silkstone, quoted in Becker 1980, p.20). 'While formulaic thinking is a vital part of such improvisation, it is just one aspect of a complex and subtle process... The main substance of a typical lesson achieves this memorisation with great efficiency' (Silkstone 1997, p.36).

Silkstone then goes on to describe how the pupils have to memorise the small melodic fragments by repetition after their teacher. Here we can see how most improvisatory traditions involve a degree of cultural background. The amount required differs widely from culture to culture and at different times within a particular culture. Who exercises control over the tradition and how tight this is is also widely variable.

Freedom and improvisation

In a beautifully prepared programme of the *Sounds of the Deep*, presented by Evelyn Glennie on BBC Radio Four (Glennie 1996), human divers discussed how they might communicate with the whales through singing. Extraordinary recordings of the whale sounds were played. One of them said that they were reputed to like the songs of UB40, but he said: 'When I got down I could not remember a single UB40 song, so I had to resort to the Beatles' *Yellow Submarine*. The whales appeared to find this interesting.' There then followed a description of how the whales' own songs were constructed and the description resembled much more the human improvisatory traditions using small motifs in a fascinating variety of ways to produce a song appropriate for every situation. How sad that the diving humans had lost their own confidence to do this so that the human diver had to revert to someone else's song for communication.

Our society has not encouraged the improvisatory powers of human beings. Parents of small children do make up songs about anything, like puddles or seeds or traffic lights. I watched an amazing lesson where a teacher of six-year-olds conducted a whole afternoon through improvised song. It was a lesson in November and was a wonderful musical dialogue about fireworks with imaginative sounds included to represent the fireworks themselves. Having young children, either as a parent/grandparent or teacher, can free that capacity for an adult if they have the courage to take it.

Improvisation in Western classical music education

Instrumental lessons in the Western classical tradition have traditionally concentrated on sight-reading as a key skill. This involves the decoding of notation which is essential to performing within the classical tradition. Improvisation is less often taught, although most children starting music lessons enjoy exploring sound. Often this is discouraged in the interest in reading the dots. I had an 11-year-old bass recorder player who said, five minutes before a concert, 'I've got some bad news for you, miss. I've forgotten my music.' It was a part of which I had no second copy and did not know what we could do. 'Don't you worry, miss. I'll busk it!' He was also the drummer for the local Assembly of God church, and so regularly improvised every Sunday for over two hours. He had both skills. He had retained both by virtue of functioning in two differing traditions.

It is likely that research would show that there is a need for greater freedom and fun in teaching the classical tradition: 'We suspect that those individuals for whom music is "all work and no play" will never achieve the highest levels of expressive performance. The achievement of the right balance of freedom and discipline is perhaps the single most challenging task for parents, teachers and young musicians' (Sloboda and Davidson 1996, p.187). It is possible for the containment of the notation to be balanced by the freedom of improvising. My own project with children with chronic anxiety showed clearly that the ability to improvise enabled some children to contain their anxiety (Boyce-Tillman 1998d).

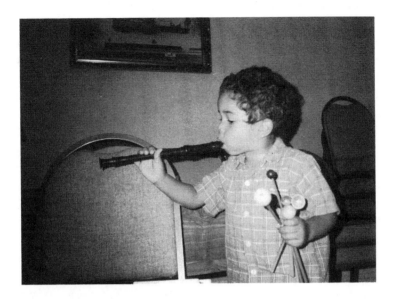

Figure 6.1 Darrell exploring music

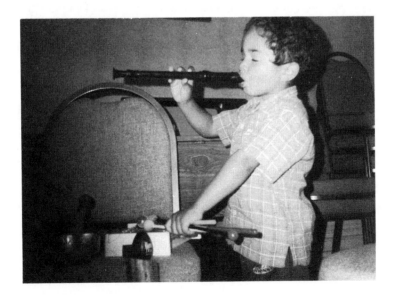

Figure 6.2 Darrell exploring music

Music and stress

In this context, people working in improvisatory forms emphasise the importance of the establishment of the right atmosphere. There needs to be, as far
as possible, a relaxed atmosphere, as people's previous musical experience
may well have been stressful and judgemental. A lightness of touch is crucial
to the success of improvisatory activities. Creative people are playful people
and creative situations need similar characteristics to safe play-grounds: they
need to be places where mistakes can be made safely and where it is safe to try
new things out. In such a situation experimenting is permitted and there is an
open atmosphere of trust. Laughter and fun, trust and openness are characteristics of the music-making situation that can contain internal and external
conflicts. Music can be a place where adults can play safely. There is an
expansiveness in the context of an accepting, trusting group. Within these,
people can discover their authentic musical voice or instrumental sound.
Eccentricity can be held within a structure that does not stifle it.

Such situations rebalance the stress of a product-based market economy.
A normalising society puts a great deal of stress on diverse human beings and
a product-based society leads to an anxiety-based perfectionism that subju-
gates human needs to product output. Human-based systems lay stress on
process, whereas in product-based systems the end justifies the means. Participating in improvisatory activities for their own sake is a useful antidote to
this and forms the basis of community music schemes linked with health
agencies.

Music and interpersonal skills

Music-making can be a place for exploring new interpersonal skills.
Matthew Sansom (1994), in approaching jazz improvisation from a psychoanalytical point of view, highlights this aspect of the work. He interviewed
Ross and Mick after an improvisatory session on electric guitar and
saxophone. Their comments include statements like:

> I was really pleased with the way it started because it was reflective – I felt
> that it was a good way to start relating to each other...

> [The other player says:] This is the first time where I made more of a
> decision to be more of a lead voice really... (p.4)

Sansom concludes from his analysis of key words in the interviews:

> It follows that the musical ideas of the improvisation represent both deci-
> sions and resources, and that degrees of feeling significant and insignifi-

cant relate to the individual's role within the dialogue... The interactions of Mick and Ross which involved the promotion of individual musical ideas gave rise to certain consequences. These were emotional and relate strongly to the sense of significance defined by the fulfilment and denial of roles. Mick experiences tension and anxiety over the roles of leading and following. He becomes concerned that he is overbearing and too dominant and that as a result Ross is not doing what he would really like to. (Sansom 1994, p.5)

Applied music

When music is used with healing intent, content takes precedence over form; musical expression will assume its own form as experience is encapsulated in sound. Applied music is characterised by relating music-making to its context. A functional approach to music leads to a greater stress on process rather than product.

This is clear in the work of Richard Bolton, a self-taught community musician in the area of popular music. He set up the Bird in Hand Activity Centre in Winchester for people who had had mental health problems. Here he runs improvisation sessions in a relaxed atmosphere, creating a sense of community through music-making. He believes in the role of music as a unique art to express both emotions and spirit and uses jazz structures to contain the music and hold people.

Questions for exploration

- How does music contain emotion/feeling in its structures? What is the relationship between the formal and expressive elements of music?

- What is the role of improvisation in this process?

- How does containment or restraint operate in improvisatory traditions? Are these musical or extra-musical?

- How can the Western classical traditions include a greater degree of freedom in their performance practice?

- How can the playful aspects of music-making be fostered?

- What is the varying relationship between process and product in music-making? How can this relationship be used therapeutically?

- What practices are useful in applied music-making in healing situations?

Maturity

The dilemma of the public and the private is a personal and cultural issue. All systems of morality and ethics address the dilemma. The balancing of the two at a personal and cultural level is a sign of maturity. The Western literature on music and creativity stresses the area of self-expression and links it with human emotion. The Western notion of the musical genius is tightly bound up with these notions. The composer must express himself regardless of the acceptance of the audience although the experience of rejection is painful.

Traditions of psychotherapy have developed ways of accessing deep areas of feeling and painful traumatic experiences but can leave people with difficult memories allied to powerful feelings, such as anger and despair; without much guidance as to what to do with them. Not only does music offer the possibility of expressing these but also of remaking them into an aesthetically satisfying object. Psychiatric practice based largely on medication and talking needs the arts to provide a medium and container for these.

The nature of the self is a fundamental conceptual problem and the presence of self-expression is less obvious in the shamanic culture when the songs and pieces are more likely to be deemed to have come from the gods, spirits, ancestors or power animals. This has been taken over into New Age thinking where it is seen as an expression of the Divine or higher self. There is, however, a notion that the process of expression is important and is the necessary fulfilment of a vocation.

There is considerable debate about the precise meaning of music, where this is situated and how it is communicated. There is clearly an element of cultural and personal interpretation in the process of decoding music. This makes it, by definition, a confidential medium as an expressive one.

Memory

Music can be used to unlock painful and pleasant areas of memory. This can be done through improvising, performing or listening. However, because of the personal aspect of meaning, it requires more of a degree of sensitive tuning on the part of the participants and more careful choice of material by the leader. Both leader and participants need to play a part in the choice of pieces, which will have different meanings for different people in any given group. The stress on calmness and order in Western society has not encouraged public expressions of grief and traditions like keening and wailing were suppressed by the Church early in Western culture. These used a wide range of human vocalisations in a ritual manner to express the grief of a community. New Age practitioners have revived interest in such practices.

The need for acceptance

Access to the process of music-making needs to be developed in educational contexts so that people can use the process of composing, improvising and performing for their personal expression. The reason for people's loss of music as a potential area for expression has frequently been their lack of confidence in their ability to use music as a medium at all. This has been created by non-acceptance – of their singing note, of the sort of patterns they are capable, of instruments and so on. In making a musical sound, we say something about ourselves in the medium of sound; if it is refused, it could be a lifetime before we offer of ourselves in that medium again. Acceptance by the group can be expressed in a variety of ways. Applause is one, and supportive discussion another.

Others find acceptance from elements in the natural world. There is the medieval story of Caedmon, a stable boy in the abbey of Hilda of Whitby, North Yorkshire. It is the custom in the evenings to pass around the harp and for each of those present – members of the religious community and pilgrims – to sing a song. Caedmon is handed the harp and is frozen with fear and unable to do anything. He races out of the refectory to the stables. Here he encounters an angel who tells him to let into his heart the natural world that he loves so much, and then sing. This he does, and the first recipients of his song are the angel and the animals. This is sufficient to empower him to tell one of the community who tells the Abbess Hilda. With her encouragement Caedmon is enabled to sing at the gathering that evening. He becomes the first English singer-poet (based on Swann 1971).

The multiple meanings of music

The capacity of music for multiple meanings – personal, cultural and inherent – needs exploring in educational and health contexts. What is clear is that music cannot be read like text and does not function at the level of specific meaning. This gives it great possibilities for use in communal situations and for the expression of things (events, experiences) that a group might find difficult in their raw (or verbal) form. There is much possibility here, especially in the area of the treatment of psychiatric illness. The New Age practitioners with less 'boundaried' concepts than those developed in verbal psychotherapeutic practice, and also drawing on shamanic practices, are exploring this area far more. People who develop musical skills are able to express painful emotions safely in a form that reveals and hides them simultaneously. In this way music could be used throughout a lifetime by people with serious traumas in their early life. Indeed, it can be the well-spring of their creative work. The work of Arts Access Aoteroa in New Zealand of establishing creative spaces in the community is part of this move. Other organisations such as REACH in the UK are experimenting with groups where 'sick' or disabled people work artistically with 'well' or 'normal' people.

Questions for exploration

- What are the processes that enable music to open up memories (both painful and joyful) and how can these be used therapeutically?

- What part can music play in the processes of grieving?

- How can we enable people to use music as a means of expression?

- What structures have we for the acceptance of musical offerings in the various traditions?

- How can the multiple levels of musical meaning be unpacked and used therapeutically?

- Can musical healing take place in more public arenas, involving more people in the processes of musical healing?

Creativity

In an age of globalisation where people will belong not to one but to a number of networks and communities, there is access to a wider variety of traditions and practices than ever before. This very diversity can be a source of individual and cultural creativity. Some of these cannot be brought together but co-exist alongside one another both in the self and in society.

All descriptions of the creative process include a phase of chaos. Notions of unity, associated with order, in the self appear on the one hand attractive; but culturally and personally they can result in a form of fascism. The encouraging of diversity or indeed chaos may appear as disintegration but can also be seen both as a necessary prelude to creative action and indeed as an end in its own right.

The notion of the integrated self that is deep in Western culture is based on the Greek notion of 'harmonia'. This runs through the classical literature, New Age practices, music therapy and shamanic practices. All such practices are designed to remove undesirable elements, whether these are perceived as troubling spirits, blockages to the expression of higher energy or power, or neuroses. It is not a once-for-all process, but a constant ebb and flow that can be seen as integration and de-integration. There is much psychological literature that links internal conflict with creativity (see Chapter One).

The arts do not merely express life as it is, but also transform it. The process of creation is a process of transformation. The flash of insight that often characterises the penultimate stage of the creative process is a moment of seeing the possibility of a new pattern not only in sound but also within the personality. Within this process lies the possibility of redeeming the damaging experiences of the past and remaking them into new ways. The creative process necessarily involves a descent into chaos. In the shamanic traditions this is regarded as another world; in music therapy and contemporary classical traditions, it is regarded as the unconscious or subconscious. The New Age includes both these interpretations within its thinking. It is from this journey that the work of art emerges. This is often clear in the workings of the composers of the classical traditions like Beethoven who left sketchbooks of their working.

De-integration and disintegration

Sometimes in a society that prizes order so highly the place of chaos is demonised and designated as 'sick'. In a society that had different values there might be better-constructed systems for understanding and handling this diversity, as in spirit possession cults. Here, diversity is applauded and regarded as a 'special' sign. The acceptance of neo-shamanism within the New Age reflects an increasing ability to accept differing frames of reference for states once considered 'sick'.

What is interesting in the descriptions of the shamanic crisis is that death and rebirth are central. In traditional societies this was regarded as very real. It was experienced as part of a journey within the context of a society with established practices and procedures for handling this process of transformation. On the other side of this process the shaman is a 'new' person. It is interesting to reflect on how this 'crisis' is viewed in Western medicine. Here, there is a notion of preventing the crisis happening, as there is no established notion of a spiritual dimension to the 'sickness'. But the characteristics of such crises in the mentally sick are often suicidal thoughts and attempts. It is interesting to reflect that such thoughts and desires for death may be transformative desires that could be dealt with by a ritual or symbolic death. In the absence of a shared religious frame, it is possible to construct transformative rituals involving music.

The Western composer as therapist or shaman

In listening we can be taken into a different world by a composer or guide who takes us through it musically. When we listen, for example, to the slow movement of Beethoven's fourth piano concerto, with its bringing together of two very contrasted elements within his self, we enter into Beethoven's experience; insofar as his journey is akin to ours we can share it and use it for own transformation. The composer, together with performer, becomes a therapist who, like the ancient shamans, has entered the Underworld on behalf of the wider community. The Underworld is now perceived as being within rather than in another realm, but the important thing is that someone has entered it and found a way through and out. The tools of the Western composer thus become akin to those of the shaman. Entering the Underworld with the bank of musical forms and structures that make up tuition of the Western classical tradition can be seen as the equivalent in this respect to the training of the shaman for his entry into the Underworld. But the response is essentially an individual response and the journey of the composer/performer must resonate with that of the listener. This shows us why pieces of music lose significance for us. We are no longer at the same place in our story. We are not just empty containers into which composers and performers pour their feelings. Each person comes with their own cultural heritage and also an individually constructed set of needs constructed as likes and dislikes. One person's musical meat is another person's musical poison.

Composing/improvising as self-transformation

When we compose or improvise we engage in the same process as the 'great' composers. A GCSE pupil was a school refuser with a number of personal problems. She spent hours alone with her recorder improvising and produced pieces of extraordinary beauty. These not only expressed her dilemmas but also resolved them by turning them into beautiful musical objects. It is in this area, par excellence, that people can transform negativity into a creation of worth and value, both for themselves and for others. In the process of writing my 1996 piece, *Healing,*[3] I had a strong sense of self-purification, completed on the day I finished the piece, which happened to be the summer solstice. The performer has a similar sensation when performing it.

Music, of all the arts, has the capacity for expressing conflicting feelings and containing them in musical structures. These can even be sung or played simultaneously. This is very clear, for example, in the big ensembles of operatic works, in which each character may be singing about a very different emotion and yet the whole fits together, as in the Finale of Act Two of Mozart's *The Marriage of Figaro*.

Multiple musical selves

The place of diversity within the self appears at first to be opposed to the notions of the unity and integration that underpin a great deal of the thinking about healing. The model of integration within the self might be better understood as the peaceful co-existence of diversity rather than its obliteration. This is more likely to be true in a globalised society when it is likely that people will belong to a number of different cultures each with different value systems.[4] This allows for a person to have a greater diversity within the self which can be expressed musically by learning different musical traditions, playing in different groups in different places and resisting the need to integrate these stylistically. In the dynamic model of the self it is likely that there are many possible shapes. As we explore the wide range of human experience, the likelihood of diversity becomes greater.

Questions for exploration

- What are the similarities between the other world of shamanic practice and Western notions of the unconscious?

- What distinguishes creative de-integration from disintegration?

- Has Western society 'demonised' de-integrative phases, which are a necessary part of growth and change at a personal and cultural level?

- Can we construct musical rituals of transformation?

3   Unpublished piece for double bass and soprano.
4   Floyd, M. (1999) Unpublished Ph.D. thesis, King Alfred's, Winchester.

- How do musical structures bring diversity into a unity or show a unity to be a diversity?

- How far does the creator of a musical event become a therapist for those who listen to it?

- How can this process be used for personal transformation?

- Does the concept of multiple musical selves enable a degree of diversity within a globalised society?

Empowerment

The balancing of challenge and nurture is central to notions of child rearing. As we become adults, it becomes our own responsibility to take on these notions for ourselves, being aware of our own needs. The notion of the heroic journey has built into it an alliance of notions of challenge and progress and tends to devalue the role of nurture. The classical tradition has been very much one of challenge, while the New Age and music therapy have been much closer to nurture. The New Age has produced a range of recordings designed for nurturing, many of them specifically for use with techniques like massage and aromatherapy. These often include the sounds of the natural world alongside instruments and voices. The development of the classical canon (a bank of familiar works) can also been seen as a nurturing phenomenon. Pieces that were once a challenge to the surrounding society have now assumed a different role when moved into a different time and place and played often. This could be seen as nurturing by the ancestors. The shamanic traditions fuse the notions of challenge and nurture. The shaman undertakes the challenge on behalf of the patient.

The healing process requires a balance between these two elements. To find this rhythm is to find a sense of empowerment. This involves self-awareness in which the dynamic model of the self can play a part. To perceive what we need at any given time may establish the rhythm of challenge and nurture necessary for living, for balance is not a once-for-all event. It is entering into a process.

Challenging procedures

Medicine has adopted and valued a number of aggressive procedures, rating surgical procedures highly in the order of healing interventions. Education has now moved to a system of testing that sees learning as a series of challenging hurdles. Western classical music has concentrated on challenge in its relationship to its audience. Classical music education too is a series of challenges with its examination systems and competitions. To acquire musical skills – technical, expressive and notational – does enable people to enter the process of musical balancing with greater insight and understanding. Musical challenge has not been part of traditional music therapy and yet there is no doubt that the acquisition of musical skills leads to empowerment (Boyce-Tillman 1998d).

Nurturing procedures

The use of music to hold people is particularly useful in community settings and in group work in music therapy. It is a capacity that can be very useful in a society where touch has become an abused area for some people. The lullaby is an area where, traditionally, children have been held musically. In child rearing there have been indications of the possibility of children taking on the songs sung to them by their parents as comforters, rather like teddy bears and comfort blankets. It is certainly true in my own experience. One of my sons had no comfort toy; I was alarmed that somehow he had missed out on an important stage in his development, until I heard him wake in the night and sing himself back to sleep with the songs with which we had sung him to sleep. A stay in hospital reinforced this at eight months, when the ward sister referred to his loud singing in the night. He had learned to comfort (and nurture) himself with song.

In a therapeutic group where a conflict had arisen, a man sang a lullaby. This was a very moving experience for all present and involved a man holding a group safely through song. I was present at a service in Gugulethu, South Africa, where people could come forward for healing. They told the pastor their problem. He relayed this to the congregation. The congregation then sang to support the healing. What was interesting here was that the songs were not the soft, gentle sounds that we associate with the nurturing of the New Age, but strong louder pieces accompanied by drumming patterns made on hymn books. The greater the need, the greater the strength of the singing of the thousand people present.

Hospitals are setting up programmes designed to produce a more nurturing environment. These include music in schemes that include art, architecture and other performing arts. The Council for Music in Hospitals, for example, sends musicians into hospitals to produce programmes tailor-made for particular situations – singers who can, for example, sing songs that patients think will be helpful.

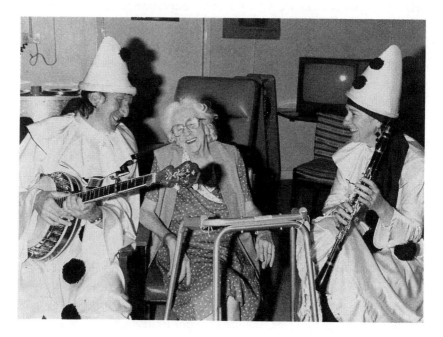

Figure 6.3 'Music is the best medicine in the world' – The Pavilion Pierrots bringing the joy of live music to a hospital audience on behalf of the Council for Music in Hospitals

Singing as empowerment

The notion that singing empowers is sometimes linked with the immune system, which is crucial to the maintenance of health at the physical level. Music is seen as influencing the body's immune system and building people's sense of self and identity. Empowerment through music takes many forms. For some people, the discovery that they can make music is a very strengthening experience, especially if they have been subjected to much discouragement and if it is enjoyed by others. The opening up of the area of composing/improvising has often been significant here. A woman who found that she was going blind just as she started learning to play the recorder discovered that now she could play her own tunes. The opening up of the area of public performing can also increase self-confidence, as in the case of a woman in her sixties who sang publicly for the first time since a parent had criticised her solo hymn-singing at the age of seven.

In the name of music education in a normalising curriculum we have sometimes cheated people out of their birthright to sing. Singing has been at the core of the music curriculum for centuries. And yet a pursuit of a falsely based excellence has meant the alienation of our birthright. If a child comes to school and doesn't speak we spend a great deal of time encouraging him or her to do so. We don't say: 'He's a non-speaker. Some people don't, you know.' And yet we do it with singing. The map of singing as presented in the average school is one of a restricted range of pitches and tone colours. We all have our own note, the note that is easiest for us to sing at any time, and this is variable. It changes at different times of the day. Our voices are often low in the morning, rise towards the middle of the day and then sink as we get more tired. Some would also say that there is a seasonal component (a yearly cycle) as well. There are also certain staging points in our lives which once would have been marked by rites of passage. The male voice changes at puberty, but so does a girl's and a woman's changes again at the menopause. Also, a trauma of some kind can be reflected in this pitch which is related to our sense of identity.

In school in the UK, if you had a choirboy-type sound and a fairly high pitch, you succeeded in singing classes. If your tone colour was dark and your pitch low it was, in general, unacceptable. The scenario went rather like this:

> Aged four, you came to school and said 'I am Jill. This is how I dress. This is how I speak. Do you like me? This is the note I sing. Do you like it?' If it conformed to the stereotype above, you found that your teacher both liked it and sang it herself. You gathered therefore that it was an acceptable sort of note to have. If, however, it wasn't, you were told not to sing. The process of the non-acceptance had begun. (Boyce-Tillman 1996b, p.215)

One man in a group with which I was working described one of his earliest school memories thus: 'I was singing in a group. We stood in rows. The teacher came down the room. If we sang out of tune he slapped us. I have never liked the sound of my own voice, even my speaking voice' (unpublished 1990 conversation with a guitarist in Gibraltar). He needed to look no further for the source of this feeling of failure.

If, however, you were allowed to sing your low note, you soon discovered that it was not in any of the songs. When you changed schools, you sang it again (or a new, lower one if you were a boy) and hoped it would feature in the new school curriculum. It seldom did, unless there was an alto or bass section in the choir and you were able to sing a separate part. However, with a diligent Head of Music, you acquired the name of a growler or groaner and you worked together in the lunch hour. He or she found the note that you sang and gradually you added others, starting with those nearest to it. If this did not happen, you might, when you left school, have been singing your note for some 11 years but it had never appeared on the map presented by your teachers. You could be forgiven for saying that you could not sing and, even worse, that you were not musical. The truth was that the map of singing that was presented to you was too small.

My friend runs a 'Can't Sing' choir at Morley College in London. Over a hundred people are prepared to give up their entire lunch hour to discovering their voice. A man of 80 came up to me and said: 'Do you know, a door has opened to me at 80 that I thought was shut for life.' It is wonderful that doors are swinging open at a time when others are shutting, but sad that it was ever shut. If he had not found where the Philippine islands were at school, would he still be looking for them? And yet he was looking for his ability to sing. He knew it was his birthright and somehow more central to his being then geographical information.

The task of the leader of singing is to find a pitch acceptable to a group, not choose one from pitched instruments like the piano. It is an individualised, intuitive process, demanding being in tune with the group. For the pitch will be lower if the group is tired, has colds, is depressed or if it is early in the day or winter time.

Singing is power, and there are remarkable stories of people who have used it in their darkest moments. From the El Mozote massacre in El Salvador in 1981 comes the remarkable story of a young girl, an evangelical Christian, who was raped several times in one afternoon. Through it all she sang:

> She had kept on singing, too, even after they had done what had to be done, and shot her in the chest. She had lain there on La Cruz [the hill on which the soldiers carried out their killings] – with the blood flowing from her chest and had kept on singing – a bit weaker than before, but still singing. And the soldiers, stupefied, had watched, and pointed. Then they had grown tired of the game and shot her again, and she sang still, and their wonder turned to fear, until they had unsheathed their machetes, and hacked her through the neck, and at last the singing stopped. (Danner 1994, pp.78–79)

It is contemporary story with echoes of the myth of Orpheus of Chapter Two.

I met a nun who felt overwhelmed by her work in a community that concerned itself with violations of human rights. After the course in which she had sung some of her songs she said to me: 'I know what I had forgotten; I had forgotten to sing. If I remember to sing I can survive the stories that our community is receiving and even transform them in some way.'

We can either sing our own songs that we make up or those of our ancestors or other strong races. Many of their songs show immense strength. In singing them we tap into that universal strength. In some cultures that would be seen as of contacting the ancestors whose role is to strengthen us in the present.

Cultural empowerment

If we read the stories of singing nations like the Jews and the black slaves we find how singing and survival are closely linked. One concerns the song *Tsvey Taybelekh*, an old Yiddish folk song which tells of two loving doves torn from one another by an unknown evil force. The song was seen as a way for the Jews to express their feelings of pain and sorrow which they couldn't do openly under the Nazis. An opera singer called Liuba Levitska sang it through her solitary confinement and all the way to her execution.

Saulius Trepekunas, a Lithuanian musician, tells the story of how Lithuania achieved its independence from the USSR by song. People gathered in the capital, Vilnius, around their campfires and sang. The Russian tanks with the television cameras of the world on them could not fire on singing citizens; so they left. His story is about the power of music to create community, particularly national identity. In this context music is an expression of national dreams and aspirations.

Music in health promotion

The increasing use of music in health-care institutions, including GPs' surgeries (see Chapter Five), shows how music can be used to promote the health of individuals in community. It can involve active music-making as well as recorded music. Advice given to patients based on surveys of lifestyle touches on music. This can involve liaison with local music-making agencies such as choirs, orchestras, rock groups, folk groups, schools, theatre groups, music teachers and community musicians and educating health promoters, such as health visitors about the possibilities. Sessions encouraging mothers to bond with their babies through music-making are already part of some programmes. (Pesek 1996)

Giving musical skills through music education of some kind can improve people's independence. I arranged music lessons for four children diagnosed with chronic anxiety as part of a treatment programme in conjunction with Winchester Child Guidance Unit. The acquisition of drumming skills by one participant enabled him to become a 'normal' teenager playing in a band and at ease with his peers who had previously bullied him; another participant learned to control the symptoms of bulimia through improvisation (Boyce-Tillman 1998b).

The Orpheus Centre, initiated by Michael Swallow and Richard Stilgoe in Surrey, is a residential centre for disabled people aged between 18 and 40. Courses vary from a three-year apprenticeship to short courses. Many aspects of the performing arts are included – music theatre, song-writing and recording, dance, lighting and sound, box-office and marketing. The participants also learn independent living skills and are given a role in the management structure with the aim of improving their confidence and enabling them to live independently in the world.

Questions for exploration

- Can music-making offer nurturing procedures alongside challenging procedures in the context of health and education?

- What relationship is there between empowerment in music and the body's immune system?

- How can we develop people's sense of self-image through singing?

- How can we encourage the empowerment of cultural groups and networks through music-making?

- How can people learn to use music as a means of self-challenge and self-nurture?

- Can we use procedures therapeutically that 'hold' people with sound? How do these work?

- How can music be linked with structures for health promotion?

Rhythm

The rhythm of the human being in micro and macro terms – like the day, year, and lifespan – necessarily involves the balancing of excitement and relaxation. Too much excitement, and the person can find no rest at all and too much relaxation and the system stagnates and atrophies. These functions of music are to be found in all traditions and appear to be linked with transcultural/physiological effects. Many people have learned to use music to establish a rhythm in their lives. The Western classical tradition has balanced them within pieces in movements and sections of different expressive characters. Shamanic cultures have used music of different characters at different stages in rituals and combined it with the use of hallucinogens under the careful supervision of the elders of the surrounding culture. In the New Age there is a stress on relaxation which appears to balance the increasing stimulation of Western society and the moods of the dominant popular and classical traditions. In music therapy, these attributes of music are used both to help patients manage their emotional state and to control pain and help in physiological procedures.

Establishing rhythm by listening

I have used a piece called the *Chinese Horseman* in many different groups and cultures. It starts with a free-flowing section with no clear pulse, high on the flute. To this, in a middle section, a walking pace beat is added. In the final section, more instruments are added, the piece gets faster and louder with a clear beat. Some people find the free-flowing first section very relaxing and freeing. They imagine open plains and high mountains. Others, however, find it unsafe and insecure. Some find the middle section with a beat much safer, while the freer spirits find it restricting and more stressful. Some people are really lifted by the final section which they see as joyful dancing. Others see it as like the rush hour in a city, worrying and stress-inducing. One person made a beautiful interpretation of it. She said:

> I am alone and sad and longing to meet someone who will heal my pain.
> It is all around me. Someone joins me and we walk together. Then we go
> together to a village where there is joyful music and dancing. I feel I
> belong and my pain is healed. (unpublished 1982 comment by a member
> of an INSET course at Reading University)

After the activity we discuss how music of different characters affect different people. People can go away and look at their CD collections in order to be aware of how they might use music to manage their own feelings.

People have developed this ability of music to establish new life rhythms in programmes to replace medication as well as drugs that are not part of the dominant tradition. The use of music is safer and more in one's personal control than drugs, and involves being aware of your personal responses to it. The process of entrainment, which means finding music that is in tune with where you are at present, is helpful here. Music cannot be prescribed on a simple cause and effect basis as the story above shows. The availability of music from other cultures makes it possible to explore a wide range of options. The effect of music from a culture with which you are familiar will be different from that from a different culture. Some accounts indicate that the effect of music from an unknown culture will be more 'pure' and free of associations (see Chapter Five).

Establishing rhythm by means of active music-making

Rouget (1985) describes how the generation of our own musical material is the subtlest way of influencing our own rhythm:

> One's internal sensitivity is also aroused by music and likewise functions as a path of reception. It is well known that when we speak, and even more when we sing, we hear ourselves from the inside. But, in fact we are doing more than hearing ourselves sing. We are *feeling* ourselves sing. We are feeling our larynx (let us say, more simply, our neck and throat) vibrate, quiver. And this is true of many other areas of the body too: the entire head, the thorax and abdomen, the pelvic region. Music is thus simultaneously an animation of things and a palpitation of the being. Both are felt more intensely when one is making music than when one is simply listening to it. We should be able to say, 'to act' music, as opposed to 'undergoing' it, for these are indeed two very different ways of experiencing it (p.120).

If people can be re-empowered to create their own songs or humming patterns they will be able to influence themselves more subtly than by using recorded music as there is a continual interaction between the music and the feelings.

Questions for exploration

- How can we best develop people's self-awareness of the effect of various types of music on their own rhythms?
- How can people be helped to generate their own music to adjust their rhythm?
- What part can music play in drug treatment programmes?
- How can interventions based on music and medication be used in an interactive way?

Wisdom

Many ancient wisdom systems see the transcendent as rooted in the body. The polarity embodiment/transcendence is concerned with the relationship of the body to feelings of transcendence, of belonging to a great cosmic whole, whether within or without a religious frame of some kind. Out of balance, the pursuit of the transcendent leads to the denial of the body, or even to an asceticism that is harmful to it. A concentration on the body and denial of the transcendent leads to an unfettered materialism.

In shamanic traditions, the body and transcendence are closely intertwined. Trance states were induced by the use of dance, music and hallucinogens. The Western classical traditions have taken on the dualistic division between body and spirit that characterised Greek spirituality and Christianity. These concentrated on the spirit and sometimes abused the body, and the link with dance was broken. Even when notions of a soul disappeared, the aesthetic was seen as appealing to the mind rather than the body.

Music therapy took on this split and developed within psychiatric medicine. Practices affecting the body have concentrated on the developing of motor skills through musical activity for people with a physical disability. There are, however, some therapists who are able to identify transcendent elements like moments of joy and wonder in their treatments: 'As a therapeutic transformation of the personality, modern psychotherapy is very much in line with these oriental religions and mysteries, without of course prescribing stages or ceremonies celebrating or imprinting these stages of transformation' (Redfearn 1992, p.183).

In the New Age, there is a very real upsurge of interest in more esoteric systems for healing the body. Practitioners find the note or sound for the kidneys or liver and encourage these to function by getting clients to sing or make the appropriate sounds. Much of the New Age uses the Eastern system of the chakras in which an energy flow through the body is thought to link us with heaven and earth.

Musical meditation and health

This forms an important part of New Age thinking and includes some notions of a change of consciousness, drawing on shamanic models. Within Christianity such chanting traditions as those developed by the Taizé religious community in France have also used the repetition of short musical phrases to induce a meditative state. The classical tradition has had a number of composers who have a meditative aspect to their compositions such as John Cage, Karlheinz Stockhausen, Olivier Messiaen and Pauline Oliveros.

Some are rediscovering pieces from the hidden classical tradition. People listening to the chants of Hildegard of Bingen, for example, find them deeply healing. When they are sung, the control of the breath required to manage the long phrases is seen as a meditation associated with the Holy Spirit. It is said to encourage hyperventilation which also induces an altered state of consciousness:

> Hildegard's compositions are incredibly physical... When she writes about the Spirit, you know she understands the Spirit as wind, as breath, because you become the wind. When she writes about Divine Mysteries, you sing out of the deepest space of your physical being from the comfort of the normal range to the extremes of your potential. (Doyle 1987, p.364)

Some music therapists have explored such techniques to relax patients and there is increasing interest in Western medicine in techniques derived from meditative traditions as an antidote to stress.

Music and the body in Western medicine

The use of music is limited in general to the development of motor skills in people with disabilities. The frames in which shamanic medicine and the New Age function are so different that to develop these ideas further is difficult. It involves the suspension of a great deal of disbelief on the part of Western medicine, a discipline constructed within the rationalistic Western culture which has devalued magic and belief as superstition. There are some doctors willing to explore such relationships (Gurukul publicity leaflet, 1999). However, they are often seen as isolated explorers, prepared to risk ridicule and marginalisation.

Music and dance

It is in Western popular music that the relationship between music and dance is at its strongest. The trance and rave music traditions have seen music and dance rejoined with notions of transcendence. In these traditions, transcendence has been made into a commodity by a capitalist value system that enables the recording industry and the drug cartels to exploit what is a fundamental human need.

The New Age thinking also uses dance in some groups. These are sometimes part of neo-shamanic rituals like Gabrielle Roth's Drumming the Five Rhythms. The circle dance has become popular as a way of cementing group cohesion.

Movement therapy is finding a place in medicine, but is often separate from music therapy. In shamanic cultures the two are inseparable with a real sense of the efficacy of music in curing physical illness. These healing systems involve trance, which is often induced by dance and music in combination.

The concert as spiritual experience

Accounts of transcendence are still found in the classical tradition but now dissociated from a religious tradition or a spiritual frame. However, the concept is still one associated with the mind. Concert halls have fixed seats and audiences are expected to sit silent and still. There is little notion that the experience will have any effect on the body. Indeed, in order to produce the spiritual experience, the performers themselves may be doing considerable harm to their own bodies (by holding their bodies in difficult positions for long periods).

Concert halls and CDs playing on a personal stereo are seen by some to be the holy spaces of the contemporary world (Boyce-Tillman 2000). The Jewish story of the origin of the Nigun (the Jewish wordless song tradition) illustrates this well. The rabbi goes to the woods, lights a fire and performs a ritual. He cannot remember the ritual but he can sing the song. God says: 'It is enough.' Next time, he goes to the wood but can no longer remember how to light the fire, so he sings the song. God says: 'It is enough.' Next time, the rabbi can no longer find the wood so he sings the song. God says: 'It is enough.' Finally he forgets the words of the song. So he sings a tune he can remember. God says: 'It is enough.'[5]

Questions for exploration

- How can musical mediation be used to promote health?
- How far can music challenge the mind/body/soul split that characterises Western medicine?
- Is there a possibility of extending the use of music in the treatment of physical illness using notions of the spiritual?
- Can the therapeutic properties of dancing to music be examined?
- How far is the concert a therapeutic spiritual experience in Western culture?

5   I am grateful to Irith Shillor for this story.

Summary

Inside all of us, there is a musician trying to get out. That musician is our own healer and potentially, through us, a healer of others. This book has set out a model of disease as imbalance – within society, within the self, within the wider cosmos. Pain can be regarded as cracks in a fabric that needs a right relatedness – a fabric in which the relatedness between all the parts is a creative one (Grey 1989). The disjunctions are the wounds – personal, cultural and cosmic. It has set out a model of how to rebalance the system using music as healing – a balance that enables each of us to explore a range of experience with safety. The music produced is a record of the process of healing. It is from the cracks that the healing music comes and to which it goes. Music offers the possibility of transformed and strengthened living. There is a beautiful Jewish story:

> A ruler had a fine diamond. It became seriously damaged. All the best jewellers were consulted to see if they could restore it to its former glory. None could do it. Eventually a jeweller came along who claimed that it could be made better than it was before. The court were astonished. After weeks of work, it was found that the jeweller had engraved around the flaw the most beautiful rose; and the place of the damage was now the place of the greatest beauty.

Music is the sounding form of the rose.

From the struggle of the individual to retain its own identity and yet belong to the community, for whom connection is the lifeblood,
from the shaping and making that enables inchoate feeling to take an audible form,
from the dilemma of making public the private and painful,
from the broken middle of contradictions in the midst of the self and society,
from the desire to rest from challenge and to free oneself from a stifling nurture,
from the finding of a rhythm of excitement and relaxation,
from the reconciliation of the ineffability of the mystic experience with the human body in its strength and weakness,
comes the music.

These are indeed:
the wounds that sing.

Musical Activities

These represent a range of activities illustrating the themes of the book. Most of them are group activities but some can be modified for individual use.

Community/individualism

Improvisation over a repeated beat – finding your role

A GROUP EXERCISE IN PAIRS

Both people in the pair have a musical instrument. It can be a simple percussion or a more complex instrument like a violin or a recorder. One person in the pair holds the beat while the other improvises freely against it. Decide how to end the improvisation without using words; simply use gesture and musical sensitivity. Change roles.

Reflect on what it felt like in each role. Did you enjoy the up-front role of the improviser or the more supportive pulse-holder role? What did each of you do when the rhythmic relationship between you foundered? Did you carry on regardless and hope that your partner found you, or did you keep changing until you found your partner? Which was more successful in the creation of ensemble? Examine how similar your musical behaviour is to your chosen role in other relationships. Are you the sort of person who prefers the anchor role, behind the scenes – holding the pulse of life for others? Or are you more of the up-front soloist who likes to have others supporting you? Explore it again taking the role that you find less easy and see if you can work at it musically.

Containment/freedom

A free improvisation group

A GROUP EXERCISE

This can be done with a group of up to about six or seven people with instruments, which can be orchestral instruments, keyboard or piano, or simple percussion. Tell the group that you are going to have a musical sharing rather like an after-dinner conversation. Everyone is free to do what they feel is right and the music should flow without any words. Sometimes one person will be more prominent than others. Sometimes two people will be having a real dialogue. Sometimes the music will be loud and challenging and at other times more peaceful and gentle. Vocal sounds can be used and anyone can challenge for the lead if they want it. People may change instruments. Most of all, you should encourage people to go with the flow. Listen to what others are doing and respond. You may or may not like to talk about what happened afterwards. It is best done with no one listening, everyone participating. The joy is in the process and the presence of a non-playing listener changes the dynamic of the exercise.

Expression and confidentiality

Conversations

A GROUP EXERCISE

Take two contrasted instruments like a drum and a woodblock. Teach the group a short phrase, such as: 'Conversations, conversations. What shall we say today?'

Say the rhyme as a group, while the instruments are passed in opposite directions around the circle. Whoever has the instruments at the end of the rhyme has a musical conversation, answering one another on the instruments. The conversations can be long or short, have balancing phrases or phrases of less-usual length. They can have dramatic changes of character or be relatively the same. One person can try to surprise the other. The group can discuss the mood afterwards if they wish, but sometimes this is very difficult as the music has so much subtlety.

Unity/diversity

Reconciling opposites

AN EXERCISE IN PAIRS

One person imagines him or herself in a wide open space with lots of freedom. There are no pressures of work and he or she is completely free to do what he or she likes. The person should spend some time there engaging in the feeling of free playing and openness, and when he or she has the expressive character of it the person should pick up an instrument and play something that represents it to his or her partner. The person should teach the partner how to play the pattern which the partner needs to remember.

The same person now imagines him or herself in a place of work. Everything is tightly under pressure. Deadlines must be met and there is a general air of order and purposefulness about the place. Again, the person should spend a few minutes there and when he or she has the expressive character of this place he or she should pick up a different instrument and play a pattern that represents this.

Working together, one partner plays the free pattern and the other the work pattern. They should play them together and see how best they will fit together.

Remember, they can be one after the other or together. Ask the pairs to keep repeating them until there appears to be some union between them. Work at bringing the patterns together into some sort of piece. Give the piece a name and try to experience the expressive character of the new piece.

Each pair should now repeat the exercise with the other person doing the visualisation.

AS AN INDIVIDUAL EXERCISE

With an instrument capable of playing two lines at once (e.g. a keyboard instrument) it is possible to do this exercise individually. It is also possible to do it on a single line instrument, but then the only possible combination will be placing one pattern after the other.

Challenge/nurture

A humming bath

A GROUP EXERCISE

Two people sit with their eyes closed in the middle of a circle of people. This can be back to back on chairs or on the ground, whatever feels most comfortable. Tell the people in the surrounding circle that they are going to hum any note that they feel comfortable with and are to carry on humming it for a long time, taking a breath whenever they need it, and that they are to try to send good thoughts to those in the middle. The circle surrounding the people starts to hum softly, standing still. Wait until the humming of the circle has settled. Then the outer circle moves gradually forward to near where the two people are sitting. They stop before they come too close and must not touch the people. They stand still in this central position and then gradually retreat until they are back where they started when the humming is gradually stopped. Ask the people in the middle to open their eyes and describe what it felt like.

Finding your note

A GROUP EXERCISE

Take a very simple phrase or verse such as:

> I am the wind that blows o'er the sea:
> I am a wave of the deep;
> I am a salmon in the water;
> I am a ray of the sun.
>
> *Adapted from a poem by Amairgen, chief poet of the Goirdelic Celts (Campbell, 1972, p.223)*

Tell the group they are going to sing a one-note song. The task is not to find out how many notes they can sing but which note is the easiest note. Say that they are going to sing the phrase on four different pitches and at the end of this they are going to be asked which was the easiest pitch. Using a fixed pitch instrument like a keyboard or recorder, play middle C. Get the group to sing the verse on that single note. Encourage them and ask them to remember what that felt like. Now do the same thing on the G below middle C; and then on the G above middle C and then on the C above middle C. Always encourage and tell people who feel they can't get that note to sing the verse on any pitch that they think they can sing. Now ask them to vote for the pitch that they found easiest, explaining how we all have our own note (see p.273).

AN INDIVIDUAL EXERCISE

Choose a quality from this list: Joy, Love, Freedom, Peace, Shalom, Calm, Truth, Strength, Wisdom, Power, Compassion, Energy (or another higher quality if one springs to mind).

Reflect on it for ten to fifteen minutes. Spend a further ten minutes allowing the quality to turn into a phrase or a short sentence such as:

I am joy

There is strength in the universe

A calm lake.

Repeat the phrase to yourself until it acquires a rhythm of the musical quality of the phrase. When you can repeat it rhythmically start softly to harmonise it with your breathing. Then sing it gently on the breath on a single note. Try various pitches until you find the one that feels really comfortable and right for you. If you have a fixed pitch instrument of some kind, find where it is.

Excitement/relaxation

A sound poem

WINTER SOLSTICE

> The earth freezes;
> The crystals sparkle in the red sinking sun;
> The trees are bare;
> The shadows slant in a blackness the soft light cannot dispel.
>
> The earth freezes;
> The ice fractures the sun's rays into rainbow colours;
> The crack of broken twigs echoes in the emptiness;
> The trees are bare;

The earth freezes;
The crystals sparkle;
There is a cool hollow spaciousness;
Under the earth, life is poised…as the year turns,
As the energy of light begins to ascend,
As Spring calls the world to leave behind its darkness
And calls us to join the beginning dance of new life.

June Boyce-Tillman

A GROUP EXERCISE

Get the group to read and absorb the poem. Ask everyone to spend time in silence visualising and absorbing various aspects of it. Let each person choose an instrument and use it to create a sound picture of one line, bearing in mind that some lines appear twice. Allow time for everyone to experiment. Check that someone has created a musical pattern for each line. This can be done without listening to the fragments, simply by a show of hands.

Read the poem leaving a space at the end of each line for the sound picture. Sometimes there will be more than one sound for each line. Encourage the group to be aware of the sounds and intuitively fit them together establishing an ending to the sound picture by common unspoken consent. At the end allow a silence, affirm the sounds and comment on particularly effective moments.

Now do the whole exercise again *without reading the poem* but using the poem as a map for the order of the sound's appearance. Encourage the group to listen sensitively to the other sounds and find how the various sections can best fit together. Allow a silence at the end and affirm the performance. You can leave it here or work on it more, maybe taking one of the more rhythmic sounds to be an ostinato to unify a section or isolating a small sound that is lost in a more dense section. Play it again and get the group to comment on possible modifications to their group piece.

This is an excellent way of unifying a group musically and getting them to feel the power of music to create a sense of group unity. The group can also be taken through a group transformation experience by such group improvisations.

AN INDIVIDUAL EXERCISE

This can be done on your own with an instrument or your own voice. Read the poem carefully to get the feel of it and create musical motifs for each line. Say the poem, playing the motifs at the end of each line.

Stop actually saying the poem, and make the piece form the musical motifs on their own. Refine the piece musically, perhaps re-arranging the ideas but always keeping the 'feel' of the original poem.

As it is then your own piece it would be possible to play or sing it as a meditation over a number of days. If you are using your voice it is possible to work at it by singing the actual words or by creating a sound picture using vocal sounds that express some of the quality of the words.

Embodiment/transcendence

Finding the silent place

A GROUP EXERCISE

Explain to everyone that they are going to make a group piece, and that the Indian cymbal means that the sound is to get quieter and that the gong means that it is to stop and that then there will be a period of silence. Get a group of people lying on the floor with their heads in the middle of the circle and their bodies pointing out like the spokes of a wheel. Each one hums his or her own sound. When the hum has settled, encourage everyone to move a little away from their own note into harmony with the group. Then encourage them to hum their own tunes, sometimes coming to rest in the harmony. Encourage them to make the humming stronger and stronger until the room is filled with sound. When the loud sound has been reached for at least a minute strike an Indian bell as a signal that the sounds are gradually to decrease. Gradually bring the sounds down till there is just a chord or a drone. Sound a deeper gong to indicate that the singing is to stop. Allow the silence that follows to last for at least three minutes.

A MODIFIED VERSION WITH VISUALISATION

Explain to the group what is going to happen as before, but say that in the silence they are journeying by singing. Ask them to imagine that they are journeying upwards or inwards (whichever feels appropriate) during the music. Say that in the silence they may meet a person, a Wise One to whom they can say anything, tell them a problem or ask a question. They should wait for an answer in the silence.

Addresses

Alfred A. Tomatis Foundation, 26 Eccleston Square, London SW1V 1NS

Arts Access Aoteroa, Level 1, 27 Dixon Street, PO Box 9828, Wellington, New Zealand. *www.suresite.com/oh/a/artsaccess*

Arts for Health, Manchester Metropolitan University, St Augustines, Upper Chatham Street, Manchester M16 5BY

Bird-in-Hand Activity Centre, 1 Priory Gardens, Parchment Street, Winchester SO23 8AJ

Celebratory Arts for Primary Health Care, 32/34 Main Street, High Bentham, Lancs. LA2 7HN

Chris Southall, Parsonage Farm, 128 Low Road, Burwell, Cambridge CB5 0EJ

Council for Music in Hospitals, 74 Queens Road, Hersham, Surrey KT12 5LW

Drake Music Project (enables disabled people to make music using technology), 79 East Road, London D1 6AH

Exeter Health Care Arts, Naomi Fabian Miller, The Royal Devon and Exeter Hospital (Wonford), Barrack Road, Exeter EX5 5DW

Guided Imagery in Music, Carole Killick, 5, Slater Bridge, Hebden Bridge, West Yorks. HX7 7DY *http://.eclipse.co.uk/pens/AIM*

Gurukul: Dr Anthea/Dr Anand, 18 Elmfield Road, Newcastle-upon-Tyne NE3 4AY *www.gurukul.org*

Hildegard Network, Kathleen Emerson, Primavera, 2 Newlands Road, Purbrook, Waterlooville, Hants, PO7 5NF

Holyrood House, Northern Churches Healing Centre, 10 Sowerby Road, Sowerby, Thirsk, N.Yorks, YO7 1HY

Isle of Wight Healing Arts, Guy Eades, St Mary's Hospital, Parkhurst Road, Newport, Isle of Wight, PO30 5TG

Music Space, The Southville Centre, Beauley Road, Southville, Bristol BS3 1QG

The Orpheus Centre, North Park Lane, Godstone, Surrey RH9 8ND *www.orpheus.org.uk*

Psychosynthesis and Education Trust, 92–94, Tooley Street, London SE1 2TH

Jill Purce, Inner Sound and Voice, 246 Colney Hatch Lane, London N10 1BD *www.jillpurce.com*

SHARE music, Angela Woolsey, 46 Markethill Road, Portadown, Co. Armagh BT62 3SH

Sound Health, Jill Rakusen, 2 St Mary's Square, Honley, Huddersfield HD7 2BA

REACH, Pinehurst People's Centre, Beech Avenue, Swindon SN2 1JT

TAPS, Traditional Arts Projects, Southill Park Arts Centre, Bracknell, Berks, RG12 7PA

Tonalis, 2 Market Place Mews, Fairford, Glos. GL7 14AB

Trust Arts Project (TAP), Belinda Sosinowicz, South London and Maudsley NHS, AMI Building, 108 Landor Road, London SW9 9NT

Waterford Healing Arts Trust, Waterford Regional Hospital, Waterford City, Ireland

Withymoor Village Surgery, Turners Lane, Brierley Hill, West Midlands DY5 2PG

References

Achterberg, J. (1985) *Imagery in Healing*. Boston: Shambhala.

Agrotou, A. (1993) 'Spontaneous ritualised play in music therapy: A technical and theoretical analysis.' In M. Heal and T. Wigram (eds) *Music Therapy in Health and Education*. London: Jessica Kingsley Publishers.

Aldridge, D. (1996) *Music Therapy Research and Practice in Medicine – From Out of the Silence*. London: Jessica Kingsley Publishers.

Alexander, J. (1994) 'Singing your way out of the blues.' *Daily Mail*, 16 July.

Armstrong, F. with Pearson, J. (1992) *As Far as the Eye Can Sing*. London: The Women's Press.

Assagioli, R. (1994) *The Act of Will*. London: Aquarian/Thorsons. (First published 1974.)

Association of Professional Music Therapists (1990) Leaflet.

Attali, J. (1985) *Noise: The Political Economy of Music* (trans. B. Massumi). Minneapolis, MN: University of Minnesota Press.

Ball, L. (1982) *Meditational Music 1*. Audio cassette, private publication.

Barkin, E. (1994) 'Four texts.' In J. Rahn (ed) *Perspectives in Musical Aesthetics*. New York: Norton.

Barthes, R. (1985a) *The Grain of the Voice: Interviews 1962–80*. (trans. L. Coverdale) New York: Hill and Wang.

Barthes, R. (1985b) *The Responsibility of Forms: Critical Essays on Music, Art, and Representation*. (trans. R. Howard) New York: Hill and Wang.

Beattie, J. and Middleton, J. (eds) (1969) *Spirit Mediumship and Society in Africa*. London: Routledge and Kegan Paul.

Becker, J. (1980) *Traditional Music in Modern Java*. Hawaii: University Press of Hawaii.

Beechwood Music (1997) *Spirit of Relaxation*, 3 audio cassettes (Littleton House, Littleton Road, Ashford, Middlesex TW15 1UU).

Belenky, M.F., McVicker Clinchy, B., Rule Goldberger, N. and Mattuck Tarule, J. (1986) *Women's Ways of Knowing: The Development of Self, Voice, and Mind*. New York: Basic Books.

Berruti, G., del Puente, G., Gatti, R., Manarola, G. and Vecchiato, C. (1993) 'Description of an experience in music therapy carried out at the Department of Psychiatry of the University of Genoa.' In M. Heal and T. Wigram (eds) *Music Therapy in Health and Education*. London: Jessica Kingsley Publishers.

Beyer, A. (ed.) (1996) *The Music of Per Norgard: Fourteen Interpretative Essays*. Aldershot: Scolar Press.

Blacking, J. (1977) *The Anthropology of the Body*. London: Academic.

Blacking, J. (1976) *How Musical is Man?* London: Faber and Faber.

Blacking, J. (1987) *A Commonsense View of All Music*. Cambridge: Cambridge University Press.

Blake, A. (1997) *The Land without Music: Music Culture and Society in Twentieth Century Britain*. Manchester: Manchester University Press.

Boddy, J. (1990) *Wombs and Alien Spirits: Women, Men and the Zar Cult in Northern Sudan*. Madison, WI: University of Wisconsin Press.

Boddy, J. (1994) 'Spirit possession revisited: Beyond instrumentality.' *Annual Review of Anthropology 23*, 407–434.

Bourgignon, E. (1965) 'The self, the behavioural environment, and the theory of spirit possession.' In M.E. Spiro (ed) *Context and Meaning in Cultural Anthropology*. London: Collins-Macmillan.

Boyce-Tillman, J.B. (1996a) 'A framework for intercultural dialogue in music.' In M. Floyd (ed) *World Musics in Education*. Aldershot: Scolar Books.

Boyce-Tillman, J.B. (1996b) 'Getting our acts together: Conflict resolution through music.' In M. Liebmann (ed) *Arts Approaches to Conflict*. London: Jessica Kingsley Publishers.

Boyce-Tillman, J. (1998a) *The Call of the Ancestors*. London: The Hildegard Press.

Boyce-Tillman, J. (1998b) *Weaving a Fragrance*. London: The Hildegard Press.

Boyce-Tillman, J. (1998c) *The Beautiful Perfumes of Goodness*. London: The Hildegard Press.

Boyce-Tillman, J. (1998d) *Music Lessons on Prescription*. Paper in the Proceedings of the Music Education as Therapy Conference of the Society for Research into the Psychology of Music and Music Education, November, King Alfred's Winchester.

Boyce-Tillman, J. (1998e) *Sharing Diversity*. Paper presented at the Early Childhood Seminar of the International Society for Music Education. Stellenbosch, South Africa.

Boyce-Tillman, J. (2000) 'The CD as sacred site.' In G. Harvey (ed) *Music in Indigenous Religion*. Aldershot: Scolar Press.

Braidotti, R. (1994) *Nomadic Subjects.* New York: Columbia University Press.

Brewer, C. (1996) 'Orchestrating learning skills.' *Open Ear 1,* 14–18.

Bright, R. (1993) 'Cultural aspects of music therapy.' In M. Heal and T. Wigram (eds) *Music Therapy in Health and Education.* London: Jessica Kingsley Publishers.

Brougham, H., Fox, C. and Pace, I. (1997) *Uncommon Ground: The Music of Michael Finnissy.* Aldershot: Ashgate.

Brown, J.E. (1989) *The Sacred Pipe: Black Elk's Account of the Seven Rites of the Oglala Sioux.??:* University of Oklahoma Press.

Bruscia, K.E. (1987) *Improvisational Models of Music Therapy.* Springfield, IL: Charles C. Thomas.

Bunt, L. (1994) *Music Therapy – An Art Beyond Words.* London: Routledge.

Caldwell, A.E. (1972) 'La Malincolia: Final movement of Beethoven's quartet op.18, No.6: A musical account of manic depressive states.' *Journal of the American Medical Women's Association 27,* 241–248.

Campbell, J. (1972) *Myths to Live by.* London: Souvenir Press.

Caplan, P. (1997) *African Voices, African Lives: Personal Narratives from a Swahili Village.* London: Routledge.

Carpenter, H. (1992) *Benjamin Britten: A Biography.* London: Faber and Faber.

Carson, C. (1986) *Irish Traditional Music.* Belfast: Appletree Press.

Castaneda, C. (1971) *A Separate Reality: Further Conversations with Don Juan.* New York: Simon and Schuster.

Chardin, T. de (1964) *The Phenomenon of Man.* London: Collins.

Chatten, C. (1997) 'A gentle way through the barrier of pain.' *Journal of Dementia Care,* May/June, 22–23.

Chopra, D. (1991) *Unconditional Life: Mastering the Forces that Shape Personal Reality.* London: Bantam Books.

Collin, M. (1997) *Altered State: The Story of Ecstasy Culture and Acid House.* London: Serpent's Tail.

Collins, D. (1994) 'Ritual sacrifice and political economy of music.' In J. Rahn (ed) *Perspectives in Musical Aesthetics.* New York: Norton.

Condon, W. (1980) 'The relation of interactional synchrony to cognitive and emotional processes.' In M. Key (ed) *The Relationship of Verbal and Non-Verbal Communication.* The Hague: Mouton.

Condon, W. and Ogston, W. (1966) 'Sound film analysis of normal and pathological behaviour patterns.' *Journal of Nervous and Mental Disorders 14,* 338–347.

Cook, N. (1987) *A Guide to Musical Analysis.* Oxford: Oxford University Press.

Cook, N. (1990) *Music, Imagination and Culture.* Oxford: Clarendon Press.

Cook, N. (1998) *Music: A Very Short Introduction.* Oxford: Oxford University Press.

Crapanzo, V. (1977) 'Mohammed and Dawia: Possession in Morocco.' In V. Crapanzo and V. Garrison (eds) *Case Studies in Possession.* New York: John Wiley and Sons.

Critchley, N. and Henson, R. (1977) *Music and the Brain: Studies in Neurology and Music.* London: Heinemann.

Csikszentmihalyi, M. (1993) *The Evolving Self.* New York: Harper and Row.

Csikszentmihalyi, M. (1997) 'Creativity: A mysterious process.' In M. Toms (ed) *The Well of Creativity.* Carlsbad, CA: Hay House.

Csikszentmihalyi, M. and Csikszentmihalyi, I.S. (1988) *Optimal Experience: Psychological Studies of Flow in Consciousness.* Cambridge: Cambridge University Press.

Danner, M. (1994) *The Massacre at El Mozote.* New York: Vintage.

De Backer, J. (1993) 'Containment in music therapy.' In M. Heal and T. Wigram (eds) *Music Therapy in Health and Education.* London: Jessica Kingsley Publishers.

Dekker, C. (1999) *Return to the Source – The Chakra Journey.* London: Return to the Source and Pyramid Records.

Densmore, F. (1943) Included in sleeve notes for *Healing Songs of the American Indians* (1965), Ethnic Folkways Library FE4251, National Sound Archive 1LP0083255.

Dewey, J. (1910) *How We Think.* New York: Heath and Co.

Dewey, J. (1934) *Art as Experience.* New York: Minton Balch and Co.

di Franco, G. (1993) 'Music therapy – A methodological approach in the mental health field.' In M. Heal and T. Wigram (eds) *Music Therapy in Health and Education.* London: Jessica Kingsley Publishers.

Diamond, J. (1980) *Your Body Doesn't Lie.* New York: Warner Books.

Dodd, V. (1989) 'Sound as tool for transformation.' *Halo,* Winter, 24–27.

Dollinger, S.J. (1993) 'Research note: Personality and music preference: Extraversion and excitement seeking or openness to experience.' *Psychology of Music 21,* 73–77.

Downes (1998) 'Meditation – its value to composers… and other musicians?' Unpublished paper.

Doyle, B. (1987) 'Introduction to the songs.' In M. Fox (ed) *Hildegard of Bingen's Book of Divine Works, with Letters and Songs.* Santa Fe, CA: Bear and Co.

Drury, N. (1984) 'The shaman: Healer and visionary.' *Nature and Health 9,* 2, 86.

Drury, N. (1989) *The Elements of Shamanism.* Shaftesbury: Element Books.

Eames, P. (1999) *The ART and Health Partnership.* Wellington: Arts Access Aotearoa.

Easton, C. (1989) *Jacqueline du Pré: A Biography.* London: Hodder and Stoughton.

Eibl-Eibesfeld, I. (1989) *Human Ethology.* New York: Aldine de Gruyter.

Ekman, K. (1946) *Jean Sibelius: His Life and Personality* (trans. E. Birse). New York: Tudor.

Eliade, M. (1951) *Le Chamanisme et les Techniques Archaïques de l'Extase.* Paris: Payot.

Eliade, M. (1964) *Shamanism: Archaic Techniques of Ecstasy.* New York: Pantheon.

Eliade, M. (1989) *Shamanism.* Princeton, NJ: Princeton University Press.

Elkin, A. P. (1977) *Aboriginal Men of High Degree.* Queensland: University of Queensland Press.

Elliott, D. (1995) *Music Matters.* Oxford: Oxford University Press.

Engel, G.L. (1977) 'The need for a new medical model: A challenge for biomedicine.' *Science 196*, 129.

Engh, B. (1993) 'Loving it: Music and criticism in Roland Barthes.' In R.A. Solie (ed) *Musicology and Difference: Gender and Sexuality in Music Scholarship*. Berkeley, CA: University of California Press.

Erdonmez, D. (1993) 'Music – A mega vitamin for the brain.' In M. Heal and T. Wigram (eds) *Music Therapy in Health and Education*. London: Jessica Kingsley Publishers.

Erlmann, V. (1982) 'Trance and music in the Hausa Bòorii spirit possession cult in Nigeria.' *Ethnomusicology*, January, 49–58.

Feder, E. and Feder, B. (1981) *The 'Expressive' Arts Therapies: Art, Music and Dance as Psychotherapy*. New Jersey: Prentice Hall.

Feng, F.M. (1973) *The Dinka and Their Songs*. Oxford: Clarendon Press.

Figueroa, A. (1977) Sleeve notes for *Love, Luck, Animals and Magic: Music of the Yurok and Tolowa Indians*. New World Records, NW297, Recorded Anthology of American Music Inc.

Fisher, K. (1996) *Moving On*. London: SPCK.

Flower, C. (1993) 'Control and creativity.' In M. Heal and T. Wigram (eds) *Music Therapy in Health and Education*. London: Jessica Kingsley Publishers.

Floyd, M. (1995) *World Musics in Education*. Aldershot: Scolar Press.

Floyd, M. (1998) 'The trouble with old men: Songs of the Maasai.' In *Change and the Performing Arts*. Proceedings of a research day of the School of Community and Performing Arts, King Alfred's, Winchester, UK.

Fordham, M. (1986) *Jungian Psychotherapy*. London: Maresfield.

Foskett, J. (1984) *Meaning in Madness – The Pastor and the Mentally Ill*. London: SPCK.

Friedman, R. (1993) *Sound Techniques for Healing*, audio cassette from Brain Sync.

Frith, S. (1987) 'Towards an aesthetic of popular music.' In R. Leppert and S. McClary (eds) *Music and Society: The Politics of Composition, Performance and Reception*. Cambridge: Cambridge University Press.

Frowen-Williams, G. (1997) *Between Earth and Sky: Explorations on the Shamanic Path*. Unpublished Dissertation for MA in ethnomusicology. University of Central England.

Fry, H.H.J. (1986) 'Overuse syndrome in musicians: Prevention and management.' *Lancet 2*, 728–731.

Fukuda, Y. (1998) 'Survey on method preferences among the ten breathing methods practised in the asthma music programme.' *Music in Health and Special Education* seminar of the International Society for Music Education, South Africa, July.

Gans, E. (1994a) 'Art and entertainment.' In J. Rahn (ed) *Perspectives in Musical Aesthetics*. New York: Norton.

Gans, E. (1994b) 'The beginning and end of aesthetic form.' In J. Rahn (ed) *Perspectives in Musical Aesthetics*. New York: Norton.

Gaertner, M. (1998) 'The sound of music in the dimming, anguished world of Alzheimer's disease.' *Music in Health and Special Education* seminar of the International Society for Music Education, South Africa, July.

Gardner, H. (1982) 'Artistry following damage to the human brain.' In A. Ellis (ed) *Normality and Pathology in Cognitive Functions*. London and New York: Academic Press.

Gardner, K. (1990) *Sounding the Inner Landscape – Music as Medicine*. Rockport, MA: Element Books.

Garfield, L.M. (1987) *Sound Medicine*. Berkeley, CA: Celestial Arts.

Gebser, J. (1973) *Ursprung und Gegenwart*. Lecture given in Munich.

Gfeller, K. (1987) 'Music therapy theory and practice as reflected in research literature.' *Journal of Music Therapy 24*, 178–194.

Ghiselin, B. (ed) (1952) *The Creative Process*. New York: Mentor Books.

Ghiselin, B. (1956) 'The creative process and its relation to the identification of creative talent.' In C.W. Taylor (ed) *The 1955 University of Utah Research Conference on the Identification of Creative Talent*. Salt Lake City, UT: University of Utah Press.

Giddens, A. (1999) *Tradition*. Third Reith Lecture. Published on the Internet.

Glennie, E. (1996) *Sounds of the Deep*, BBC Radio 4, 23 April.

Godwin, J. (1987) *Music, Magic and Mysticism: A Sourcebook*. London: Arkana.

Goehr, L. (1992) *The Imaginary Museum of Musical Works: An Essay in the Philosophy of Music*. Oxford: Clarendon Press.

Goldman, J. (1992) *Healing Sounds – The Power of Harmonics*. Shaftesbury: Element Books.

Gooch, S. (1972) *Total Man: Towards an Evolutionary Theory of Personality*. London: Allen Lane, Penguin Press.

Goodchild, C. (1993) *The Naked Voice*. London: Rider.

Grainger, R (1995) *The Glass of Heaven: The Faith of the Dramatherapist*. London: Jessica Kingsley Publishers.

Green, L. (1988) *Music on Deaf Ears: Musical Meaning, Ideology and Education*. Manchester and New York: Manchester University Press.

Green, L. (1997) *Music, Gender, Education*. Cambridge: Cambridge University Press.

Grey, M. C. (1989) *Redeeming the Dream: Feminism, Redemption and Christian Tradition*. London: SPCK.

Grimes, R.L. (1982) *Beginnings in Ritual Studies*. London: University Press of America.

Grimm, D. and Pefley, P. (1990) 'Opening doors for the child "inside".' *Paediatric Nursing 16*, 4, 368–369.

Grof, S. with Bennett, H.Z. (1993) *The Holotropic Mind*. London: HarperCollins.

Guilford, J.P (1962) 'Creativity: Its measurement and development.' In S.J. Parnes and H.F. Harding (eds) *A Source Book of Creative Thinking*. New York: Charles Scribners Sons.

Hassan, S.Q. (1975) *Les Instruments de Musique en Irak et leur Role dans la Société Traditionelle*. Paris: Mouton Editeur.

Hadfield, J. (ed) (1960) *A Book of Pleasures: An Anthology of Words and Pictures*. London: Vista Books.

Halifax, J. (1979) *Shamanic Voices.* New York: Dutton.

Hamel, P. (1978) *Through Music to the Self – How to Appreciate and Experience Music Anew.* (trans. P. Lemusurier) Tisbury: Compton Press.

Hamilton, P. (1998) *Old Harry's Game.* Radio play broadcast on BBC Radio Four, 23 April.

Harner, M. (1990) *The Way of the Shaman* (third edition). London: HarperCollins.

Harrer, G. and Harrer, H. (1977) 'Music, emotion and autonomic function.' In M. Critchley and R.A. Henson (eds) *Music and the Brain.* London: Heinemann Medical Books.

Hart, M. and Lieberman, F. (1991) *Planet Drum.* London: HarperCollins.

Haworth, J.T. (1997) *Work, Leisure and Well-Being.* London: Routledge.

Hekmat, H. and Hettel, J. (1993) 'Attenuating effects of preferred versus non-preferred music interventions.' *Psychology of Music 21,* 2, 163–173.

Heline, C. (1964) *Color and Music in the New Age.* Marina del Ray, CA: De Vorss.

Helman, C.G. (1994) *Culture, Health and Illness.* London: Butterworth/Heinemann.

Hills, P. and Argyle, M. (1998) 'Musical and religious experiences and their relationship to happiness.' Chapter in book in preparation entitled *Personality and Individual Differences.*

Hindemith, P. (1952) *A Composer's World.* New York: Doubleday and Co.

Howe, M.J.A. and Sloboda, J.A. (1991) 'Young musicians' accounts of significant influences in their early lives. 1. The family and their musical background.' *British Journal of Music Education 8,* 16–18.

Illich, I. (1976) *Deschooling Society.* Harmondsworth: Penguin.

Illich, I. (1977) *Limits to Medicine: Medical Nemesis: The Expropriation of Health.* Harmondsworth: Penguin.

Jaërvinen, T. (1997) 'Tonal dynamics in jazz improvisation.' *Third Triennial ESCOM Conference Proceedings.* Uppsala.

Jahoda, M. (1982) *Employment and Unemployment: A Social Psychological Analysis.* Cambridge: Cambridge University Press.

James, J. (1993) *The Music of the Spheres: Music, Science and the Natural Order of the Universe.* London: Abacus.

James, W. (1900) *Talks to Teachers on Psychology.* New York: Rhinehart and Winston.

Jamison, R. (1993) *Touched with Fire: Manic-Depressive Illness and the Artistic Temperament.* New York: Free Press.

Janzen, J. (1982) *Lemba: A Drum of Affliction in Africa and the New World.* New York and London: Garland Publishers.

Janzen, J. (1987) 'Therapy management: Concepts, reality, process.' *Medical Anthropology Quarterly 1,* 1, 68–84.

Jennings, S. (1985) 'Temiar dance and the maintenance of order.' In P. Spencer (ed) *Society and the Dance: The Social Anthropology of Process and Performance.* Cambridge: Cambridge University Press.

Jennings, S. (1999) *Introduction to Developmental Play Therapy: Playing and Health.* London: Jessica Kingsley Publishers.

Jensen, F. (1982) *C.G. Jung, Emma Jung and Toni Wolff.* San Francisco, CA: The Analytical Club.

Jordan, J.V., Kaplan, A.A., Baker Miller, J., Stiver, I.B. and Surrey, J.L. (1991) *Women's Growth in Connection: Writings from the Stone Centre.* New York: The Guilford Press.

Jorgensen, E. (1996) 'The artist and the pedagogy of hope.' *International Journal for Music Education 27,* 36–50.

Jung, C.G. (1964a) *The Development of Personality.* (collected works, volume 17, trans. R.F. Hull). London: Routledge and Kegan Paul.

Jung, C.G. (1964b) *Man and His Symbols.* London: Aldus Books, Jupiter Books.

Keyes, L.E. (1973) *Toning: The Creative Power of the Voice.* Marina del Ray, CA: De Vorss and Co.

Kelly, G. (1955) *The Psychology of Personal Constructs, Volumes One and Two.* New York: Norton.

Kemp, A.E. (1996) *The Musical Temperament.* Oxford: Oxford University Press.

Kirby, E.T. (1975) 'Shamanistic theatre: Origins and evolution.' In E.T. Kirby *Ur-Drama: The Origins of Theatre.* New York: New York University Press.

Koestler, A. (1964) *The Act of Creation.* London: Hutchinson.

Koestler, A. (1981) 'The three domains of creativity.' In D. Dutton and M. Krausz (eds) *The Concept of Creativity in Science and Art.* Boston, MA: Martinus Nijhoff Publications.

Kortegaard, H.M. (1993) 'Music therapy in the psychodynamic treatment of schizophrenia.' In M. Heal and T. Wigram (eds) *Music Therapy in Health and Education.* London: Jessica Kingsley Publishers.

Kristeva, J. (1989) *The Language of the Unknown: An Initiation into Linguistics.* (trans. A.M. Menke) New York: Columbia University Press.

Kubler Ross, E. (1983) A broadcast talk in *The Listener 110,* 19 September, 2828.

Langer, S. (1953) *Feeling and Form: A Theory of Art.* London: Routledge and Kegan Paul.

Leach, E. (1996) *Levi-Strauss.* London: Fontana Press.

Lee, S.C. (1995) *The Circle is Sacred: A Medicine Book for Women.* Tulsa, OK: Council Oak Books.

Leonard, G. (1978) *The Silent Pulse.* New York: E.P. Dutton.

Levine, S.K. (1997) *Poiesis: The Language of Psychology and the Speech of the Soul.* London: Jessica Kingsley Publishers.

Levi-Strauss, C. (1970) *The Raw and the Cooked.* (trans. J. and D. Weightman) London: Cape.

Lewis, C.S. (1955) *The Magician's Nephew.* Harmondsworth: Penguin Books.

Lewis, I.M. (1966) 'Spirit possession and deprivation cults.' *Man 1,* 3, 307–329.

Lewis, I.M (1985) Programme Notes to the *Ancestral Voices* programme, at the Commonwealth Centre's Third Festival of Folk and Traditional Arts, London.

Li, L. (1993) 'Mystical numbers and manchu traditional music: A consideration of the relationship between shamanic thought and musical ideas.' *British Journal of Ethnomusicology 2*, 99–115.

Lieberman, J.N. (1967) 'A developmental analysis of playfulness as access to cognitive style.' *Journal of Creative Behaviour 1*, 4, Fall, 391–397.

Lifetime Cassettes (1993) *Sea So Serene.* PO Box 101244, Nashville, TN 37210, US.

Lingerman, H.A. (1983) *The Healing Energies of Music.* Wheaton, IL: The Theosophical Publishing House.

Loane, B. (1984) 'Thinking about children's compositions.' *British Journal of Music Education 3*, November, 205–231.

Lodewijks, T. (1998) 'Zoomzim a-zoomba: Musical mini-plays for the physical side of blind and cerebral palsy children.' Demonstration at the *Music in Health and Special Education* seminar of the International Society for Music Education, South Africa, July.

Lovelock, W. (1952) *The Examination Fugue.* London: A. Hammond and Co.

McClary, S. (1991) *Feminine Endings.* Minnesota, MS: University of Minnesota Press.

McDonnell, L. (1983) 'Music therapy: Meeting the psychosocial needs of hospitalised children.' *Children's Health Care 12*, 1, 29–33.

Maranto, C.D. (1993) 'Applications of music in medicine.' In M. Heal and T. Wigram (eds) *Music Therapy in Health and Education.* London: Jessica Kingsley Press.

Marshall, L. (1969) 'The medicine dance of the !Kung bushmen.' *Africa 39*, 347–380.

Maslow, A.H. (1958) *Creativity in Self-Actualising People.* Lecture for Creativity Symposium, Michigan State University, East Lansing, 28 February.

Maslow, A.H. (1962a) *Towards a Psychology of Being.* Princeton, NJ: D. van Nostrand Company Incorporated.

Maslow, A.H. (1962b) 'Emotional blocks to creativity.' In S.J. Parnes and H.F. Harding (eds) *A Source Book of Creative Thinking.* New York: Charles Scribners Sons.

Maslow, A.H. (1967) 'The creative attitude.' In R.L. Mooney and T.A. Razik (eds) *Explorations in Creativity.* New York: Harper and Row.

Maslow, A.H. (1987) *Motivation and Personality* (third edition). New York: Harper and Row.

Menuhin, Y. (1972) *Theme and Variations.* New York: Stein and Day.

Messenger, J. (1958) 'Esthetic talent.' *Basic College Quarterly 4*, 20–24.

Meyer, L. (1956) *Emotion and Meaning in Music.* Chicago: University of Chicago Press.

Meyer, L. (1967) *Music – The Arts and Ideas.* Chicago: University of Chicago Press.

Middleton, R. (1990) *Studying Popular Music.* Milton Keynes: Open University Press.

Miller, A. (1987) *For Your Own Good – The Roots of Violence in Child-Rearing.* London: Virago.

Moltmann, J. (1967) *Theology of Hope.* (trans. J. Leitch) London: SCM Press.

Moore, J.G. (1979) 'Religious worship in Jamaica.' In J. Blacking and J. Kealinohomoku (eds) *The Performing Arts: Musical Dance.* The Hague: Mouton.

Morrison, J. (1997) 'Is it music to their ears?' *Journal of Dementia Care*, May/June, 18–19.

Myers, I.B. (1993) *Gifts Differing: Understanding Personality Type* (original edition 1980). Palo Alto, CA: Consulting Psychologists Press.

Myers, I.B. and McCaulley, M.H. (1985) *Manual: A Guide to the Development and Use of the Myers–Briggs Type Indicator* (second edition). Palo Alto, CA: Consulting Psychologists Press.

Newham, P. (1997) *Therapeutic Voicework.* London: Jessica Kingsley Publishers.

Newham, P. (1998) Publicity leaflet for voice movement therapy.

Nietzsche, F., edited Tanner, M. *et al.* (1994) *The Birth of Tragedy:Out of the Spirit of Music.* Harmondsworth: Penguin.

Nketia, J.H. (1957) 'Possession dances of African societies.' *International Folk Music Journal 9*, 4–9.

Nkosi, W. (1992) Sleeve notes to *The Rhythm of Healing.* National Sound Archive 1CD004251.

Nordoff, P. and Robbins, C. (1977) *Creative Music Therapy.* New York: John Day.

Obeyesekere, G. (1970) 'The idiom of demonic possession: A case study.' *Social Science and Medicine 4*, pp.97–111.

Oldfield, A. (1993) 'Music therapy with families.' In M. Heal and T. Wigram (eds) *Music Therapy in Health and Education.* London: Jessica Kingsley Publishers.

The Orb (1996) *Auntie Aubrey's Excursions beyond the Call of Duty – The Orb Remix Project.* London: Deviant.

Ortiz, J.M. (1997) *The Tao of Music, Sound Psychology: Using Music to Change Your Life.* Dublin: New Leaf.

Panoramic Sound (1988) *Visions – American Indian Flute.* PO Box 5812, Houston, Texas, TX 77258, US.

Pavlicevic, M. (1997) *Music Therapy in Context: Music, Meaning and Relationship.* London: Jessica Kingsley Publishers.

Paynter, J. (1977) 'The role of creativity in the school music curriculum.' In M. Burnett (ed) *Music Education Review I.* London: Chappell.

Perry, F. (1988) Sleeve notes to the audio-cassette *Deep Peace.* Mountain Bell BEL 001.

Pesek, A. (1996) 'Music as a tool to help refugee children and their mothers: The Slovenian case.' In R.N. Kirin and M. Povrzanovic (eds) *War, Exile and Everyday Life – Cultural Perspectives.* Zagreb: Institute of Ethnology and Folklore Research.

Pinkola Estes, C. (1992) *Women Who Run with the Wolves.* London: Rider.

Pruett, K.D. (1990) 'Coping with life on a pedestal.' In F.R.Wilson and F.L.Roehmann (eds) *Music and Child Development.* St Louis, Missouri: MMB Music.

Purce, J. (1998) Publicity leaflet for *The Healing Voice*. (see Appendix II.)

Rahn, J. (1994a) 'Introduction: The aesthetics of perspectives.' In J. Rahn (ed) *Perspectives in Musical Aesthetics*. New York: Norton.

Rahn, J. (1994b) 'What is valuable in art, and can music still achieve it?' In J. Rahn (ed) *Perspectives in Musical Aesthetics*. New York: Norton.

Raijmaekers, J. (1993) 'Music therapy's role in the diagnosis of psycho-geriatric patients in The Hague.' In M. Heal and T. Wigram (eds) *Music Therapy in Health and Education*. London: Jessica Kingsley Publishers.

Rakusen, J. (1992) *Imagine*. Self-published publicity leaflet. (see Sound Health in Appendix II.)

Redfearn, J. (1992) *The Exploding Self: The Creative and Destructive Nucleus of the Personality*. Wilmette, IL: Chiron Publications.

Reti, R. (1961) *The Thematic Process in Music*. London: Faber and Faber.

Rider, M.S. and Welin, C. (1990) 'Imagery, improvisation and immunity.' *The Arts in Psychotherapy 17*, 3, 211_216.

Rigler, M. (1998) *You Bet It's Good Medicine*. Handout: Withymoor Surgery, West Midlands.

Ristad, E. (1982) *A Soprano on Her Head*. London: People Press.

Robbins, C. (1993) 'The creative processes are universal'. In M. Heal and T. Wigram (eds) *Music Therapy in Health and Education*. London: Jessica Kingsley Publishers.

Roberts, K. (1997) 'Work and leisure in young people's lives.' In J.T. Haworth (ed) *Work, Leisure and Well-Being*. London: Routledge.

Robertson, P. (1996) *Music and the Mind* (booklet). London: Channel Four Television.

Robertson, P. (1998) 'The case for music.' *Yamaha Education Supplement 28*, Spring/Summer, 19–21.

Rochlitz, R. (1994) 'Language for one, language for all.' In J. Rahn (ed) *Perspectives in Musical Aesthetics*. New York: Norton.

Rogers, C. (1970) 'Towards a theory of creativity.' In P.E. Vernon (ed) *Creativity*. Harmondsworth: Penguin.

Rogers, C. (1976) *On Becoming a Person*. London: Constable.

Rooley, A. (1990) *Performance: Revealing the Orpheus Within*. Shaftesbury: Element Books.

Roose-Evans, J. (1994) *Passages of the Soul*. Shaftesbury: Element Books.

Ross, M. (1978) *The Creative Arts*. London: Heinemann.

Roth, G. (1992) *Swaying My Prayers – An Interview with Alex Fisher* (sleeve notes).

Rouget, G. (1985) *Music and Trance: A Theory of the Relations between Music and Possession*. (trans. B. Biebuyck) Chicago, IL. and London: University of Chicago Press.

Ruddick, S. (1989) *Maternal Thinking: Towards a Politics of Peace*. New York: Ballantine Books.

Sansom, M. (1994) 'Musical meaning: A psychoanalytical look at improvisation.' Paper presented at the *29th Annual Research Students' Conference*, Royal Holloway College, London.

Schraig, C. (1997) *The Self after Postmodernity*. Yale, CT: Yale University Press.

Scruton, R. (1983) 'Understanding music.' *Ratio 25*, 97–120.

Shepherd, J. (1991) *Music as Social Text*. Cambridge: Polity Press.

Shepherd, J. and Wicke, P. (1997) *Music and Cultural Theory*. Cambridge: Polity Press.

Shostak, M. (1983) *Nisa: The Life and Works of a !Kung Woman*. New York: Vintage Books.

Silkstone, F. (1997) 'The more you play it, the more it comes out differently: Improvisation and composition in Thai tradition.' *Resonance, Structure and Freedom 6*, 1, 35–37.

Sloboda, A. (1993) 'Individual therapy with a man who has an eating disorder.' In M. Heal and T. Wigram (eds) *Music Therapy in Health and Education*. London: Jessica Kingsley Publishers.

Sloboda, J. (1985) *The Musical Mind*. Oxford: Clarendon Press.

Sloboda, J. and Davidson, J. (1996) 'The young performing musician.' In I. Deliege and J. Sloboda (eds) *Musical Beginnings: Origins and Development of Musical Competence*. Oxford: Oxford University Press.

Smeijsters, H. and van den Hurk, J. (1993) 'Research in practice in the music therapeutic treatment of a client with symptoms of anorexia nervosa.' In M. Heal and T. Wigram (eds) *Music Therapy in Health and Education*. London: Jessica Kingsley Publishers.

Smithsonian Folkways (recorded 1982) Sleeve notes to *Dreamsongs and Healing Sounds in the Rainforests of Malyasia*. J995. National Sound Archive 1CD0094813.

Sorel, G. (1945) *La Poésie Moderne et la Sacré*. Paris: Gallimard.

Sparshott, F.E. (1981) 'Every horse has a mouth: A personal poetics.' In D. Dutton and M. Krausz (eds) *The Concept of Creativity in Science and Art*. Boston, MA: Martinus Nijhoff Publications.

Spender, N. (1980) 'Music therapy.' In S. Sadie (ed) *New Grove Dictionary of Music and Musicians*. London: Macmillan.

Starhawk (1991) Sleeve notes to *The Way to the Well – A Trance Journey for Empowerment*. Harmony Network Cassette STAR 1, P.O. Box 2550, Guerneville, CA 95446, US.

Stebbins, R.A. (1992) *Amateurs, Professionals and Serious Leisure*. Montreal/Kingston: McGill/Queen's University Press.

Steckel, R. (1973) *Herz der Wirhlichkeit*. Wuppertal: Judie-Taschenbuch.

Stein, M. A. (1967) 'Creativity and Culture.' In R.L.Mooney and T. A. Razik (eds) *Explorations in Creativity*. New York: Harper and Row.

Steiner, R. (1970) *Theosophy*. New York: Anthroposophic Press.

Stern, D., Jaffe, J., Bebbe, B. and Bennet, S. (1975) 'Vocalizing in unison and in alternation: Two modes of communication within the mother–infant dyad.' *Annals of the New York Academy of Science 263*, 89–100.

Stewart, R.J. (1987) *Music and the Elemental Psyche: A Practical Guide to Music and Changing Consciousness.* Wellingborough: The Aquarian Press.

Stockhausen, K. (1968) *Auf den Sieben Tagen.* Vienna: Universal Edition.

Storr, A. (1992) *Music and the Mind.* London: HarperCollins.

Subotnik, R.R. (1996) *Deconstructive Variations: Music and Reason in Western Society.* Minneapolis, MN: University of Minnesota Press.

Swann, D. (1971) *The Song of Caedmon.* London: Stainer and Bell.

Swanwick, K. and Tillman, J.B. (1986) 'The sequence of musical development.' *British Journal of Music Education 3*, 3, 305–337.

Tagg, P. (1982) 'Analysing popular music: Theory, method and practice.' *Popular Music 2*, 37–68.

Tame, D. (1984) *The Secret Power of Music – The Transformation of Self and Society through Musical Energy.* Rochester, VT: Destiny Books.

Temmingh, K. (1998) 'Music in communication and healing of autistic children.' Demonstration at the *Music in Health and Special Education* seminar of the International Society for Music Education, South Africa, July.

Tillman, J.B. (1976) *Exploring Sound.* London: Stainer and Bell.

Tillman, J.B. (1987) *Towards a Model of the Development of Musical Creativity: A Study of the Compositions of Children aged 3–11.* Unpublished Ph.D. Thesis, University of London Institute of Education.

Tomatis, A. (1991) *The Conscious Ear: My Life of Transformation through Listening.* London: Station Hill Press.

Topp-Fargion, J. (1992) *Closer to the Gods.* Programme on BBC Radio 3, 24 September. National Sound Archive H693, British Library.

Torrance, E.P (1970) *Creative Learning and Teaching.* New York: Dodd, Mead.

Towse, E. and Flower, C. (1993) 'Levels of interaction in group improvisation.' In M. Heal and T. Wigram (eds) *Music Therapy in Health and Education.* London: Jessica Kingsley Publishers.

Tubbs, N. (1998) 'What is love's work?' *Women: A Cultural Review 9*, 1, 34–46.

Tucek, G.K. (1994) *Traditional Oriental Music and Art Therapy: The Oriental Approach to Heal Disease with Artistic Media and Its Status Today* (English translation). Academy for Traditional Central Asian Music and Art Therapy, study texts no. 7.

Turner, V.W. (1968) *The Drums of Affliction: A Study of Religious Process among the Ndembu of Zambia.* Oxford: Clarendon.

Underwood, B. (1999) *Plato's Methodology in His Construction of the Musical Subject.* Paper presented at Feminist Musicological Theory Conference, London, July.

Van der Weyer, R. (ed) (1997) *Hildegard in a Nutshell.* London: Hodder and Stoughton.

Van Nieuwenhuijze, D.O. (1998) 'The simplicity of complexity.' Conference Paper at Fourteenth World Conference of Sociology, Montreal.

Vander, J. (1986) 'Ghost dance songs and religion of a wind River Oshone woman.' *Monograph Series in Ethnomusicology 4.* Los Angeles, CA: University of California.

Vernon, P.E. (1970) *Creativity.* Harmondsworth: Penguin.

Vitebsky, P. (1995) *The Shaman* DBP quoted in Frowen-Williams, p.51.

Vitz, P. (1979) *Psychology as Religion: The Cult of Self-Worship.* London: Lion.

Walker, A. (1996) *The Same River Twice: Honoring the Difficult.* London: The Women's Press.

Walker, S. (1972) *Ceremonial Spirit Possession in Africa and Afro-America.* Leiden: E.J. Brill.

Wallas, C. (1926) 'The art of thought.' In P.E. Vernon (ed, 1970) *Creativity.* Harmondsworth: Penguin.

Walser, R. (1993) *Running with the Devil: Power, Gender, and Madness in Heavy Metal Music.* Hanover, NH: University Press of New England.

Walsh, R.N. (1990) *The Spirit of Shamanism.* Mandala.

Walters J. and Gardner, H. (1992) 'The crystallizing experience: Discovering an intellectual gift.' In R.S. Albert (ed) *Genius and Eminence* (second edition). Oxford: Pergamon.

Warr, P. (1987) *Work, Unemployment and Mental Health.* Oxford: Clarendon Press.

Wheeler, B.L (1988) 'An analysis of literature from selected music therapy journals.' *Music Therapy Perspectives 5*, 94–101.

Wigram, T. (1993) 'Music therapy research to meet the demands of health and educational services – Research and literature analysis.' In M. Heal and T. Wigram (eds) *Music Therapy in Health and Education.* London: Jessica Kingsley Publishers.

Wilensky, H.L. (1960) 'Work, careers and social integration.' *International Science Journal 4*, 32–56.

Wilson, G.D. (1994) *Psychology for Performing Musicians: Butterflies and Bouquets.* London: Jessica Kingsley Publishers.

Wilson, P.J. (1967) 'Status ambiguity and spirit possession.' *Man 2*, 366–378.

Witherspoon, G. (1977) *Language and Art in the Navajo Universe.* Ann Arbor, MI: University of Michigan Press.

Wrawicker, J. (1996) Sleeve notes to *Textures.* London: Trance Europe Express.

Yalom, I.D. (1985) *The Theory and Practice of Group Psychotherapy.* London: Basic Books.

Young, S. (ed) (1993) *An Anthology of Sacred Texts by and about Women.* New York: Crossroad.

Zuckerkandl, V. (1956) *Sound and Symbol: Music and the External World.* (trans. W.R. Task) Princeton, NJ: Princeton University Press.

Subject Index

Author
Index

Achterberg, J. 15–16
Adorno, T. 48, 79, 85, 90, 113
Agrotou, A. 244
Akstein, D. 195
Aldridge, D. 17–18, 30, 32, 159, 205–6, 212–13, 221–2, 239
Alexander, J. 177
Alvin, J. 203, 245
Amairgen 285n
Anand, Dr. and A. 214
Apollo 69, 83
Aristotle 24n, 62
Armstrong, F. 42, 160, 162, 167
Artaud, A. 104
Assagioli, R. 27, 61–2
Association of Professional Music Therapists 207
Attali, J. 79

Bach, J. S. 63, 224
Baker Miller, J. 35
Ball, L. 106
Barkin, E. 49
Barthes, R. 93
Bastide, R. 126
Bayeazid II 148
Beatles 159, 242, 259
Beattie, J. and Middleton, J. 128
Beaulieu 173
Becker, J. 259
Beethoven, L. van 50, 77, 96–7, 105–6, 139n, 268
Belenky, M. F., McVicker Clinchy, B., Rule Goldberger, N. and Mattuck Tarule, J. 11
Bembo, P. 83
Benedetti 212
Berendt, J. 159
Berruti, G., del Puente, G., Gatti, R., Manarola, G. and Vecchiato, C. 209, 219, 223, 232
Besson, M. 102
Beyer, A. 99, 112, 116
Black Elk 131–3, 150
Blacking, J. 36–7, 63–4, 118
Blake, A. 70, 90, 82, 105
Blois, T. 220–1
Boddy, J. 145
Bode, B. 19
Boethius 74, 107–8
Bolton, R. 263
Bonny, H. 46, 234
Bourgignon, E. 138
Boyce-Tillman, J. 20, 21, 75, 187, 254, 257, 260, 271, 273, 276, 281, 286–7
Brahms, J. 90
Braidotti, R. 11, 49–50
Brewer, C. 58
Bright, R. 223–4, 231
Britten, B. 45
Brougham, H., Fox, C. and Pace, I. 78, 80, 88
Brown, J. E. 150
Bruscia, K. E. 206
Bunt, L. 33–4, 203, 206, 207, 210–11, 217, 218–19, 220,

223, 226, 230, 234, 236–7, 238–9, 244

Caedmon 265
Cage, J. 52, 115, 279
Caldwell, A. E. 96–7
Callas, M. 194
Calliope 69
Campbell, J. 285n
Caplan, P. 123, 152
Carpenter, H. 45
Carson, C. 37
Castaneda, C. 123
Castoriadis, C. 80
Cattell 89
Chardin, T. de 172
Chatten, C. 233
Cherry, D. 159
Chopin, F. 22
Chopra, D. 28
Clynes, M. 63
Collin, M. 188–9
Collins, D. 79, 80
Coltrane, J. 159
Condon, W. 212
Condon, W. and Ogston, W. 62
Cook, N. 72, 76, 81, 85, 86, 89, 93, 112, 255
Counts, G. 19
Crapanzo, V. 138
Critchley, N. and Henson, R. 239
Csikszentmihalyi, M. 11, 13–14, 36

Danner, M. 274
De Backer, J. 218, 219, 222, 227–8, 229
Deason Barrow, M. 65–6
Dekker, C. 187–8
Deleuze 50
Densmore, F. 143, 145
Derrida, J. 48
Dewey, J. 18
di Franco, G. 38, 219
Diamond, J. 175, 183–4
Dodd, V. 192
Dollinger, S. J. 232
Donnars, J. 195
Dowland, J. 98
Downes, A. 80–1, 116
Doyle, B. 280
Drury, N. 132–3, 147
du Pré, J. 100–1

Eades, G. 214
Eames, P. 215, 224, 254
Easton, C. 101
Eibl-Eibesfeld, I. 57
Ekman, K. 98
El-Farabi, H. 148
El-Kindi 148
Eliade, M. 124, 130, 145, 150
Elkin, A. P. 140
Elliot, D. 72
Emerson, D. 180
Engh, B. 93
Epstein, D. 58
Erdonmez, D. 44, 208, 241
Erlmann, V. 139, 146
Eurydice 69

Feder, E. and Feder, B. 204–5
Feng, F. M. 129, 142, 147–8
Ficino, M. 75, 111, 112
Figueroa, A. 126–7
Finnissy, M. 78, 80, 88

Fisher, K. 34
Flackus, E. 242–3
Flower, C. 219, 229
Floyd, M. 72, 129, 269n
Fludd, R. 71
Fordham, M. 48, 228
Foskett, J. 17, 35
Fowler, J. 100
Francesco do Milano 110–11
Freire, P. 55
Freud, S. 40, 48, 204
Friedman, R. 192–3
Frith, S. 72
Fromm, E. 19
Frowen-Williams, G. 189–91, 195
Fry, H. H. J. 62
Fukuda, Y. 241

Gaertner, M. 219–20
Gans, E. 36, 113
Gardner, K 71, 162, 163, 170
Gardner 177, 186–7, 191–2
Garfield, L. M. 170
Gebser, J. 172, 184
Gergis, S. 250
Gfeller, K. 237
Ghiselin, B. 19
Giddens, A. 15
Gigli, B. 194
Girard, R. 79
Glass, P. 116
Glennie, E. 259
Godwin, J. 71, 74, 108, 114, 115, 158
Goehr, L. 76
Goldman, J. 157, 167, 173, 175, 187, 192, 193, 194, 198
Gooch, S. 10–11
Goodchild, C. 162, 169
Govinda, L. 184
Graf Durckheim 48
Grainger, R. 226–7
Green, L. 91–2
Grey, M. 35, 282
Grimes, R. L. 148–9
Grimm and Pefley 221
Grof, S. with Bennett, H. Z. 140
Guilford, J. P. 19

Halifax, J. 140
Hamel, P. 49, 65, 98, 116, 143, 147, 161, 167, 169–70, 172, 173, 174, 181, 182, 183, 184, 197, 231, 234, 242, 243
Hamilton, P. 202–3
Handel, G. F. 158, 244
Harford, Canon 203
Harner, M. 147
Harrer, G. and Harrer, H. 57
Hart, M. and Lieberman, F. 191
Hassan, S. Q. 125
Haworth, J. T. 13, 14, 39
Haydn, F. J. 97
Hegel, G. W. F. 47
Heidegger, M. 47–8, 111–12
Hekmat, H. and Hettel, J. 233
Heline, C. 158, 185
Helman, C. G. 16–17, 186
Hengesch, G. 231
Hermes 70
Hermes Trismegistus 74, 157
Hero, B. 186–7
High Eagle, J. C. 181
Hilda, Abbess 265